ALLE ZEIT WACH
SJ
1842

TERATOLOGY
Trends and Applications

Edited by
C. L. Berry and D. E. Poswillo

With Contributions by
R. M. Atkinson · S. M. Barlow · K. Benirschke
A. Bentovim · C. L. Berry · K. S. Brown · J. Burn
T. A. Connors · J. P. Germain · A. Gropp
M. C. Johnston · J. Langman · I. R. Phillips
D. E. Poswillo · R. M. Pratt · D. F. Roberts
P. Rodier · D. Sopher · F. M. Sullivan · W. Webster

With 78 Figures

Springer-Verlag
Berlin Heidelberg New York 1975

C. L. Berry, M. D., Ph. D. (Lond.), M. R. C. Path., University Reader in Pathology, Guy's Hospital Medical School, Hon., Consultant Pathologist, Guy's Hospital, London, SEI 9RT, England

D. E. Poswillo, D. Sc., F. D. S. R. C. S., F. D. S. R. C. S., M. R. C. Path., Professor of Teratology, Royal College of Surgeons of England, Lincoln's Inn Fields, London, and Consultant Oral and Maxillo-facial Surgeon, Queen Victoria Hospital, East Grinstead, England

ISBN-13: 978-3-642-66174-7 e-ISBN-13: 978-3-642-66172-3
DOI: 10.1007/978-3-642-66172-3

Library of Congress Cataloging in Publication Data Main entry under title:
Teratology. Bibliographie: p. Includes index. 1. Deformities-Genetic aspects.
2. Teratogenic agents. I. Berry, Colin Leonhard, 1937 —
II. Poswillo D., 1927 — [DNLM: 1. Abnormalities.
QS675 N532] RB155. T47 616'.043 75-20069

Softcover reprint of the hardcover 1st edition 1975

Foreword

In the fifteen years since the thalidomide disaster teratology has become a science in its own right, distinct from its progenitors, experimental embryology and developmental biology, but bearing many of the familiar features of both parents. In this growth period there have been contributions from many different scientific disciplines as diverse as molecular biology and obstetrics, which have united in the field of study of congenital malformations.

Scientists in academic departments, government research institutes and industrial pharmacology have all explored ways of evaluating the potential of drugs and chemicals to damage the embryo; strict methods of screening for teratogenicity have become mandatory in most parts of the world. Despite a wealth of basic information in the fields of genetics and embryology, there is little concrete knowledge of the causal mechanisms of malformation in Man, and even less concerning the relevance to Man of those laboratory and animal tests which decide the fate of potentially useful drugs. It is timely, therefore, that in 1975 a group of young and active scientists and clinicians concerned with the broader implications of teratology should review the past and look to the future of this emerging speciality.

In this volume the editors have blended the opinions of teratologists; their message presages change in many of the old and accepted areas of investigative teratology. The scope of their contributions is such that there is much to offer the academic embryologist and teratologist, the obstetrician and pediatrician, and the toxicologist or teratologist advising industry or government. In the past the applied sciences, such as teratology, have tended to lag behind the achievements of the pure sciences on which they were based. Here, for the first time in this new speciality, both academic and applied scientists look into the future and discuss the areas which may soon undergo radical change.

W. J. Hamilton
Professor emeritus of Anatomy
University of London

Table of Contents

List of Contributors

R. M. Atkinson, Ph. D., M. B., Ch. B., B. Sc., Head of Toxicology Department, Glaxo Research Limited, Breakspear Road South, Uxbridge, Middlesex, England.

Susan M. Barlow, B. Sc., Ph. D. (Lond.), Research Assistant, Department of Pharmacology, Guy's Hospital Medical School, London, SEI-9RT, England.

K. Benirschke, M. D., Professor, Department of Reproductive Medicine, University of California, P. O. Box 109, La Jolla, California, 92037, USA.

A. Bentovim, M. B., B. S., F. R. C. Psych., Consultant Psychiatrist, The Hospital for Sick Children, Gt. Ormond Street, London, WCIN-3JH, England.

C. L. Berry, M. D., Ph. D. (Lond.), M. R. C. Path., University Reader in Pathology, Guy's Hospital Medical School, Hon., Consultant Pathologist, Guy's Hospital, London, SEI-9RT, England.

K. S. Brown, M. D., Division of Developmental Biology, National Institute of Dental Research, National Institutes of Health, Bethesda, USA.

J. Burn, B. Med. Sci., Medical Student, Department of Human Genetics, 19, Claremont Place, Newcastle-upon-Tyne, NE2-4AA, England.

T. A. Connors, D. Sc., Ph. D. (Lond.), Reader in Biochemical Pharmacology, Chester Beatty Research Institute, Fulham Road, London, SW3-6JB, England.

Jocelyn P. Germain, F. I. M. L. T., Senior Technician, Department of Dental Science, Royal College of Surgeons, London, England.

A. Gropp, Professor Dr., Klinisch-Theoretisches Zentrum, Abteilung für Pathologie, 24 Lübeck 1, Kronsforder Allee 71/73, W. Germany.

M. C. Johnston, Ph. D., D. D. S., Division of Developmental Biology, National Institute of Dental Research, National Institutes of Health, Bethesda, USA.

J. Langman, M. D., Ph. D., Professor and Chairman, Department of Anatomy, University of Virginia, 1300, Jefferson Park Avenue, Charlottesville, Virginia, 22901, USA.

I. R. Phillips, B. Vet. Med., M. R. C. V. S., Royal College of Surgeons Research Establishment, Downe, Kent, England.

D. E. Poswillo, D. Sc., F. D. S. R. C. S., F. D. S. R. C. S., M. R. C. Path., Professor of Teratology, Royal College of Surgeons of England, Lincoln's Inn Fields, London, England.

R. M. PRATT, Ph. D., Division of Developmental Biology, National Institute of Dental Research, National Institutes of Health, Bethesda, USA.

D. F. ROBERTS, M. A. (Cantab.), D. Phil. (Oxon.), Reader in Human Genetics, University of Newcastle-upon-Tyne, 19, Claremont Place, NE2-4AA, England.

PATRICIA RODIER, Ph. D., Assistant Professor, Department of Anatomy, University of Virginia, Charlottesville, Virginia, 22901, USA.

DINAH SOPHER, B. Sc. (Hons.), M. I. Biol., Royal College of Surgeons Research Establishment, Downe, Kent, BR6 7JJ, England.

F. M. SULLIVAN, B. Sc., Senior Lecturer in Pharmacology, Department of Pharmacology, Guy's Hospital Medical School, London, SEI-9RT, England.

W. WEBSTER, B. Sc., Ph. D. (Lond.), Research Assistant, Department of Anatomy, University of Virginia, Charlottesville, Virginia, 22901, USA.

New Attitudes to Experimental Teratology

The study of the mechanism of malformation requires an understanding of the normal processes of development. Thus, it is difficult to separate experimental teratology from experimental embryology. While many animal systems have been used to demonstrate the effects of specific environmental agents on morphogenesis, the induction of chromosomal abnormalities resulting in well defined syndromes is an exciting new field of investigation, and offers hope of a pathway towards an understanding of the relationship of genetic control to morphogenesis. Tools such as radiation and radiomimetic agents have been widely used, often unselectively, to damage the developing embryo. Knowledge of the specific effects of cytotoxic agents enables a more selective approach to be made. Each of these approaches contributes to a better understanding of those errors of morphogenesis which lead to recognised patterns of malformations in man.

1. A Developmental Approach to Teratology

M. C. JOHNSTON and R. M. PRATT

With 1 Figure

This chapter examines some of the more recent information on normal development and considers the potential of this information for application to problems of abnormal development. Some theoretical and practical problems relating to a developmental approach to teratology are reviewed and ways are suggested in which they may be more effectively dealt with.

While the topics discussed here may at times touch upon material presented in other chapters, developmental aspects will always be emphasized. Consideration of genetic and environmental factors, for example, will be limited to the manner in which they may alter development.

Current Concepts of Development Related to Teratology

General Features of Embryonic Development

In order to put into proper context current concepts of individual developmental phenomena (e. g. cell migration) and the manner in which they are altered in abnormal development, some general features of embryonic development will first be described. These general features are now well accepted and greater detail may be found in standard texts (LANGMAN, 1969; BALINSKY, 1970; HAMILTON and MOSSMAN, 1972).

Gastrulation is the first massive movement of embryonic cells and even by this stage of development specific alterations often lead to malformations without resulting in death of the embryo. Gastrulation leads to the formation of the middle germ layer (mesoderm) and sets the stage for the first major tissue interaction, the induction of neural plate formation in the ectoderm by cells migrating to form the mesoderm (Fig. 1). The ectoderm must be competent to respond and once the stimulus has been transmitted the continued presence of the inductive influence is no longer necessary.

Subsequent changes in the neural plate illustrate additional, relevant, developmental phenomena (Fig. 1). These include differential growth of the neural plate and the onset of regional specialization. For example, major components of the brain, spinal cord and eye differentiate in different areas of the neural plate or tube. At the margin of the tube, and apparently also dependent on the same initial inductive influences, neural crest cells differentiate (Fig. 1). After migration, crest cells form such as extensive series of derivatives (only some of which are neural) that it has been suggested they be designated a fourth germ layer (WESTON, 1970 for review). Development continues in a step-by-step fashion until the organ systems are laid down and final differentiation begins. The time during development at which each level of maturity is reached differs considerably in different tissues and organs and these variations are of critical importance for the action of teratogenic influences. For example, cell migration and differentiation in different portions of the brain continue until very late stages (see Chapter 11, LANGMAN *et al.*).

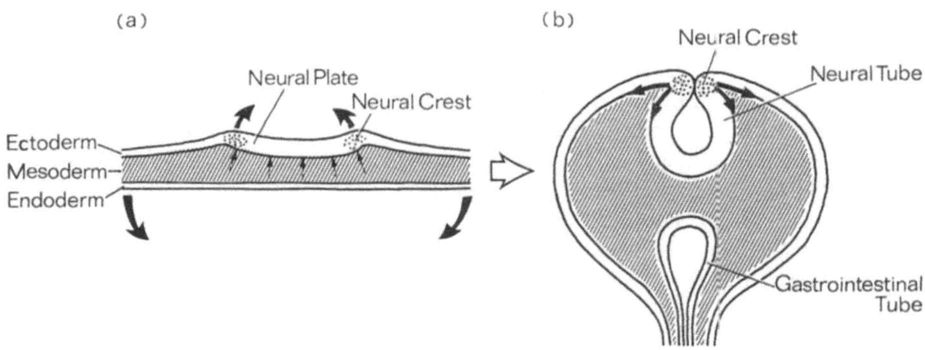

Fig. 1. (a) Cross-section through three germ layer embryo. The neural plate has been induced by an inductive stimulus passing from underlying mesoderm (broken arrows). The initiation of neural plate and lateral wall folding processes is indicated by solid arrows. (b) Following fusion processes the neural tube and gastrointestinal tubes will separate from the embryo's surface. The directions of neural crest migration are indicated by arrows

Specific Developmental Phenomena

Although teratological influences frequently alter more than one aspect of development, it is useful first to review current knowledge about some selected phenomena and to examine ways in which they may be altered in abnormal development.

Cell Migration

Many of the massive embryonic cell migrations take place in a matrix (TOOLE, 1973; PRATT *et al.*, 1975 b). In all systems they have studied, TOOLE and TRELSTAD (1971) have shown that migration is preceded by hyaluronate (hyaluronic acid) production. Further evidence (TOOLE and TRELSTAD, 1971; PRATT *et al.*, 1975 b) indicates that the major area of increased production is along the migration path and, perhaps with other matrix components, provides a suitable substratum for the migrating cells. TOOLE (1973) has suggested that the hyaluronate inhibits potential inductive interactions between the migrating cells and their environment until they reach their final location, where condensation and differentiation are preceded by removal of the hyaluronate through hyaluronidase production. There is also some evidence that collagen is present in very young embryos in basement membranes and possibly as a matrix component. Such collagen may serve as a site for the attachment of migrating cells (HAY, 1973).

Premature removal or interference with the production of matrix components would be expected to influence cell migration. Preliminary studies by FITZHARRIS and MARKWALD (1974) do, in fact, indicate that experimental interference with the synthesis or secretion of collagen or glycosaminoglycan (mucopolysaccharide) results in the inhibition of migrating embryonic heart cells.

There is considerable controversy regarding the mechanisms of cell migration. Several may operate depending on the cell type and developmental age. Many prospective neuroblasts appear to migrate individually, utilizing glial cells as a substratum (RAKIC and SIDMAN, 1973). Gastrulating cells in sea urchin embryos appear to move by extending long filopodia which, after making contact and attachments, contract and pull the cell body along (GUSTAFSON and TONEBY, 1971; KARP and SOLURSH, 1974). Embryonic cells migrating in a matrix, frequently adopt an essentially bipolar form somewhat similar to fibroblasts in a collagen gel (BARD and ELSDALE, 1973). Scanning electron micrographic studies (REVEL, 1974; STEFFEK *et al.*, 1975) indicate that filopodia are extended from the leading edges of such cells and that they apparently do not often make contact with structures other than matrix components. ROTH *et al.* (1975) have suggested that interaction between migrating cells and matrix components may be mediated through cell surface glycosyl transferases and carbohydrate components of the matrix.

A considerable amount of evidence now indicates that new membrane is produced at the cell's migration front (ABERCROMBIE *et al.*, 1972) and there is also some evidence that the new membrane is translocated over the subsurface cytoplasm to be taken back into the cell in the "cap" region (HARRIS, 1973). Studies on migrating lymphocytes show that the "cap" in these cells occurs at the posterior pole (DE PETRIS and RAFF, 1973) suggesting that some cells may migrate by a "tractor-tread" system. Actin and myosin has now been found in numerous cell types and the motive force for cell migration may be exerted through an actin-myosin complex located in subsurface cytoplasm (WESSELS *et al.*, 1973).

SPIEGELMAN and BENNETT (1974) have attributed the accumulation of mesoderm cells in the primitive streak region of T-locus mutant embryos to a migration failure. Lobopodia extending from these abnormal cells lack the subsurface (actin?) microfilament lattice and this could account for the lack of motive force. They also suggested that failure to form attachments might be a factor, in line with DE HAAN'S (1958) conclusion that EDTA interferes with migrating cardiac cells by altering intercellular attachments.

It has been suggested (MORRISS, 1973; HASSELL *et al.*, 1975) that part of the teratogenic activity of vitamin A may result from its action on migrating cells. HASSELL *et al.* (1975) postulated that the inhibition of palate shelf development which resulted from vitamin A administration may have been due to an inhibition of mesenchyme cell migration related to maxillary process formation. There is also some indication that vitamin A may interfere with crest cell migration (JOHNSTON, 1975) or with the migrations of prospective neuroblasts in the brain at very late stages of development (LANGMAN and WELCH, 1967). Intramuscular injection of vitamin A-palmitate into pregnant rats at the time of gastrulation results in large spaces between gastrulating mesoderm cells and MORRISS (1973) postulates that the separation of the cells may have interfered with their ability to migrate. Known effects of vitamin A on glycosaminoglycan synthesis (KOCHAR and JOHNSON, 1965; SOLURSH and MEIER, 1973) and/or direct effects on cell membranes (MORRISS, 1973) could be among the mechanisms by which vitamin A interferes with migrating cells.

Other Morphogenetic Movements

Actin-myosin complexes appear also to be involved in the closure of the neural tube and the invagination of glandular epithelia (BURNSIDE, 1971; WESSELS *et al.*, 1973; KARFUNKEL, 1974). Cytochalasin B causes disaggregation of actin filaments (YAMADA, 1975) and both LINVILLE and SHEPPARD (1972) and KARFUNKEL (1974) have been able to prevent neural tube closure with cytochalasin B. Microtubles appear also to be involved in neural tube closure and other morphogenetic movements (YAMADA, 1975) and it is possible to inhibit their formation with drugs such as colchicine. Microtubule-inhibiting drugs also interfere with cell mitosis, complicating interpretation of their effects (e. g. failure of tube closure after injection of colchicine in the hamster: FERM, 1963).

Inductive Interactions and Differentiation

During development cells become increasingly diversified by passing through a series of discrete stages of differentiation. The progressive differentiation of neural crest cells provides examples (WESTON, 1970). Apparently as a result of neural plate induction, crest cells differentiate as distinct cell types in the neural fold. Crest cells are at that time endowed with migratory ability and the competence to respond to a limited number of inductive stimuli. For example, pharyngeal endoderm induces crest cells that migrate to its vicinity to become chondroblasts. An additional interaction with oral ectoderm is involved in the differentiation of crest cells into odontoblasts. Presumably at each stage, specific inductive interactions are involved with the responding cell producing RNA's appropriate to its new role.

Classical studies (HOLTFRETER and HAMBURGER, 1955; SAXÉN and TOIVONEN, 1962) have outlined the principles involved in inductive interactions. Induction differs from other influences, such as hormones, that affect cell differentiation in that once the inductive stimulus has been transmitted and the responding tissue has become committed to the new line of differentiation ("determination"), the continued presence of the inducing tissue is no longer necessary. The responding tissue shows competence to respond to an inductive influence for a limited time only and many extraneous influences can replace the normal inductor. In some instances reciprocal inductive interactions are involved where each tissue acts as inducer and responder, e. g. eye cup and lens (COULOMBRE and COULOMBRE, 1975) or enamel organ and tooth papilla (SLAVKIN, 1974).

The interposition of Millipore or Nucleopore filters between interacting tissues *in vitro* has shown that some interactions can occur without contact over a considerable distance (GROBSTEIN, 1975) while others seem to require contact of cell surfaces (SAXÉN, 1975). An interesting recent observation has been the induction of scleral cartilage by matrices synthesized by pigmented retina (NEWSOME, 1975).

HOLTZER and MAYNE (1973) have argued that determination requires a particular type of cell division which they term a "quantal" division. As supporting evidence, they cite the failure of numerous studies to show that induction is possible without cell division. The determination event presumably involves the activation of appropriate sets of genes. Considerable time may elapse before there is overt evidence of the differentiated state. It is possible that differentiation (after determination) may be suppressed in some cell types such as hypoglossal myoblasts which must undergo very long migrations before overtly expressing their phenotype (HAZELTON, 1970). Some cell types, such as the exocrine cells of the mouse pancreas (RUTTER *et al.*, 1968) remain for a long time in a "protodifferentiated" state, and proliferation continues at a rapid rate until just before birth when the amount of secretory product increases dramatically.

In genetically defective interactions either the inducing tissues (neural tube for somite induction; DUNN and BENNETT, 1964) or the tissues being induced (ectodermal scales by mesoderm; GOETINCK and ABBOTT, 1964) may be defective. Abnormal positional relationships may result in failed or incomplete induction as in the induction of lens by a defective eye cup (CHASE and CHASE, 1941). The narrow time periods during which inducing tissues are capable of induction and responding tissues are capable of response suggests that defects in timing should be of critical importance, but little evidence is available to confirm or deny this suggestion (SAXÉN, 1973; COULOMBRE and COULOMBRE, 1975).

Cell Proliferation

The normal controls for embryonic cell proliferation are poorly understood. There is some evidence (FUJITA, 1962; MARCHOK and HERMANN, 1967) that many, if not most, relatively undifferentiated embryonic cell populations are dividing at almost maximal rates (i. e. every 8 or 9 hrs in homiotherms). Increasing density of cell populations (e. g. of mesenchyme cells associating with epithelia as in limb bud or facial process development) is frequently seen but in such cases it is difficult to distinguish increased proliferation from aggregation. Evidence for a growth promoting effect of mesenchyme on epithelia has been shown repeatedly and RUTTER *et al.* (RUTTER *et al.*, 1973; LEVINE *et al.*, 1974) have isolated a protein from mesenchyme that is capable of stimulating proliferation of pancreatic glandular epithelial cells by acting at the cell surface.

Other factors involved in the regulation of proliferation have been proposed (MOSS, 1972) such as neurotrophic stimuli, but supporting evidence is limited. Nerve and epidermal growth factors have been studied extensively (ANGELETTI *et al.*, 1965; HOOPER and COHEN, 1967) but there is still no evidence that they play a significant role in normal development. In mammals, it is possible that maternal humoral factors may influence rates of cell proliferation. Thyroxin, for example, might have an overall stimulatory effect as it does on amphibian embryos (CHIBON and BRUGAL, 1969). That such humoral support is necessary for normal development is suggested by studies in which ocular and other defects result from maternal partial thyroidectomy (LANGMAN and VAN FASSEN, 1955) or ear defects from thiouracil administration (DEOL, 1973).

Direct evidence for altered proliferation rates in abnormal development has been obtained and may be particularly important in the genesis of spontaneous defects. There is some evidence, for example, that reduced proliferation of facial tissue is responsible for the spontaneous cleft lip associated with either the Dancer gene or the administration of 6-aminonicotinamide in mice (TRASLER and LEONG, 1974). In other types of cleft lip more complex imbalances between the growth rates of forebrain and frontonasal processes may be involved (ROSS and JOHNSTON, 1972; JOHNSTON *et al.*, 1975).

Cell Death

Cell death plays an extensive role in normal embryonic development (GLUCKSMANN, 1950; SAUNDERS, 1966). It is the usual method of eliminating organs and tissues that are useful only during embryonic or larval life. It is also involved in the morphogenesis of organs and tissues as in the remodelling of limbs, cartilage and bone and accompanies the formation of folds and confluence of anlage (e. g. during fusion of palatal shelves). Cell death also occurs as part of what might be termed a "redundancy phenomenon" seen in the loss of excess cells in the primordia of spinal cord and brain stem nuclei (HAMBURGER and LEVI-MONTALCINI, 1956; ROGERS and COWAN, 1972) or of mesoderm cells remaining in the visceral arches after blood-vessel development (JOHNSTON and LISTGARTEN, 1972).

Cells are induced to die (programmed cell death) well before the time of death. In the rat secondary palate, for example, the medial-edge epithelial cells cease DNA synthesis 24—36 hrs prior to death (SHAPIRO and SWEENY, 1969; PRATT *et al.*, 1975 a). Although the biochemical basis of programmed cell death is far from clear, mediation of epithelial cell death in the secondary palate by elevated cyclic AMP has recently been proposed (PRATT and MARTIN, 1975).

Excessive loss of cells at locations where cell death normally occurs may lead to abnormal development as in the "wingless"-chick mutant (HINCHCLIFFE and EDE, 1973) or in the extension of cell death in knee joint development following the application of insulin (ZWILLING, 1959). Conversely, failure of cell death leads to polydactyly and/or syndactyly in the talpid^3 mutation (HINCHCLIFFE and EDE, 1967).

Cell death unrelated to normal degenerative processes is often seen in abnormal development. Ionizing radiation was among the earliest teratogenic influences employed (for review, see HICKS and D'AMATO, 1966; RUSTAD, 1972) and while it has major effects on proliferating cells, differentiating cells may be even more sensitive. At the molecular level, breaks are found to occur in the DNA backbone after exposure of chromosomes to ionizing radiation and abnormal cross-linking between nucleotide bases occurs. Cross-linking between chromosomes may lead to cell death through non-disjunction at subsequent cell division. Some of the effects of ionizing radiations are not understood, including the well established mitotic delay (RUSTAD, 1972).

A number of other antimetabolites affect primarily the DNA synthesizing capability of cells (e. g. FUdR) and also cause cell death (SCHWEICKEL and MERKER, 1973). Increased cell death can also be caused by other substances (see Chapter 4, CONNORS).

Finally some additional comments regarding the sensitivity of embryonic cells to lethal injury are in order. The explanation of many unusual observations must await increased knowledge of certain phenomena such as determination and developmental clocks. It is known, for example, that determined cells prevented from expressing their differentiated phenotype may die. An example is the death of prospective neuroblasts unable to migrate to their definitive location because of abnormalities in the glial cells which normally guide their migrations (RAKIC and SIDMAN, 1973). Inability of defective cells to migrate in a normal environment could presumably also lead to cell death. It is possible that the excessive cell death in T-locus mouse mutants may in some way be related to migration problems (DUNN and BENNETT, 1964; SPIEGELMAN and BENNETT, 1974).

Groups of cells involved in both inductive and proliferative interactions appear to be particularly sensitive to a wide range of teratogens. For example, massive cell death is seen in the olfactory placode and surrounding condensing mesenchyme after administration of either hadicidin (LEJOUR, 1970), an antibiotic thought to have antifolate activity, or X-irradiation (ETO *et al.*, 1975).

Some Theoretical and Practical Problems

Examples of developmental alterations used in the previous section were selected for relative simplicity. Frequently analysis of abnormal development is made more difficult by a number of complicating factors. At any period of development, a number of processes may undergo simultaneous alterations at one developmental stage often leading to a sequence of changes that may be difficult to analyze. A number of procedures have been developed to reduce complexity and examples will be given in the following discussion.

The Primary Biochemical or Physiological Action of a Teratogen is Frequently Unknown

Environmental Agents

Many of the most popular experimental teratogens were initially selected either because of clinical observations (e. g. thalidomide) or through empirical testing on experimental animals (e. g. X-irradiation, cortisone, vitamin A). Although they have dramatic and reproducible effects on developmental phenomena, their primary action on embryonic cells is often not known. The primary biochemical and physiological actions of some of these agents on a number of cells and tissues is now undergoing intensive study (DE LUCA *et al.*, 1973) with considerable success; many of the procedures utilized in these experiments can be adapted in order to study their action on embryonic cells.

Genetic Factors

As more is learned about normal development it should become increasingly feasible to discover genetically determined malformations in earlier stages, even in man

(NISHIMURA, 1971). It may then be possible to construct hypotheses as to the nature of the primary defect (SPIEGELMAN and BENNETT, 1974) and to test these hypotheses through the use of experimental teratogens which lead to phenocopies. Examples of the utilization of experimental agents which interact with genetic factors in either positive or negative fashion may be very useful. These will be illustrated by examples below.

Simultaneous Alterations of Multiple Developmental Processes

β-aminopropionitrile (BAPN) has been shown to induce cleft palate in the rat by a specific inhibition of collagen cross-linking (PRATT and KING, 1972). Although collagen in a number of oral-facial structures is affected by BAPN, the defective palatal collagen is presumed to prevent palatal shelf elevation and induce cleft palate. As more is learned about normal development and the ways in which it may be altered, it should become feasible to apply selected agents as probes that will interfere, with single development processes. For example, it should be possible to interfere with matrix components during specified periods of development in order to examine the effects of altering selected cell migrations.

Some technical comments related to the use of experimental teratogens in such studies are in order. Although chronic exposure may sometimes be desirable, a relatively short exposure with controlled dose levels greatly simplifies the study of altered development. The action of some analogues such as 6-aminonicotinamide can be overcome by a subsequent injection of nicotinic acid, thus giving a more closely defined period of exposure. Methotrexate and folinic acid may be used in the same way (BERRY *et al.*, 1972). Such pin-pointing of developmental time is difficult for mammalian embryos which show considerable variation both within and between litters. *In vitro* procedures, e. g. whole embryo culture, or the use of easily accessible non-mammalian embryos, such as that of the chick, may be useful for some processes.

The problems of interaction between simultaneously altered developmental processes may be lessened through use of techniques for the isolation and/or recombination of cells or tissues. Some examples of these have been given in previous sections dealing with inductive and other interactions.

Organ culture procedures are extensively used. Examples include *in vitro* culture of secondary palate shelves in studies related to secondary palate elevation and fusion (SMILEY and KOCH, 1971; PRATT *et al.*, 1975 a; BRINKLEY and AVERY, 1975). SAXÉN and KATILA (1974) have utilized organ-culture procedures to examine the mechanism of action of tetracycline on mineralizing embryonic tissues.

Rapid advances have been made in the use of cell culture for the study of abnormal function. In particular, the culture of fibroblasts from individuals with connective tissue disorders, accompanied by chemical analysis of synthesized extracellular material has shown that these cultured cells continue to synthesize abnormal collagen (ORKIN *et al.*, 1975). Many other possible applications suggest themselves such as testing migratory cell populations under standardized conditions and examination of embryonic cells for defects in proliferation.

A common complicating factor in many instances of developmental alterations is breakdown of fluid compartments such as the vascular and cerebrospinal systems and the less completely separated fluid compartments of different tissues (GRABOWSKI, 1970, for review). Such breakdown has the potential for simultaneously affecting many developmental phenomena such as cell migration and tissue interactions. Examples include breakdown of tissue compartments with excess vitamin A (MORRISS, 1973), genetically determined blebbing (subepidermal fluid accumulation; BONNEVIE, 1934), vascular edema and hemorrhage following thalidomide administration (POSWILLO, 1973) and alterations in cerebrospinal fluid production or resorption leading to brain abnormalities (COULOMBRE and COULOMBRE, 1958; GRABOWSKI, 1970).

Interaction of Causative Factors

As noted in an earlier section, many of the common human malformations appear to result from the interactions of multiple genetic and environmental factors. Consequently, considerable interest has been shown in the influence of such interaction on developing embroys. Presumably, much smaller environmental disturbances, would be sufficient to push a genetically predisposed embryo over a threshold leading to developmental breakdown. Also, environmental factors may exert an ameliorating influence on genetically determined abnormality and some examples will be presented below (see also BERRY and GERMAIN, 1972 and Chapter 5). An exhaustive analysis of the interaction of causative factors is not warranted, however, and the reader is referred to SAXÉN and RAPPOLA (1969) for further examples.

There is considerable evidence that the critical factor in the embryogenesis of many types of cleft lip is insufficient mesenchyme at the point of fusion between median and lateral nasal processes (ROSS and JOHNSTON, 1972; TRASLER and LEONG, 1974). TRASLER (1968) has provided evidence that this results from an alteration in the configuration of the facial processes in A/Jax mouse embryos (10—15% of which eventually develop cleft lip) as compared to control C57Bl6 mouse embryos. BHAKDINARONK and JOHNSTON (1973) have observed that the threshold dose for radiation-induced cleft lip in C57Bl6 embryos produces a pronounced increase in the frequency of cleft lip in A/Jax embryos when applied at the same developmental stage. Preliminary evidence (unpublished) indicates that mesenchyme deficiency in the A/Jax primary palatal processes is exaggerated by X-irradiation.

The direction of genetically determined abnormal development may be reversed through environmental alterations. In a well documented study deficiency of a specific substance, manganese, produced a phenocopy of the morphological defect of the ear of "pallid" mice. Manganese supplementation in this mouse was then found to eleminate the spontaneous otolith defect (ERWAY *et al.*, 1971).

Sequences of Developmental Alterations

Knowledge of normal development is essential for sorting out the sequence of events following the primary developmental alteration or alterations. Some complex associations of malformations can be sorted out if it is known that they are defects in the derivatives of a common defective primordium. Special consideration needs to be given to the events preceding and following developmental "breakdown".

Derivatives of a Common Primordium

Interference with neural plate development by x-irradiation (BHAKDINARONK *et al.*, unpublished) and, presumably, other similar teratogenic influences (BINNS *et al.*, 1963; FERM and CARPENTER, 1968; DE MYER, 1964), results in associated malformations of the brain, eye and face. Major components of the most-affected structures are derived from the anterior neural plate (JOHNSTON, 1975).

Developmental Breakdown

Frequently, a developmental process fails to be completed, as in cleft lip formation, or a previously formed structure breaks down, as in vascular hemorrhage leading to limb defects (POSWILLO and SOPHER, 1971). Sometimes, complex sequences of developmental alternations may result from, or be followed by, such instances of developmental failure.

For a single developmental event, the point of breakdown can usually be reached in many ways. For example, superficially similar cases of cleft lip may result either from defective neural plate development (see above) or from late interference with mesenchyme proliferation in the frontonasal processes (LEJOUR, 1970; TRASLER, personal communication). In both cases the critical point would be whether or not sufficient mesenchyme is present in the median and lateral nasal processes at the time they normally fuse to form the lip primordium. As noted in the previous section the effects of two (or more) causative factors may "summate" to reduce the amount of mesenchyme to a sufficiently low level for cleft lip formation.

Breakdown at one stage frequently interferes with development at later stages. While this is true for cleft lip formation (ROSS and JOHNSTON, 1972), a more interesting example is provided by a series of heart malformations found in Keshland dogs (PATTERSON *et al.*, 1972). All these malformations, which vary from subclinical septal defects to the tetralogy of Fallot, can be related to variations in the degree of underdevelopment of the septum of the conus arteriosis. Development of this septum represents a critical stage in early development of the heart including the separation of the great arteries. Severe failure affects many subsequent morphological changes.

Concluding Remarks

Despite considerable progress in understanding normal morphogenesis, a developmental approach to teratology still presents complex problems. Some of these will be resolved as more is learned about basic mechanisms of development but the fact that many alterations lead to complex developmental interactions will tend to slow progress. However, increased utilization of a developmental approach appears to be the only way that teratology can be put on a firmer, less empirical basis (WILSON, 1973).

Finally, the possible contribution of teratological studies to the understanding of normal development should be stressed. Attempts to analyze mammalian (including human) malformations in terms of mechanisms learned primarily from nonmammalian species should help to determine to what extent mammalian embryos develop by similar mechanisms. Careful analysis of developmental alterations resulting from teratogens known to interfere with specific functions or with synthesis or secretion of specific substances may provide evidence as to the role they may play in normal development processes. These are new and exciting approaches to unresolved problems, and they can be utilized in the inseparable combination of developmental biology and teratology.

References

Abercrombie, M., Heaysman, J. E. M., Pegruin, S. M.: Locomotion of fibroblasts in culture. V. Surface marking with concanavalin A. Exp. Cell Res. **73**, 536 (1972).

Angeletti, P. U., Gandini-Artard, D., Toschi, G., Levi-Montalcini, R.: Metabolic aspects of the effect of nerve growth factor on sympathetic and sensory ganglia. Protein and RNA synthesis. Biochem. biophys. Acta (Amst.) **95**, 111 (1965).

Balinsky, B. I.: An Introduction to Embryology, Ed. 3. Philadelphia: W. B. Saunders Co. 1970.

Bard, J., Elsdale, T.: The three-dimensional culturing of fibroblasts in collagen gels. Biology of the Fibroblast, E. Kulonen and J. Pikkarrinen, Eds. New York: Acad. Press 1973.

Berry, C. L., Germain, J.: Absence of the third molar in the mouse: Its relevance to human malformation. J. Path. **108**, 35 (1972).

Berry, C. L., Germain, J., Looker, T.: The effect of methotrexate on DNA synthesis and its reversal by folinic acid. J. Embryol. exp. Morph. **28**, 601 (1972).

Bhakdinaronk, A., Johnston, M. C.: Interaction of X-irradiation and genetic predisposition for cleft lip in mice. J. dent. Res. **52 A**, 112 (1973).

Binns, W., James, L. F., Shupe, J. L.: A cyclopian-type malformation in lambs induced by maternal ingestion of a range plant, Veratrum Californicum. Am. J. vet. Res. **24**, 1164 (1963).

Bonnevie, K.: Embryological analysis of gene manifestation in Little and Bagg's abnormal mouse tribe. J. exp. Zool. **67**, 443 (1934).

Brinkley, L., Avery, J. K.: Mechanical intervention with the cranial base during palatal shelf elevation *in vitro*. J. dent. Res. **75 A**, 80 (1975).

Burnside, B.: Microtubules and microfilaments in amphibian neurulation. Amer. Zool. **13**, 989 (1973).

Chase, H. B., Chase, E. B.: Studies on an anophthalmic strain of mice. I. Embryology of the eye region. J. Morph. **68**, 279 (1941).

Chibon, M., Brugal, G.: Étude autoradiographique de l'action de la temperature et de la thyroxine sûr la durée des cycles mitotiques dans l'embryon âgé et la jeune larve de *Pleurodeles Waltlii Micah* (Amphibien Urodèle). C. R. Acad. Sci. (Paris) D, **269**, 70 (1969).

Coulombre, A., Coulombre, J.: The role of mechanical factors in brain morphogenesis. Anat. Rec. **130**, 289 (1958).

Coulombre, A., Coulombre, J.: Abnormal organogenesis of the eye. Handbook of Teratology, J. G. Wilson and F. C. Fraser, eds. New York: Plenum Press 1975 (In press).

De Haan, R. L.: Cell migration and morphogenetic movements. The Chemical Basis of Development, W. D. McElroy and B. Glass, eds. Baltimore: Johns Hopkins Press 1958.

De Luca, L. M., Rosso, G., Wolf, G., Maestri, M.: Retinol glycolipids. J. biol. Chem. **245**, 641 (1973).

De Meyer, W.: Cleft lip and jaw induced in fetal rats by vincristine. Arch. Anat. Histo. Emb. **48**, 179 (1964).

Deol, M. S.: An experimental approach to the understanding and treatment of hereditary syndromes with congenital deafness and hypothyroidism. J. med. Genet. **10**, 235 (1973).

De Petris, S., Raff, M. C.: Fluidity of the plasma membrane and its implications for cell movement. Locomotion of Tissue Cells, M. Abercrombie, ed. Amsterdam: Elsevier 1973.

DUNN, L. C., BENNETT, D.: Abnormalities associated with a chromosome region in the mouse. I. Transmission and population genetics of the T-region. II. Embryological effects of lethal alleles in the T-region. Science **144**, 260 (1964).

EDE, D. A., BELLAIRS, R., BANCROFT, M.: A scanning electron microscope study of the early limb-bud in normal and talpid^3 mutant chick embryos. J. Embryol. exp. Morph. **31**, 761 (1974).

ERWAY, L. C., FRASER, A. S., HURLEY, L. S.: Prevention of congenital otolith defect in pallid mutant mice by manganese supplementation. Genetics **67**, 97 (1971).

ETO, K. E., BHAKDINARONK, A., KING, C. T. G., JOHNSTON, M. C.: Decreased frequency of cleft lip in A/Jax embryos following application of X-irradiation and cyclophosphamide on gestational day 10. Teratology, 1975.

FERM, V. H.: Colchicine teratogenesis in the hamster embryo. Proc. Soc. exp. Biol. (N.Y.) **112**, 775 (1963).

FERM, V. H., CARPENTER, S. J.: The relationship of cadmium and zinc in experimental mammalian teratogenesis. Lab. Invest. **18**, 429 (1968).

FITZHARRIS, T. P., MARKWALD, R. R.: Structural components of cardiac jelly. J. cell Biol. **80**, 235 (1974).

FUJITA, S.: Kinetics of cellular proliferation. Exp. cell Res. **28**, 52 (1962).

GLUCKSMANN, A.: Cell death in normal vertebrate ontogeney. Biol. Rev. **26**, 59 (1951).

GOETINCK, P. F., ABBOTT, V. K.: Tissue interactions in the scaleless mutant and the use of scaleless as an ectodermal marker in studies of normal limb differentiation. J. exp. Zool. **155**, 161 (1964).

GRABOWSKI, C. T.: Embryonic oxygen deficiency — a physiological approach to analysis of teratological mechanisms. Adv. Teratol. **4**, 125 (1970).

GROBSTEIN, C.: Developmental Role of Intercellular Matrix: Retrospection and Prospection. Second International Santa Catalina Conference, p. 9, H. C. SLAVKIN and R. C. GREULICH eds. New York: Acad. Press 1975.

GRUNEBERG, H.: The Pathology of Development. A Study of Inherited Skeletal Disorders in Animals. Oxford: Blackwell (1963).

GUSTAFSON, T., TONEBY, M.: How genes control morphogenesis. The role of serotonin and acetylcholine in morphogenesis. Amer. Scientist **59**, 452 (1971).

HAMBURGER, V., LEVI-MONTALCINI, R.: Some aspects of neuroembryology. Genetic Neurology. P. WEISS, ed. Chicago: University of Chicago Press 128, 1950.

HAMILTON, W. J., MOSSMAN, H. W.: Human Embryology. W. HEFFER, ed. 2. Cambridge, England, 1972.

HARRIS, A. K.: Cell surface movements related to cell locomotion. Locomotion of Tissue Cells, M. ABERCROMBIE, Ed. North-Holland: Elsevier 1973.

HASSELL, J. R., PRATT, R. M., KING, C. T. G.: Growth of the secondary palate during normal and abnormal development, 1975, (In preparation).

HAY, E. D.: Origin and role of collagen in the embryo. Amer. Zool. **13**, 1088 (1973).

HAZELTON, R. D.: A radioautographic analysis of the migration and fate of the occipital somites of the chick embryo with specific reference to the hypoglossal musculature. J. Embryol. exp. Morph. **24**, 455 (1970).

HICKS, S. P., D'AMATO, C. J.: Radiosensitivity at various stages of the mitotic cycle and cellular differentiation. Adv. Teratol. **1**, 215 (1966).

HINCHLIFFE, J. R., EDE, D. A.: Limb development in the polydactylous talpid mutant of the fowl. J. Embryol. exp. Morph. **17**, 385 (1967).

HINCHLIFFE, J. R., EDE, D. A.: Cell death and the development of limb form and skeletal pattern in normal and winglesas (WS) chick embryo. J. Embryol. exp. Morph. **30**, 753 (1973).

HOLTFRETER, J.: Mesenchyme and epithelia in inductive and morphogenic processes. Epithelial Mesenchyme Interactions, E. FLEISCHMAJER and R. BILLINGHAM, Eds. Baltimore: Williams and Wilkins 1968.

HOLTFRETER, J., HAMBURGER, V.: Amphibians. Analysis of Development. B. H. WILLIER, P. A. WEISS, V. HAMBURGER, eds. Philadelphia: Saunders 1955.

Holtzer, H., Mayne, R.: Experimental Morphogenesis: the induction of somite chondrogenesis by embryonic spinal cord and notochord. Pathobiology of Development, E. V. Perrin and M. J. Feingold, eds. Baltimore: Williams and Wilkins 1973.

Hooper, J. K., Cohen, S.: Epidermal growth factor. I. The stimulation of protein and ribonucleic acid synthesis in chick embryo epidermis. Biochim. biophys. Acta (Amst.) **138**, 347 (1967).

Johnston, M. C.: The neural crest in abnormalities of the face and brain. Brain and Face Malformation, J. Langman, ed. Nat. Fdn. 1975 (In press).

Johnston, M. C., Hassell, J. R., Brown, K. S.: The embryology of cleft lip and cleft palate. Plastic Surg. Clinics North Amer. **2**, 95 (1975).

Johnston, M. C., Listgarten, M. A.: The migration interaction and early differentiation of oro-facial tissues. Developmental Aspects of Oral Biology, p. 55, H. C. Slavkin and L. A. Bavetta, Eds. New York: Acad. Press 1972.

Karfunkel, P.: The mechanisms of neural tube formation. Int. Rev. Cytol. **38**, 245 (1974).

Karp, G. C., Solursh, M.: Acid mucopolysaccharide metabolism, the cell surface, and primary mesenchyme cell activity in the sea urchin embryo. Develop. Biol. **41**, 110 (1974).

Kochhar, D. M., Johnson, E. M.: Morphologic and autoradiographic studies of cleft palate induced in rat embryos by maternal hypervitaminosis A. J. Embryol. exp. Morphol. **14**, 223 (1965).

Langman, J.: Medical Embryology. Ed. 2. Baltimore: Williams & Wilkins Co. 1969.

Langman, J., Faassen, F. van: Congenital defects in rat embryos after partial thyroidectomy of the mother animal. A preliminary report on the eye defects. Amer. J. Ophthal. **40**, 65 (1955).

Langman, J., Welsh, G. W.: Effect of vitamin A on the development of the central nervous system. J. comp. Neurol. **128**, 1 (1966).

Lejour, M.: Cleft lip induced in the rat. Cleft Palate J. **7**, 169 (1970).

Levine, S., Pictet, R., Rutter, W. J.: Control of cell proliferation and cytodifferentiation by a factor reacting with the cell surface. Nature (Lond.) **246**, 49 (1973).

Linville, G. P., Shepard, T. H.: Neural tube closure defects caused by cytochalasin B. Nature (Lond.) **236**, 246 (1972).

Marchok, A. C., Herrman, H.: Studies of muscle development. I. Changes in cell proliferation. Develop. Biol. **15**, 129 (1967).

Menkes, B., Sandor, S., Ilies, A.: Cell death in teratogenesis. Adv. Teratology **4**, 170 (1970).

Morriss, G. M.: The ultrastructural effects of excess maternal vitamin of the primitive steak stage rat embryo. J. Embryol. Rap. Morph. **30**, 219 (1973).

Morriss, G. M., Steel, C. E.: The effect of excess vitamin A on the development of rat embryos in culture. J. Embryol. exp. Morph. **32**, 505 (1974).

Moss, M. L.: Neurobiology of oro-facial growth. Acta Biotheoretica **22**, 236 (1972).

Newsome, D. A.: Collagen synthesis in cultured neural crest cells, their derivatives and retinal pigmented epithelium: Stimulation of cartilage collagen production. Effects of Extracellular Matrix on Gene Expression. Second International Santa Catalina Conference, H. C. Slavkin and R. C. Greulich, eds. New York: Acad. Press 1975.

Nishimura, H.: Incidence of malformations in abortions. Congenital Malformations. F. C. Fraser and V. A. McKusick, eds. Amsterdam, New York: Excerpta Medica Press 1969.

Orkin, R. B. W., Ketley, J. N., Pope, M., Penttinen, R., Martin, G. R.: Function of the genetically distinct collagens. Aberrations in Developmental Processes. Second International Santa Catalina Conference, p. 195, H. C. Slavkin and R. C. Greulich, eds. New York: Acad. Press 1975.

Patterson, D. F., Pyle, R. L., Buchanan, J. W.: Hereditary cardiovascular malformations of the dog. Birth Defects: Original Articles Series, Cardiovascular Systems, D. Bergsma, ed. Baltimore: Williams and Wilkins 1972.

Poswillo, D.: The pathogenesis of the first and second branchial arch syndrome. Oral Surg. **35**, 302 (1973).

Poswillo, D., Sopher, D.: Malformation and deformation in the animal embryo. Teratology **4**, 498 (1971).

PRATT, R. M., GREENE, R. M., HASSELL, J. R., GREENBERG, J. H.: Epithelial cell differentiation during secondary palate development. In Proceedings of the 2nd International Santa Catalina Island Colloquium on the role of the extracellular matrix in gene expression, H. C. SLAVKIN and R. C. GREULICH, eds. New York: Academic Press 1975 a.

PRATT, R. M., KING, C. T. G.: Inhibition of collagen crosslinking associated with β-aminoproprionitrile-induced cleft palate in the rat. Develop. Biol. **27**, 322 (1972).

PRATT, R. M., LARSON, M. A., JOHNSTON, M. C.: Migration of cranial neural crest cells in cell-free hyaluronate-rich matrix. Develop. Biol. **44**, 298 (1975 b).

PRATT, R. M., MARTIN, G. R.: Epithelial cell death and elevated cyclic AMP during palatal devlopment. Proc. nat. Acad. Sci. (Wash.) **72**, 814 (1975).

RAKIC, P., SIDMAN, R. L.: Weaver mutant mouse cerebellum: Defective neuronal migration secondary to abnormality of Bergmann glia. Proc. nat. Acad. Sci. (Wash.) **70**, 240 (1973).

REVEL, J. P.: Some aspects of cellular interactions in development. The Cell Surface in Development. A. A. MOSCONA, ed. New York: Wiley 1974.

ROGERS, L., COWAN, W. M.: The development of the mesencephalic nucleus of the trigeminal nerve in the chick. J. comp. Neurol. **147**, 291 (1973).

ROSS, R. B., JOHNSTON, M. C.: Cleft Lip and Palate. Baltimore: Williams & Wilkins 1972.

ROTH, S., BERBERA, A. J., SHUR, B. D., MARCHASE, R. B.: The location and nature of molecules potentially involved in morphogenesis of the developing nervous system. Outer cell surface specificities and cell interactions. Second International Santa Catalina Conference, p. 413 H. C. SLAVKIN and R. C. GREULICH, eds. New York: Acad. Press 1975.

RUSTAD, R. C.: Radiation responses during the mitotic cycle of the sea urchin egg. Cell Proliferation and Development. I. L. CAMERON, ed. New York: Acad. Press 1972.

RUTTER, W. J., KEMP, J. D., BRADSHAW, W. S., CLARK, W. R., RONZIO, R. A., SANDERS, T. G.: Regulation of specific protein synthesis in cytodifferentiation. J. cell. comp. Physiol. Suppl. **1**, 72 (1968).

RUTTER, W. J., PICTET, R. L., MORRIS, P. W.: Toward molecular mechanisms of developmental processes. Ann. Rev. Biochem. **42**, 601 (1973).

SAUNDERS, J. W.: Cell death in embryonic systems. Science **154**, 604 (1966).

SAXÉN, L.: Tissue interactions in teratogenesis. Pathobiology of Development, E. V. D. PERRIN and M. J. FEINGOLD, Eds. Baltimore: Williams and Wilkins 1973.

SAXÉN, L.: Transmission and spread of kidney tubule induction. Epithelial-mesenchymal interactions. Second International Santa Catalina Conference, p. 523, H. S. SLAVKIN and R. C. GREULICH, eds. New York: Acad. Press 1975.

SAXÉN, L. S., KAITILA, I.: The effect and mode of action of tetracycline on bone development *in vitro*. Advanc. exp. Med. **27**, 205 (1972).

SAXÉN, L., RAPOLA, J.: Congenital Defects. New York: Holt, Rhinehart and Winston 1969.

SAXÉN, L. S., TOIVONEN, S.: Primary Embryonic Induction. London: Acad. Press 1962.

SCHWEICKEL, J. V., MERKER, H. J.: The morphology of various types of cell death in prenatal tissues. Teratology **1**, 253 (1973).

SHAPIRO, B. L., SWEENY, L.: Electronmicroscopic and histochemical examination of oral epithelial-mesenchymal interaction (programmed cell death). J. dent. Res. **48**, 652 (1969).

SLAVKIN, H. C.: Embryonic tooth formation. Oral Sci. Rev. **4**, 1 (1974).

SMILEY, G. R., KOCH, W. E.: An *in vitro* and *in vivo* study of single palatal processes. Anat. Rec. **173**, 405 (1972).

SOLURSH, M., MEIER, S.: The selective inhibition of mucopolysaccharide synthesis by vitamin A treatment of cultured chick embryo chondrocytes. Calc. Tissue Res. **13**, 131 (1973).

SPIEGELMAN, M., BENNETT, D.: Fine structural study of cell migration in early mesoderm of normal and mutant mouse embryo (T-locus: t^9/t^9). J. Embryol. exp. Morph. **32**, 123 (1974).

STEFFEK, A. J., MUJUID, D. K., JOHNSTON, M. C.: Scanning electron microscopy (SEM) of cranial neural crest migration. J. dent. Res. **54 A**, 165 (1975).

TOOLE, B. P.: Hyaluronate and hyaluronidase in morphogenesis and differentiation. Amer. Zool. **13**, 1961 (1973).

TOOLE, B. P., TRELSTAD, R. L.: Hyaluronate production and removal during corneal development in the chick. Develop. Biol. **26**, 28 (1971).

TRASLER, D. G.: Pathogenesis of cleft lip and its relation to embryonic face shape in A/Jax and C57BL mice. Teratology **1**, 33 (1968).

TRASLER, D. G., LEONG, S.: Face shape and mitotic index in mice with 6-aminonicotinamide-induced and inherited cleft lip. Teratology 9, a-39 (1974).
WEBSTER, D. A., GROSS, J.: Studies on possible mechanisms of cell death in the chick embryo. Develop. Biol. 22, 157 (1970).
WESSELLS, N. K., SPOONER, B. S., LUDUENA, M.: Surface movements microfilaments and cell location. Locomotion of Tissue Cells, M. ABERCROMBIE, ed. Amsterdam: Elsevier 1973.
WESTON, J. A.: The migration and differentiation of neural crest cells. Advanc. Morph. 8, 41 (1970).
WILSON, J. G.: Environment and Birth Defects. New York: Acad. Press 1973.
YAMADA, K. M.: Cell morphogenetic movents. Handbook of Teratology. J. G. WILSON and F. C. FRASER, eds. New York: Plenum Publishers 1975 (In press).
ZWILLING, E.: Micromelia as a direct effect of insulin. Evidence from *in vitro* and *in vivo* experiments. J. Morph. 104, 159 (1959).

2. Chromosomal Animal Model of Human Disease. Fetal Trisomy and Developmental Failure

A. GROPP

With the Assistance of B. PUTZ

With 14 Figures

An important consequence of recent studies on abortion in man is the recognition of the considerable frequency of chromosomal abnormalities of the zygote which cause abnormal development and early or late developmental breakdown. Among the prenatally lethal chromosomal aberrations, three types seem to be more important (Fig. 1): the XO constitution, autosomal trisomy and triploidy. Their respective proportions differ to a certain extent when the data presented by individual laboratories are compared. However, these differences depend mainly on the source and the selection of the material (early or later abortions). The largest group of abnormalities is represented in all surveys by the autosomal trisomies. There is, therefore, great interest in answering the question of how triplicate chromosomes affect differentiation and development.

While it has been possible in man to assign particular specific chromosomal aberrations of abortuses (mainly triploidy or perhaps XO) to certain pathologic patterns of development (PHILIPPE, 1973), it is far more difficult, if not impossible, to detect such relationships in cases of autosomal errors. These usually display severe retardation which may hide more or less specific profiles of abnormal development. In addition, secondary processes, mainly maceration, can cause considerable alterations of an aborted embryo impeding or precluding morpho-embryological analyses. Recently, a mouse model has been worked out (GROPP *et al.*, 1974 a, b; 1975), which permits the specific experimental induction of autosomal trisomies. This model should provide suitable conditions for the systematic study of the detrimental effect of the autosomal errors which lead to developmental abnormality and eventually to developmental breakdown.

Biological and Cytogenetic Premises of the Animal Model

The experimental mouse system is based on the observation that structural heterozygosity of the Robertsonian type may enhance irregular meiotic segregation and thus produce chromosomally unbalanced gametes and aneuploidy of the embryo.

Robertsonian changes (Rb) involve centric fusion (or translocation) which unites the arms of two acrocentric chromosomes to form one metacentric. In the mouse, whose normal karyotype shows 40 acrocentric chromosomes, metacentrics (Fig. 2 a) have been observed in exceptional cases in laboratory mouse strains (LÉONARD and

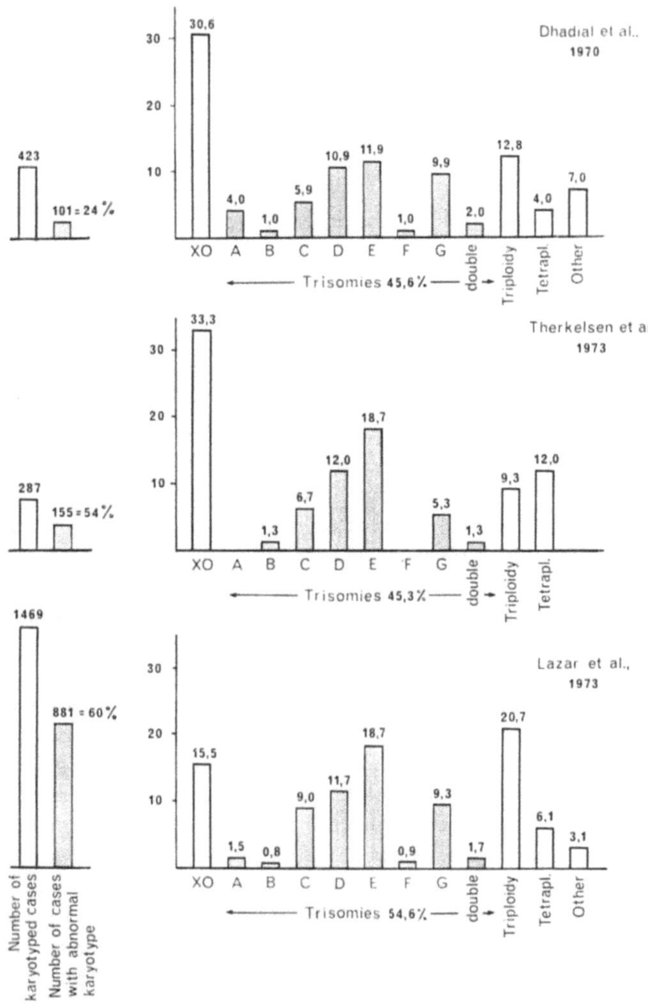

Fig. 1. Incidence of lethal chromosomal abnormalities causing developmental failure (abortion) in man. Results of three surveys

DEKNUDT, 1967; EVANS *et al.*, 1967; WHITE and TJIO, 1968; BARANOV and DYBAN, 1971) and in greater number in some feral populations of the domestic mouse from south-eastern Switzerland (GROPP *et al.*, 1970; 1972) and Italy (CAPANNA *et al.*, 1975). Table 1 records the established metacentrics of the mouse to date, the identity of their arms and, as far as possible, the assignment of known linkage groups. Some of the metacentrics of feral origin designated with the symbol Rb1 to 10Bnr (cf. Fig. 2) have been introduced by breeding procedures in laboratory mouse strains (CATTANACH *et al.*, 1972; GROPP and ZECH, 1973). The Rb1 to 7Bnr are derived from *M. poschiavinus*, whose karyotype includes seven pairs of metacentrics. Single or double metacentric male and female heterozygotes produce variable, some-

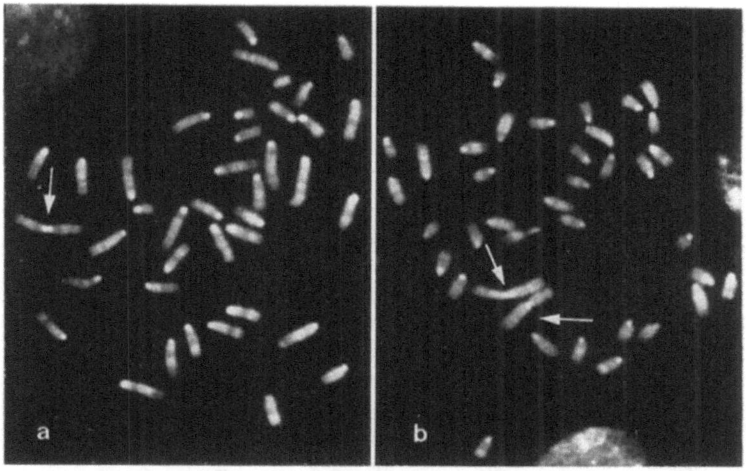

Fig. 2 a and b. Somatic metaphases (from fetal tissue); mixed C- and Q-type band staining with the fluorochrome "33258" (HILWIG and GROPP, 1971). — (a) Presence of Rb9Bnr metacentric in a heterozygous individual (Rb9/+) — (b) Trisomy, 41 chromosome arms, two metacentrics: Rb5 and Rb9Bnr

Table 1. Metacentrics — derived from Robertsonian fusion

Designation of metacentric	Arms designated according to the numbering system for mouse chrom.	Linkage group assigned to individual chrom. arm	Origin of metacentric
Laboratory mouse strains			
Rb1Ald	15/6	VI/XI	LÉONARD and DEKNUDT (1967)
Rb163H	19/9	XII/II	EVANS *et al.* (1967)
Rb1Wh	19/5	XII/XVII	WHITE and TJIO (1967)
Rb1IeM	17/8	IX/XVIII	BARANOV and DYBAN (1971)
Feral mouse origin			
Rb1Bnr	3/1	—/XIII	Valle di Poschiavo (Rb1—7) and adjacent regions of South-Eastern Switzerland, GROPP *et al.* (1972)
Rb2Bnr	6/4	XI/VIII	
Rb3Bnr	15/5	VI/XVII	
Rb4Bnr	13/11	XIV/VII	
Rb5Bnr	12/8	XVI/XVIII	
Rb6Bnr	14/9	III/II	
Rb7Bnr	17/16	IX/—	
Rb8Bnr	11/10	VII/X	
Rb9Bnr	12/4	XVI/VIII	
Rb10Bnr	10/1	X/XIII	
Rb1Rma	6/1	XI/XIII	Central Italy (Apennines), CAPANNA *et al.* (1975)
Rb2Rma	8/3	XVIII/—	
Rb3Rma	11/7	VII/I	
Rb4Rma	15/4	VI/VIII	
Rb5Rma	10/9	X/II	
Rb6Rma	18/2	XV/V	
Rb7Rma	17/5	IX/XVII	
Rb8Rma	14/12	III/XVI	
Rb9Rma	16/13	—/XIV	

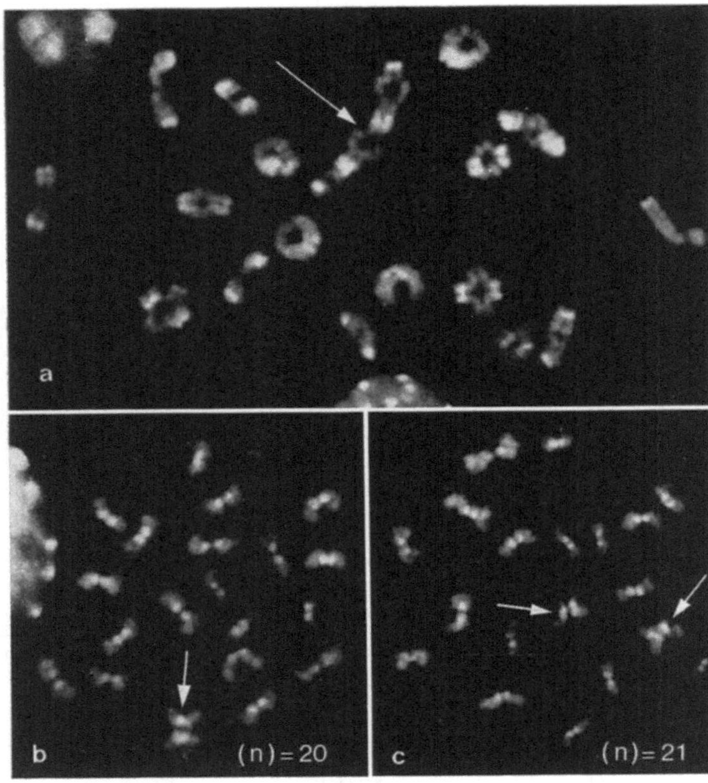

Fig. 3 a—c. Meiotic divisions (testis), C-type band staining with the fluorochrome "33258 H" — (a) Diakinesis (metaphase I) of Rb6Bnr/Rb163H double metacentric heterozygote forming a quadrivalent (→). — (b) Metaphase II with one metacentric (→); modal haploid number of chromosome arms (=20). — (c) Metaphase II with two metacentrics (→); hypermodal number of arms (=21)

times considerable rates of meiotic anaphase I non-disjunction. They can be assessed by chromosome counts of the haploid products of the 1st meiotic division, i. e. in metaphase II figures (TETTENBORN and GROPP, 1971; CATTANACH and MOSELEY, 1973). In a general way, irregular meiotic anaphase I segregation seems to be more important in female than in male gametogenesis. The incidence of this error is rather high in double metacentric heterozygotes with monobrachial homology which, in meiosis I, exhibit a quadrivalent formed by the two partially homologous metacentrics (Fig. 3 a). Non-disjunction generally involves the elements building up this quadrivalent. Its formation is thus responsible for the increased rates of malsegregation which in the male, may lead to 13—22% (Table 2) metaphase II figures (Fig. 3 c vs. b.).

The data shown in Table 2 should be considered from the viewpoint that anaphase I double non-disjunction of acrocentrics (Fig. 4, left-hand rectangles) produces metaphases II with a pseudomodal, doubly unbalanced number of chromosome arms. Thus, the true proportion of balanced M II cells is distinctly lower than represented in the column of "normal" arm counts. On the other hand, according to the design proposed for the induction of trisomy (Fig. 4), relevance need to be attributed only to the hypermodal M II which, by non-disjunction, are endowed with both metacentrics (Fig. 3 c; Fig. 4 rectangle with heavy black line). Theoretically, trisomy could also result from nondisjunction of one of the acrocentrics involved in the formation of the quadrivalent figure, while the metacentrics segregate normally. However, this type has not been observed (GROPP *et al.*, 1975).

Table 2. Incidence of meiotic anaphase I malsegregation in double metacentric heterozygotes as shown by chromosome counts in meiotic metaphase II [a]

Designation of double heterozygote [b]	sharing a chromosome arm which corresponds to mouse chrom. no.	Percentage of Metaphase II cells with		
		hypomodal (n<20) counts %	normal (n=20) %	hypermodal (n>20) %
Rb1/Rb10	1	12	74	14
Rb2/Rb1Ald	6	18	63	19
Rb5/Rb1IeM	8	19	62	19
Rb6/Rb163	9	15	70	15
Rb8/Rb10	10	18	69	13
Rb4/Rb8	11	18	65	17
Rb5/Rb9	12	21	58	21
Rb3/Rb1Ald	15	21	57	22
Rb7/Rb1IeM	17	19	64	17

[a] cf. GROPP *et al.*, 1975.
[b] For metacentrics of the series Rb1 to 10Bnr the symbol Bnr is omitted.

Probably the majority of unbalanced precursor cells resulting from meiotic malsegregation can develop to morphologically normal gametes, e. g. spermatozoa (STOLLA and GROPP, 1974). Fertilization may then cause monosomy or trisomy of the zygotes. Considerable selective elimination of aneusomics occurs at implantation. A selective effect with regard to the individual types of aneusomy (monosomy and trisomy) is documented in Table 3 from a study of the fetal backcross progeny of *Mus poschiavinus* × laboratory mouse F_1-hybrids heterozygous for seven metacentrics (FORD, 1971; GROPP, 1971). Thus, monosomics (or combined monosomics and trisomics) only occasionally survive beyond day 8 or 9 of development. In contrast, trisomic mouse embryos remain viable for longer and develop until a later fetal period, but eventually are eliminated before the end of gestation. In this respect, the mouse is different from man, in whom at least some types of trisomy may survive into postnatal or even adult life.

Experimental Design

Fig. 4 shows in the upper part the main types of segregants produced by irregular anaphase I distribution in double metacentric heterozygotes with monobrachial homology. The heterozygous mice are crossed with partners of an "all acrocentric" laboratory strain (Fig. 4 lower part), and the females are sacrificed at different times

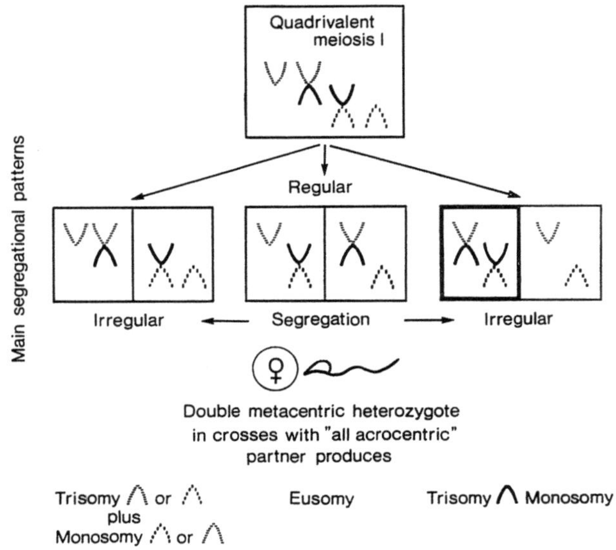

Fig. 4. Experimental breeding design for the induction of individual trisomies

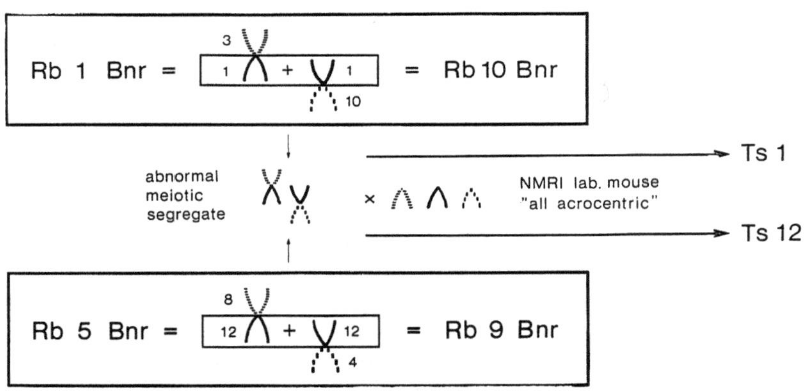

Fig. 5. Specific experimental design for the induction of Ts 1 and Ts 12

between day 8 and 17 of pregnancy for the analysis of the fetal progeny. If it is correct to assume that the resulting monosomics and the combined aneusomics do not survive day 8 or 9, then trisomy (no. of chromosome arms = 41) is the only unbalanced combination found after this developmental stage. This condition, if induced by joint non-disjunction of the metacentrics, is marked by the presence of both metacentrics (Fig. 2 b) and is therefore easy to ascertain by simple cytogenetic procedures. For example, karyotypes may be prepared directly from the cells of fetal membranes after previous maternal Colcemid injection. This allows the embryos to be saved for morphological, biochemical or other analyses.

Following this experimental design, the specific nature of trisomy in the fetal progeny may then be determined by the choice of the special double heterozygote combination.

Thus, the Rb1/Rb10 heterozygote is used for inducing the trisomy of chromosome no. 1 (Fig. 5 a), because the two metacentrics Rb(*1*.3)1 and Rb(*1*.10)10 share a chromosome arm corresponding to the mouse chromosome no. 1. Similarly, the Rb(8.*12*)5/Rb(4.*12*)9Bnr heterozygote (Fig. 5 b) is suitable for the induction of trisomy no. 12. The combinations, at present available (Table 2) allow the study of Ts nos. 1, 6, 8, 9, 10, 11, 12, 15 and 17. The induction of the remaining autosomal trisomies depends on the breeding of other double heterozygotes with the respective homology desired (Table 1). So far Ts 1, 6, 8, 10, 11, 12, 15, 17 (GROPP *et al.*, 1974 1975) and 19 (WHITE *et al.*, 1972, 1974) have been investigated.

In the experimental design shown in Fig. 4, male or female heterozygotes might be used for the crosses with "all acrocentric" mice. Yet WHITE *et al.* (1974) reported that male Rb(5.*19*)1Wh/Rb(9.*19*)163H produced more trisomics than female hybrids. On the other hand, it has been observed (DÖRING *et al.*, 1975) that a postmeiotic maturation arrest in spermatogenesis may occur, of uncertain aetiology, and thus cause complete male sterility in some double heterozygote combinations (Rb5/Rb1IeM and Rb7/Rb1IeM are examples). The respective females are fertile and can be used for the induction of trisomic offspring.

Incidence, Biologic Features and Developmental Profiles of Fetal Trisomy

General Observations. The occurrence of trisomy is regularly associated with many dead or resorbed implantations. These probably represent the remnants of the nonviable aneuploids of which the monosomics are the first to be eliminated (day 5 to 9, cf. Table 3). With the further progression of pregnancy, the frequency of resorptions increases to the same extent as trisomics decay.

Table 3. Backcrosses (*M. poschiavinus* [a] × lab. mouse) F_1 ♀ [b] × NMRI ♂

Stage of development	Total No. of implantations	No. of chromosome arms (N.F.) hypomodal ← euploid → hypermodal				
		37< 38	39	40	41	42 >43
Blastocysts	79	7	17	38	14	3
10th day	51	—	—	34	15	2
15th day	38	—	1	32	5	—
20th day	23	—	—	22	1	—
Live born	18	—	—	18	—	—

[a] *M. poschiavinus*, 2n=26 chrom., including the metacentrics Rb1—7Bnr (Table 1).
[b] F_1 : 2n=33 chrom., heterozygous for Rb1—7Bnr (N.F.=40).

The actual frequency of trisomic implants in the progeny of double heterozygotes differs depending on the individual metacentric combinations. It probably also depends on whether the heterozygote is the male or the female progenitor (WHITE *et al.*, 1974). Furthermore, the sequential elimination of trisomic embryos (cf. Table 3) explains their greater frequency early in gestation than, for example, after day 15. From our own studies (GROPP *et al.*, 1975), the mean frequency between day 10—14

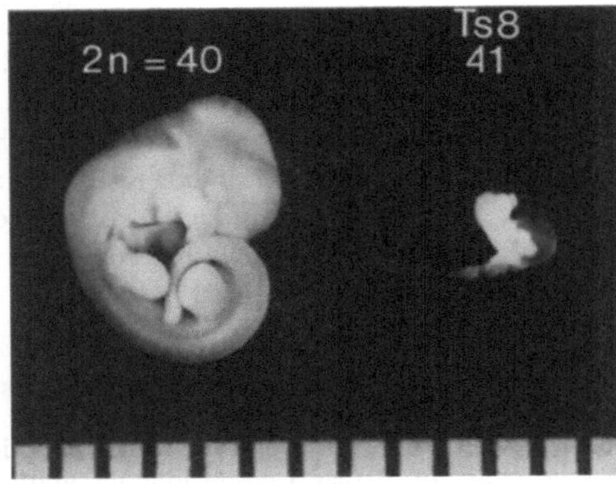

Fig. 6. Ts 8 and normal litter mate, day 12. Extreme retardation and hypoplasia of trisomic embryo (caudal part damaged). Embryos on mm scale

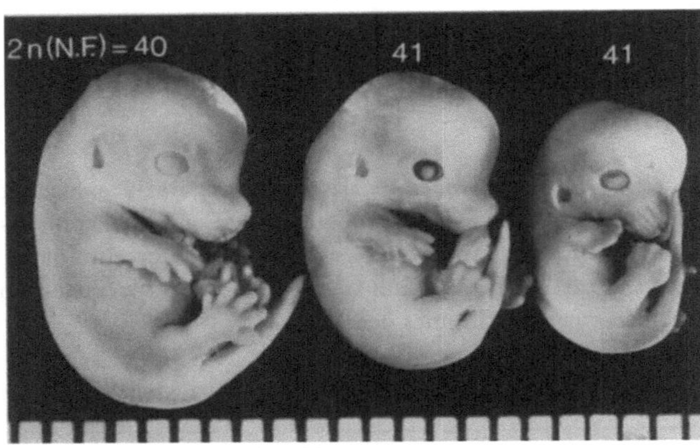

Fig. 7. Three embryos from same pregnancy, day 15. Center and right: Ts 1 displaying variable, slight to moderate, retardation and hypoplasia; left: normal embryo. Embryos on mm scale

is 16.6% for Ts 1 (progeny of male Rb1/Rb10Bnr), 8.1% for Ts 11 (prog. of male Rb4/Rb8Bnr), 14.5% for Ts 12 (prog. of male Rb5/Rb9Bnr), 7.6% for Ts 8 (prog. of female Rb5/Rb1IeM), and 5.4% for Ts 17 (prog. of female Rb7/Rb1IeM). Comparable data from WHITE *et al.* (1974) on Ts 19 from stages between day 12½ to 15½ are 27.2% (prog. of male heterozygote) and 7.9% (prog. of female heterozygote). The respective frequencies for other trisomics have not yet been established.

It is obvious that the developmental profiles in autosomal trisomy may differ considerably according to which individual autosome is involved. In a general way, autosomal trisomy in the mouse is — as mentioned before — almost invariably connected with earlier (day 10 to 13) or later (day 14 to 17) prenatal death. However, it is noteworthy in this respect that Ts 19 (WHITE *et al.*, 1974) sometimes seems to allow brief post partum survival.

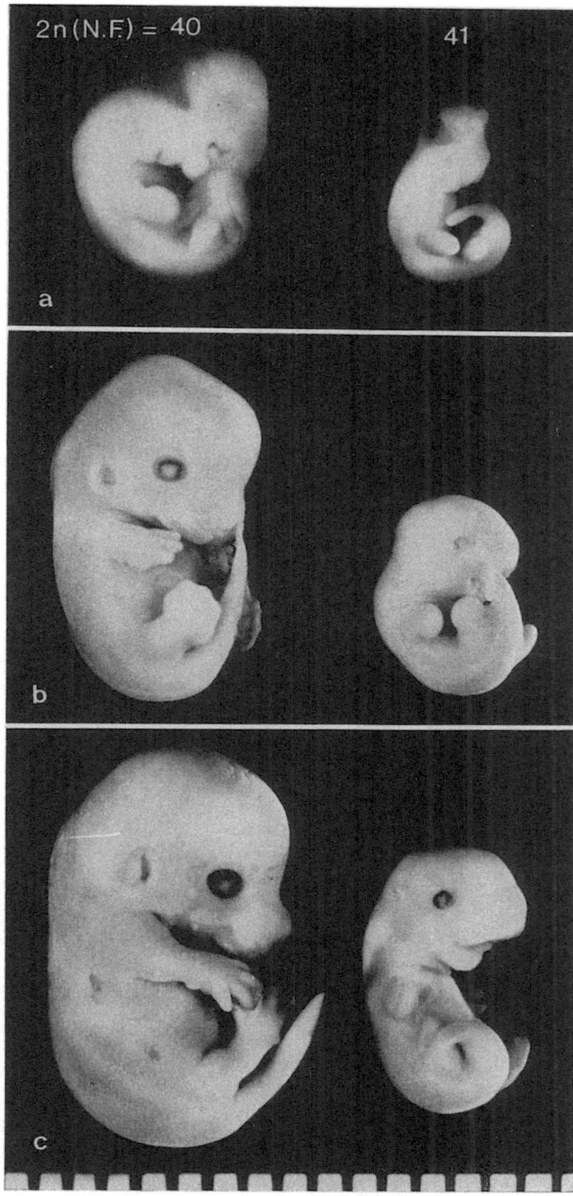

Fig. 8 a—c. Ts 1 at day 12 (a), day 13 (b) and day 14³/₄ (c), showing more severe retardation and hypoplasia, compared with normal litter mate (left)

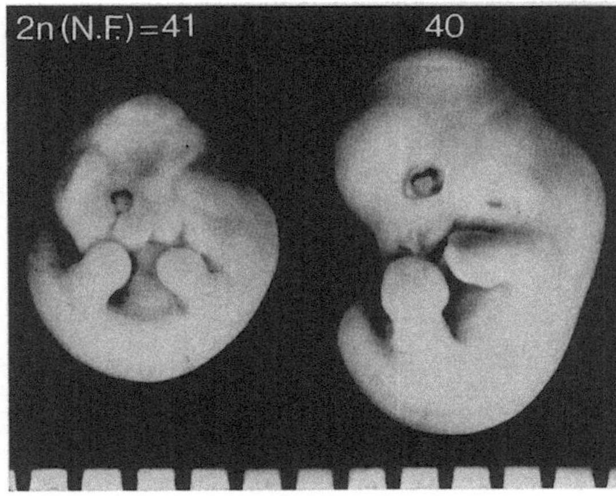

Fig. 9. Ts 10 and normal litter mate, day $12^1/_2$. Slight retardation of the trisomic embryo

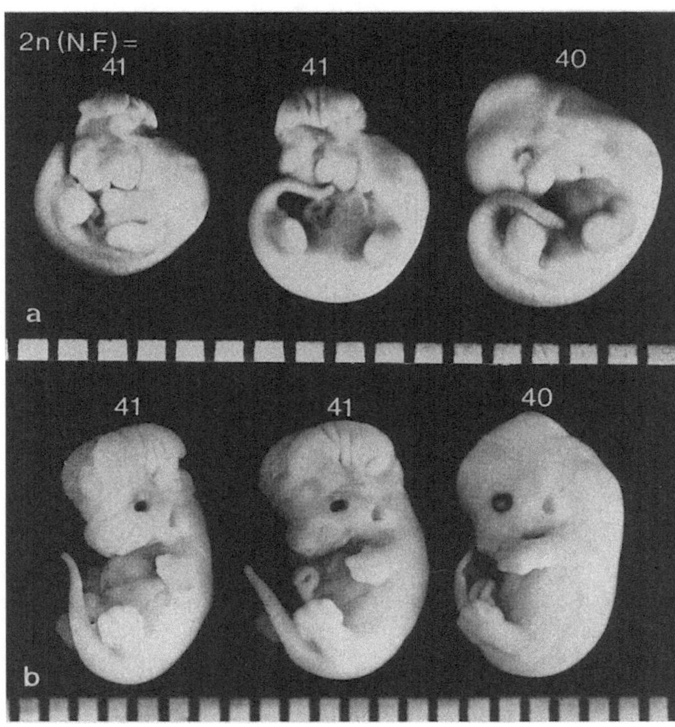

Fig. 10 a and b. Ts 12. Left and center: affected embryos, right: normal litter mate; day 12 (a) and day 13 (b). Trisomic embryos showing exencephaly and microphthalmia

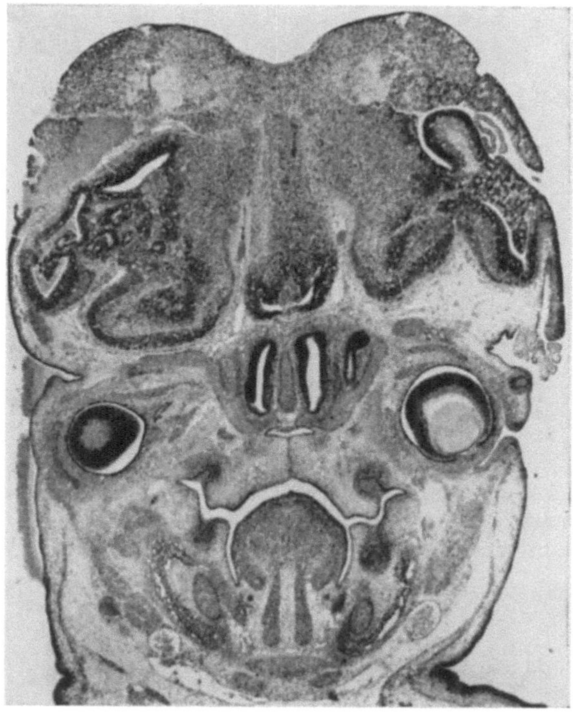

Fig. 11. Histological section of the head of an embryo with Ts 12, day 16 (see text)

Some specific trisomies are characterized by severe hypoplasia and extreme developmental retardation or inhibition. This is true for Ts 8, 11, 15 and 17. Trisomic implants corresponding to these types seldom survive longer than day 11 or 12 of fetal development. They usually form a minute unorganized mass (Ts 11 and 15) or an extremely retarded embryo (Fig. 6), sometimes with the external signs of initial differentiation of the encephalic vesicles (Ts 8 and 17). Rare specimens of these types of trisomy found still later (e. g. day 14) only show an empty sac.

Trisomies with a Syndrome of Prevalent Developmental Retardation and Hypoplasia. Some of the trisomies of the fetal mouse known to date are mainly characterized by a syndrome of generally slight or moderate, occasionally severe retardation and hypoplasia. Ts 1, Ts 6 and Ts 10 belong to this category.

The different manifestations of developmental impairment, as depicted in Figs. 7 and 8 for Ts 1, result from the allelic heterogeneity of mouse lines generally used in our own experiments (as well as in those of White *et al.*, 1974). Thus, two examples of slight or moderate retardation and hypoplasia are shown in Fig. 7, while Figs. 8 a to c show embryos with Ts 1 at day 12, 13 and 15 exhibiting a rather severe impairment of fetal development. The more severely affected embryos usually also exhibit variable degrees of craniofacial hypoplasia or dysmorphy. This particular expression of Ts 1 (Figs. 8 b and c) becomes more frequent with the progression of

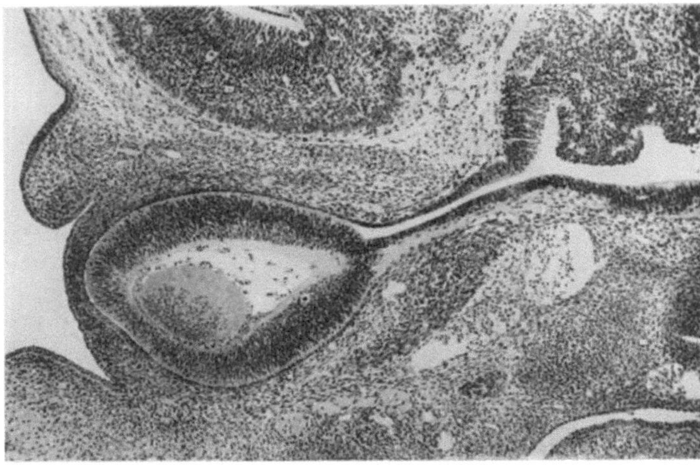

Fig. 12. Histological section with the orbita of an embryo with Ts 12, day 14. Smallness, dysplasia and abnormal downward inclination of the eye

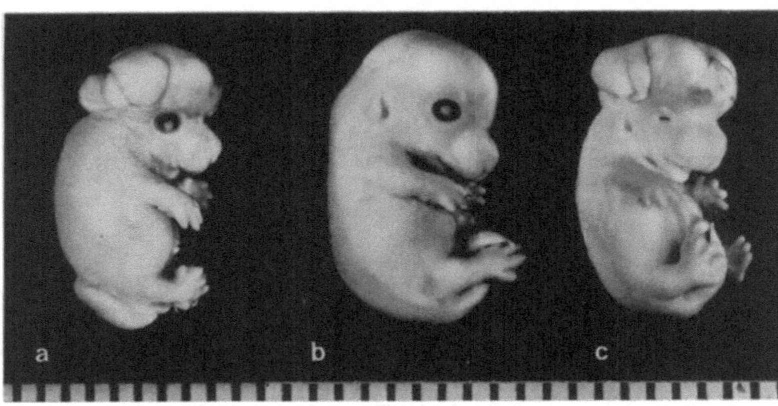

Fig. 13 a—c. Ts 12 (c) and normal litter mate (b) at day 14$^1/_2$ compared with embryo (a) day 15 after treatment of the mother with Vitamin A, 12 500 U (see text). In (a) exencephaly and spina bifida, but no microphthalmia

fetal development, i. e. usually until day 15 when developmental breakdown and death affects the embryos with this trisomy. However, some rare instances of a cyclopia-like malformation were noted in Ts 1. Not infrequently, more severe degrees of developmental impairment were also observed in Ts 6 and Ts 10 (Fig. 9). Death usually occurs in these two trisomies before day 15.

In all these cases the placenta displays concomitant changes of retardation and hypoplasia. In general, the more retarded and smaller the affected embryo the smaller is the placenta.

Trisomies with Syndromes of Malformation. Ts 19 (WHITE *et al.*, 1972, 1974) and Ts 12 (GROPP and KOLBUS, 1974) are the only trisomies of the fetal mouse in which specific gross malformations have been observed. These are cleft palate in Ts 19 and exencephaly/microphthalmia in Ts 12. Both have a longer prenatal survival span, Ts 12 until day 17, Ts 19 to term or beyond.

Isolated cleft palate was consistently associated with Ts 19 only under the condition of a special cytogenetic constitution (Rb1Wh/Rb163H/Rb163H triple metacentric), thus demonstrating the effects of the genetic background upon the expression of trisomy. A significant decrease of fetal and placental weights at all stages of development has been found in Ts 19, but the only specific change found in the viscera was degeneration of oocytes in some of the ovaries.

In contrast, exencephaly and accompanying microphthalmia are constant features of Ts 12 (Figs. 10 and 13 c). Its expression is rather uniform. Fig. 10 demonstrates isolated exencephaly and microphthalmia, but very slight or moderate hypoplasia. So far these changes have been seen only in heterogeneic breeding systems. Occasionally in later stages, subcutaneous, mostly dorsal oedema may become prominent. Histologically (Fig. 11), the basiphenoid is slightly hypoplastic. There is evidence that its abnormal downward inclination, causing a size reduction and a shift of the angle of the orbita together with a concomitant hypoplasia of the bulb, is responsible for the microphthalmic malformation (Fig. 12).

It is interesting to note that the exencephaly-microphthalmia-syndrome of Ts 12 can be clearly distinguished from exencephaly induced by exogenous factors. Thus, in experiments (B. PUTZ, unpubl.) in which vitamin A (12 500 U, injected i.p., day 9) was used as a teratogen in mice with the same genetic background as in the breeding experiments for trisomy, exencephaly was usually accompanied by spina bifida, while microphthalmia was not observed (Fig. 13 a). Moreover, vitamin A induced exencephaly permits a longer survival than Ts 12.

Conclusions and Prospects for a Systematic Study of Experimental Trisomy

Taking advantage of the availability of 23 metacentrics with different arm composition (Table 1) providing a great choice of double metacentric combinations, and using the experimental approach described in this chapter, it should be theoretically possible to induce almost all 19 autosomal trisomies of the mouse (with the exception of Ts 2, 7 and 18). At present our own observations allow the depiction of the phenotypes and the developmental profiles of 9 of these trisomic conditions. Considering the selection against monosomics and trisomics in the early stages of embryogenesis (FORD, 1971; GROPP, 1971) and the fate of trisomy in later stages, a general picture emerges which is characterized by sequential steps of developmental failure, ending up with death and elimination of the chromosomally abnormal progeny (Fig. 14). It is interesting to note that sometimes the developmental breakdown sets in suddenly (Ts 6, 10, 12), while in other cases it evolves after a short period of slowing down of growth and differentiation (Ts 8, 11, 15, 17, and some cases of Ts 1).

From a genetical point of view, it might be thought surprising that trisomy of a large chromosome like Ts 1 or Ts 4, allows relatively long survival and development, whereas Ts 11, 15

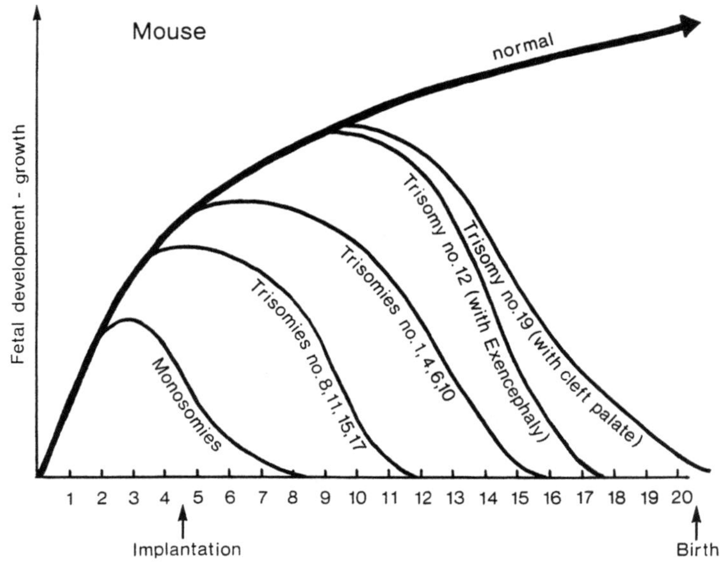

Fig. 14. Developmental characteristics of some fetal trisomy syndromes of the mouse

and 17 are eliminated at an early developmental stage. Obviously, the phenotypic expression of trisomy depends on the presence and dosage effects of important genes and on the total amount of genetically active chromatin in the extra chromosome.

The longer span of survival of Ts 12 and Ts 19 compared, for example, with Ts 1, 6 or 10, supports the assumption that gross morphological malformation per se is not the major cause of developmental breakdown. This failure may be, at least in part, due to factors causing impairment and slowing down of growth. In fact, an increased doubling time of trisomic tissues has been found in Down's syndrome by Schneider and Epstein (1972) and in other trisomic and triploid conditions by Cure *et al.* (1973). From preliminary labelling studies of mouse tissues *in vitro,* there is no evidence that slower growth rates of trisomic cells (Ts 1 and Ts 12) might be caused by a lower proportion of cells taking part in the growth pool. Moreover, the length of the S-phase and of the total cell cycle does not depart significantly from the normal (P. Citoler, pers. comm.). However, many questions concerning these observations are still open, and offer points of departure for future studies. Thus, it would seem important to examine the growth kinetics of trisomic embryos and of individual organs at different stages along the curves of the developmental profiles (Fig. 14). Moreover, the observation that the trisomic placenta is also involved in the impaired growth and differentiation, raises the question of whether a corresponding or even a disproportionate manifestation of such effects in the placenta could initiate the developmental breakdown of the embryo perhaps via an inadequate fetal blood supply.

A systematic survey of trisomy in the mouse embryo affords a prospect of considerable value in developmental pathology and teratology. It also provides a method by which the genotype-phenotype relationship in gross genome unbalance may be examined. Ts 1, for example, can be regarded as a syndrome of proportionate or disproportionate hypoplasia and retardation, offering a model for the study of hypoplasia and runting in fetal development. In contrast, the Ts 12-syndrome lends itself as a suitable model for the analysis of aetiological factors and of the teratological processes involved in the origin and the pathogenesis of the "anencephaly-exencephaly complex" (cf. MARIN-PADILLA, 1970) and of microphthalmia.

Probably, the endogenous chromosomal cause of craniorhachischisis in Ts 12 does not have a counterpart in man, despite isolated observations as in a case of WRIGHT *et al.* (1974) with partial trisomy. It has been suggested that other genetic disorders, e. g. autosomal recessive inheritance (PENROSE, 1957; FUHRMANN *et al.*, 1971) may also play a role in the genesis of neural tube defects in man. It can be assumed, however, that the aetiology of this malformation is complex and multifactorial involving environmental agents (cf. GIROUD and MARTINET, 1960; MURAKAMI and KAMEYAMA, 1963; POSWILLO *et al.*, 1972) as well as genetic factors. Thus, a more extensive comparison of the chromosomal animal model of Ts 12 (Figs. 10 and 13) with the changes produced by exogenous agents (cf. Fig. 13 a), and experimental designs allowing the analysis of the possible interaction of endogenous and exogenous factors, represent an interesting task for future investigators.

A *mouse* model for the study of genetically determined abnormal development has the advantage that a huge body of knowledge about gene mutants is available in this species, and that most of the gene linkage groups can be assigned to individual chromosomes (Table 1). It is tempting therefore, to study the expression of triplicate genes not only in complex phenotypes, but also at the level of single gene products. For example, the phenotype of iso-citrate-dehydrogenase in Ts 1 is at present under investigation (C. P. CLAUSSEN and A. GROPP, unpubl.), inasmuch as the coding gene for this enzyme belongs to L.G. XIII located at chromosome no. 1 (see Table 1). However, systematic analyses of gene-dose relationships of genomes with triplicate autosomes are far from complete. It is important for this purpose that trisomy should be induced within a genetically defined (inbred) mouse system. It is to be expected that the results of such studies which should clarify the consequences of genome unbalance may shed considerable light on the genetic regulation of normal developmental processes. The failure of this regulation in abnormal development and malformation may also be studied.

Summary

We have established an experimental model in the mouse allowing the detailed study of the principles governing the expression of a triplicate autosome and of genome-phenotype relationships in trisomy syndromes. Trisomy, in this model, results from irregular meiotic disjunction of double metacentric heterozygotes, provided that the two metacentrics are partially homologous but segregate together. A choice of metacentrics in mouse lines is available which permits the induction of almost all autosomal trisomies except Ts 2, 7 and 18. All trisomic conditions described to date cause early or late fetal death, and are thus eliminated before term or less commonly shortly post partum. Trisomy no. 1 exhibits developmental retardation and moderate or severe hypoplasia. The affected embryos die between day 14 and 15. Similar but often less severe changes characterize Ts 6 and Ts 10. In contrast, embryos with trisomy no. 12 show exencephaly and microphthalmia, mostly without developmental retardation. They may survive until day 17. Cleft palate has been observed in Ts 19. Trisomy of chromosome no. 8, 11, 15 and 17 causes gross developmental retardation and extreme smallness. Characteristically death occurs at day 12. As a rule, hypoplasia of the placenta can be found in the trisomic syndromes of the mouse. Thus far the cause of fetal death in the trisomic syndromes remains obscure. It is improbable that malformation per se is a major causative factor.

The inferences drawn from studies of chromosomal factors causing developmental failure have complementary aspects to those related to environmental disturbances. It is possible to discover more of the mechanisms by which genes and environment interact by studies in systems of this type.

Acknowledgements. The work done in the laboratory of the author has been generously supported by the Deutsche Forschungsgemeinschaft, Bonn-Bad Godesberg. I am grateful to Mrs. U. Kolbus and to Miss G. Noack for their technical help, and to Mrs. E. Hüttenhain for her help in preparing the manuscript.

References

Baranov, V. S., Dyban, A. P.: Disturbance of embryogenesis in trisomy of autosomes arising in offspring of mice with Robertsonian translocation (centric fusion) of T1IeM. Arch. Anat.-Histol. Embryol. **113**, 67—77 (1972).

Capanna, E., Cristaldi, M., Perticone, P., Rezzoni, M.: Identification of chromosomes involved in the 9 Robertsonian fusions of the Appennine mouse with a 22-chromosome karyotype. Experentia (Basel) **31**, 294—296 (1975).

Cattanach, B. M., Moseley, H.: Nondisjunction and reduced fertility caused by the tobacco mouse metacentric chromosomes. Cytogenet. Cell Genet. **12**, 264—287 (1973).

Cattanach, B. M., Williams, C. E., Bailey, H.: Identification of the linkage groups carried by the metacentric chromosomes of the tobacco mouse *(Mus poschiavinus)*. Cytogenet. Cell Genet. **11**, 412—423 (1972).

Cure, S., Boué, A., Boué, J.: Consequence of autosomal anomalies on cell multiplication. Compte rendue du colloque organisé sous la patronage de I.N.S.E.R.M. Ed.: A Boué et Ch. Thibault. Paris 1973, 12.—14. Septembre 1973. S. 255—269.

Dhadial, R. K., Machin, A. M., Tait, S. M.: Chromosomal anomalies in spontaneously aborted human foetuses. Lancet **1970 II**, 20—21.

Döring, L., Gropp, A., Aechter, J., Winking, H.: Genetically determined maturation arrest in spermatogenesis (Studies on a mouse model), in prep.

Evans, E. P., Lyon, M. F., Daglish, M.: A mouse translocation giving a metacentric marker chromosome. Cytogenet. Cell Genet. **6**, 105—119 (1967).

Ford, C. E.: Gross genome unbalance in mouse spermatozoa: Does it influence the capacity to fertilize? Proc. Int. Symp. The Genetics of Spermatozoon. Edinburgh Aug. 16—20, 1971. S. 359—369.

Fuhrmann, W., Seeger, W., Böhm, R.: Apparently monogenic inheritance of anencephaly and spina bifida in a kindred. Humangenetik **13**, 241—243 (1971).

Giroud, A. et Martinet, M.: Anencephalie expérimentale chez la souris et comparaisons avec l'anencephalie chez l'homme. Acta anat. (Basel) **44**, 358—370 (1960).

Gropp, A.: Reproductive failure due to fetal aneuploidy in mice. Proc. of the 7th World Congress on Fertility and Sterility Oct. 17—25, 1971. Tokyo and Kyoto. S. 326—330.

Gropp, A., Giers, D., Kolbus, U.: Trisomy in the fetal backcross progeny of male and female metacentric heterozygotes of the mouse I. Cytogenet. Cell Genet. **13**, 511—535 (1974).

Gropp, A., Kolbus, U.: Exencephaly in the syndrome of trisomy no. 12 of the fetal mouse. Nature (Lond.) **249**, 145—147 (1974).

GROPP, A., KOLBUS, U., GIERS, D.: Systematic approach to the study of trisomy in the mouse, II. Cytogenet. Cell Genet. **14**, 42—62 (1975).

GROPP, A., TETTENBORN, U., LEHMANN, E. von: Chromosomenvariation vom Robertson'schen Typus bei der Tabakmaus, *M. poschiavinus*, und ihren Hybriden mit der Laboratoriumsmaus. Cytogenet. Cell Genet. **9**, 9—23 (1970).

GROPP, A., WINKING, H., ZECH, L., MÜLLER, H. J.: Robertsonian chromosomal variation and identification of metacentric chromosomes in feral mice. Chromosoma (Berl.) **39**, 265—288 (1972).

LAZAR, P., GUEGUEN, S., BOUÉ, J., BOUÉ, A.: Epidémiologie des avortements spontanés précoses a propos de 1469 avortements caryotypes. Compte rendue du colloque organisé sous la patronage de I.N.S.E.R.M. Ed.: A. BOUÉ et CH. THIBAULT. Paris 1973, 12.—14. Septembre 1973. S. 317—331.

LÉONARD, A., DEKNUDT, G. H.: A new marker for chromosome studies in the mouse. Nature (Lond.) **214**, 504—505 (1967).

MARIN-PADILLA, M.: Morphogenesis of anencephaly and related malformations. In: "Current Topics in Pathology", Berlin-Heidelberg-New York: Springer. **51**, 145—174 (1970).

MURAKAMI, U., KAMEYAMA, Y.: Vertebrate malformation in the mouse foetus caused by maternal hypoxia during early stages of pregnancy. J. Embryol. exp. Morphol. **11**, 107—118 (1963).

PENROSE, L. S.: Genetics of anencephaly. J. ment. Defic. Res. **1**, 4 (1957).

PHILIPPE, E.: Consequences des anomalies chromosomiques sur le developpement. Compte rendue du colloque organisé sous la patronage de I.N.S.E.R.M. Ed.: A. BOUÉ et CH. THIBAULT. Paris 1973, 12.—14. Septembre 1973. S. 119—126.

POSWILLO, D., SOPHER, D., MITCHELL, S.: Experimental induction of fetal malformation with "blighted" potato: a preliminary report. Nature (Lond.) **239**, 462—464 (1972).

SCHNEIDER, E. L., EPSTEIN, CH. J.: Replication rate and lifespan of cultured fibroblasts in Down's syndrome (36940). Proc. Soc. exp. Biol. (N.Y.) **141**, 1092—1094 (1972).

STOLLA, R., GROPP, A.: Variation of the DNA content of morphologically normal and abnormal spermatozoa in mice susceptible to irregular meiotic segregation. J. Reprod. Fertil. **38**, 335—346 (1974).

TETTENBORN, U., GROPP, A.: Meiotic nondisjunction in mice and mouse hybrids. Cytogenet. Cell Genet. **9**, 272—283 (1970).

THERKELSEN, A. J., GRUNNET, N., HJORT, T. et al.: Studies on spontaneous abortions. Compte rendue du colloque organisé sous la patronage de I.N.S.E.R.M. Ed.: A. BOUÉ et CH. THIBAULT. Paris 1973, 12.—14. Septembre 1973. S. 255—269.

WHITE, B. J., TJIO, J.-H.: A mouse translocation with 38 and 39 chromosomes but normal N.F. Hereditas **58**, 284—296 (1968).

WHITE, B. J. TJIO, J. H. WATER, L. C. van de, CRANDALL, C. Trisomy for the smallest autosome of the mouse and identification of the T1Wh translocation chromosome. Cytogenet. **11**, 363—378 (1972).

WHITE, B. J., TJIO, J.-H., WATER, L. C. van de, CRANDALL, C.: Trisomy 19 in the laboratory mouse. I. Frequency in different crosses at specific developmental stages and relationship of trisomy to cleft palate. II. Intra-uterine growth and histological studies of trisomics and their normal littermates. Cytogenet. Cell Genet. **13**, 217—245 (1974).

WRIGHT, Y. M., CLARK, W. E., BREG, W.: Craniorachischisis in a partially trisomic 11 fetus in a family with reproductive failure and a reciprocal translocation 1(6p +; 11q −). J. med. Genet. **11**, 69—75 (1974).

3. Animal Models of Major Gene Defects

K. S. Brown

With 1 Figure

Malformations inherited by simple dominant or recessive patterns have been well recognized in the literature of teratology and human genetics (McKusick, 1966, 1969; Saxén and Rapola, 1969; Stern, 1973; Wilson, 1973; Motulsky and Lenz, 1974). Much of the literature on man is based on very small pedigrees and detailed studies of the genetics and the embryology have not been done. Many malformations in man have not been susceptible to genetic analysis due to lack of adequate pedigree data. Embryological studies of malformation have been limited by the rarity of the defects and the lack of fetal specimens. Only recently has an extensive series of normal human embryos been examined (Nishimura *et al.*, 1968).

The purpose of this chapter will be to discuss practical aspects of genetic methodology as applied to animal model systems of malformation and to illustrate directions that the use of genetic models point out for future research on aetiology and prevention of birth defects. Four general areas of developmental physiology under genetic control will be selected for discussion: metabolic limits on cell growth and differentiation, special responses to hormones, cell surface factors in relation to development and programmed cell death. No attempt will be made to list or categorize defects as this has been done *in extenso* in the works mentioned below.

Sources of Data on Animal Defects

The occurrence of malformation syndromes as inherited traits in domestic species has been reviewed (Mulvihill, 1972; Patterson, 1974). The morphological defects of mice that are inherited as simple genetic traits have been recorded in monographs (Gruneberg, 1952; Green, 1966) and many new defects are recorded regularly in Mouse News Letter (Searle, 1975).

The literature on defects in domestic and laboratory species is regularly abstracted (Excerpta Medica). The World Health Organization has recently instituted a bibliographic listing of congenital defects in animals (Beveridge, 1974). For the mouse, listing of titles is also available as a supplement to Mouse News Letter (Staats, 1975).

The Implications of Simple Inheritance Patterns

Since vertebrate species share much of their genome, their general body plan and the processes by which it develops, it is to be expected that many hereditary defects are homologous between the species. This homology is particularly evident among mammals in which reproductive tracts, endocrinology and chromosome organization are similar.

The homology between hereditary defects of man and other species is the basis for the importance assigned to hereditary malformations that occur in experimental and domestic animals. Observations of the etiology and pathogenesis of defects of development in fetuses of lower animals permits inferences to be drawn about homologous malformations in man. For example, hereditary heart defects seen in human kindreds, such as tetralogy of Fallot, show strain specific inheritance among inbred dogs (PATTERSON, 1974). Such animal models provide insight into human disease by allowing experimental investigations not possible in man. Preventive or corrective therapies that are successful in lower animals provide a rational basis for similar interventions in human pregnancies with high risk of homologous defects.

Those malformations that are inherited by patterns which suggest the action of a *single gene*, whether it be dominant or recessive, are of particular value in the study of the mechanisms of development because of the implication contained in the concept of single gene action; this is best summarized in the phrase "one gene—one enzyme, or one gene—one polypeptide chain". When a trait, however complex or pleotropic, is inherited in a strict pattern of single gene transmission, then it may be concluded either, that there is one single primary enzymatic defect, which may be identified as acting at a particular time and place during development and from which all subsequent changes follow by the normal rules of developmental physiology and biochemistry, or alternatively, that a primary defect has occurred in the control mechanism for a group of related metabolic processes which are under a unified control. Such a principle has been used to identify the primary defect in a wide variety of biochemical diseases (STANBURY *et al.*, 1966).

Because of the great significance of the conclusion that there is one single primary defect in such malformations, it is essential to specify the conditions under which the conclusion is justified and also those under which it is not. The conclusion is justified when all of the individuals that have the trait do in fact have the same defective gene. To be sure of the identity of the gene a defined pedigree must be known in which its transmission can be traced.

For *dominantly inherited malformations*, in which every individual with the defective gene demonstrates a characteristic phenotype and in which the phenotype is not changed by the presence of other genes or environmental factors during development, the definition of the pedigree and the identification of the individuals at risk is relatively easy. Such conditions are rare in nature because of the strong selection pressure against malformations inherited in the dominant pattern.

In most *domestic species* both natural and human selection have acted to remove from breeding stock genes which tended to reduce the number, growth rate and viability of the young. Only in species where economic benefit has not been a consideration, such as pets or laboratory animals, e. g. dogs, cats, rats and mice, has selection been relaxed or even reversed by human interference to preserve animals with reduced viability such as miniature, achondroplastic, and neurologically abnormal types, and color or form phenotypes which have reduced survival value compared to the wild type (PATTERSON, 1974; STANBURY *et al.*, 1966).

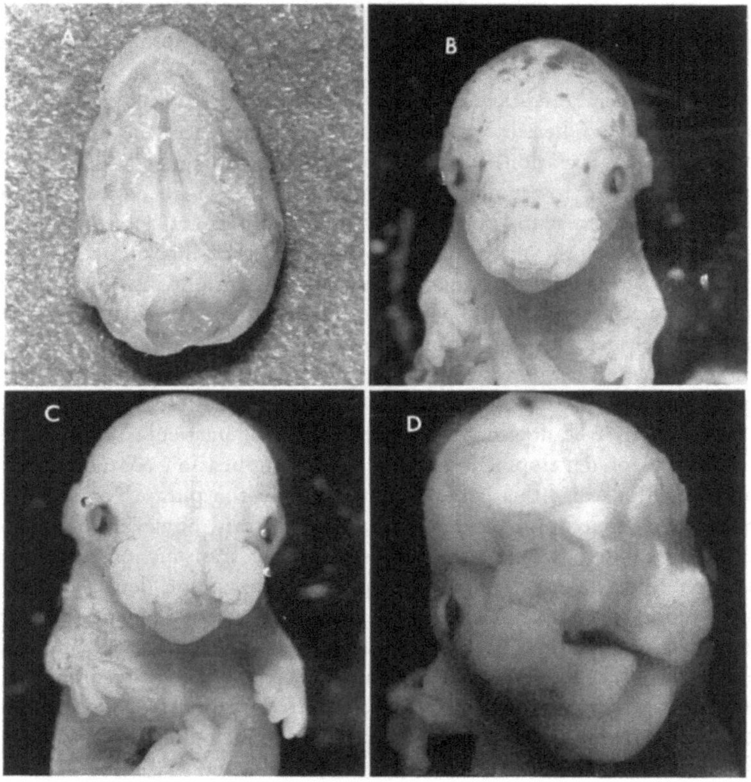

Fig. 1. A—D. Heterogeneity of malformations in the homozygous Tw/Tw mouse. (A) Isolated cleft palate in a day 16 embryo (looking at roof of mouth with jaw removed). (B) Bilateral cleft lip with cleft palate in day 15 embryo. (C) Bilateral cleft lip with nose cleft and cleft palate in day 15 embryo. (D) Bilateral cleft nose with reduced nasal process, cleft lip and cleft palate in day 15 embryo. (Photos courtesy Dr. LEENA SEDERLOF)

In domesticated species programs of selective breeding have resulted in the rapid evolution of the entire genotype of domestic breeds or strains so that particular phenotypes are favored, for example the modern breeds of dairy and beef cattle. Phenotypes may be expressed in a pattern of inheritance indicating that only one major gene is acting but it is essential to remember that selection works on the entire genotype, not just on the gene of particular interest, unless unusual efforts are made to isolate the effect of a single gene by special breeding plans. Thus when we consider the effects of even the most sharply defined inherited trait we must remain aware of the influence of the background genotype in which it expresses itself.

The concept of *dominant inheritance* implies that the individual with one defective gene and one wild, or normal, gene (heterozygote) at a particular locus will have the same phenotype as the individual that has two defective genes (homozygote) given that background genes and environment are equal. In practice perceived phenotype has often proved to be dependent on the mode of examination and it may be said that true dominance does not exist. For defects of morphological development reported dominant inheritance is frequently associated with early embryonic death in the homozygote so that the usage of the term dominant has come to mean an expressed phenotype in the heterozygote. For example, the genes *Dc* (Dancer), and *Tw* (Twirler) in the mouse are both dominant in that the heterozygote of each *Dc*/+ and *Tw*/+ shows a behavior pattern due to vestibular abnormalities (GREEN, 1966). However, both of these genes result in lethal homozygotes Dc/Dc and Tw/Tw which die either at birth or in utero with cleft lip and palate of various degrees of severity (Fig. 1). Thus if the phenotype of cleft lip is the trait of interest each of these genes would be thought of as a recessive. Similarly for *recessive inheritance* the absolute criteria of the textbooks become less sharp in the living animals and in practical usage. The recessive abnormal gene usually results in some effect on phenotype when heterozygous, although this may be minimal.

When homozygous, the recessive gene is recognized by a characteristic phenotype. This may be the result of an abnormal positive gene action but is often the result of the lack of action by the missing normal allele.

When a recessive gene has a viable phenotype in the homozygous state mating of two homozygous animals can only result in homozygous offspring, thus a "true breeding" stock is easy to achieve. When the homozygous recessive is lethal or sterile, the homozygous state can only be produced by mating two heterozygous carriers. Heterozygous animals then must be identified by the production of abnormal offspring after mating with proven heterozygous mates. This is "progeny testing" and is the standard way of maintaining a recessive lethal trait in which no phenotype has been recognized for the heterozygous carrier.

Inbred Strains

The production of highly defined domestic animal lines by special breeding programs has had different effects on malformation rates depending on the objectives and success of the breeding schemes employed. For the economically important domestic species such as cattle, pigs and chickens the selection against malformation, lethality and growth retardation has been rigorous and more directed than natural selection, while simultaneous selection for size and metabolic characters of economic interest has also been carried out (WIESNER, 1960; BREWBAKER, 1964).

In the laboratory rat, in which uniformity and reproductive vigor were the desirable traits, highly inbred lines were established by "a purging of bad genes", in which many lines were lost (HUTT, 1964). Similar selection for fertility in mouse strains was an obligatory part of the development of the highly inbred uniform lines frequently used in teratology research today.

To some extent these are artificial creations of human selection and may give responses different from a natural animal population. On the other hand the restricted environmental variability, rich diet and lack of predation may permit survival of lineages with less adaptive genotypes that would have been eliminated in nature. An example of such breeds in dogs is the miniatures, while the white blue eyed or heterochromic cats have reduced survival value (BERGSMA and BROWN, 1971) and albino strains are generally at a disadvantage (WITKOP *et al.*, 1974).

One consequence of inbreeding is that different inbred lines may vary as much from one to another as would individuals in a wild population. Thus differences in responses among inbred lines may be an indication of the degree of genetic variation in response to a teratogen or as background for the action of a particular gene. Mice strains vary greatly in their response to both the action of major genes and teratogens. Thus although the genetic expectations for single locus inheritance are met in small samples of data with limited genetic variability of background the simulation of mendelian frequencies by polygenic inheritance must be considered a possibility. Only guidance from tests for major gene action permit the conclusion that monogene control is operating. Polygenic determination of certain characteristics will be considered in other chapters of this book (See Chapter 12, Roberts and Burn, and Chapter 5, Berry and Germain).

Tests for Action of Major Genes

To prove major gene action in the inheritance of a trait several criteria must be satisfied. The least important of these are the *genetic proportions among the offspring of parents of defined type.* Because the entire genotype of the strain or subspecies may be significantly involved in producing the phenotype, any one particular segregating locus may provide the limiting step and thus appear to be all important.

A more important indication of major gene action is *transfer of a trait to different genetic backgrounds or sublines* with maintenance of the phenotypic character and the genetic proportions. This can be accomplished by crossing the strain with the trait to one without it and then selectively backcrossing individuals that manifest the trait and/or the ability to transmit it, to the strain that had previously lacked the trait. By repeated backcrossing with selection for the trait the total genetic contribution of the original affected parent is reduced by nearly half in each succeeding backcross generation although the particular gene of interest is maintained by selection. After three generations of backcrossing the original parent would contribute about 1/16 of the genes and after nine generations about 1/1000 of the genes in the next generation. If the trait remains constant during such a process the evidence that it is due to one gene is considerably strengthened. Pairs of strains differing at only one locus are called "congenic".

The most convincing proof of single gene action is obtained by the *establishment of a genetic linkage* between the trait in question and a marker gene or chromosome. Sex-linkage is the best known example of proof that a gene is on the X chromosome of mammals. In some species all the chromosomes are known to have marker genes which can be used to test for linkage to a particular chromosome. The recent development of metacentric chromosomes in mice, as discussed in another chapter of this book (Chapter 2, Gropp) makes cytological detection of linkage a practical possibility that will rapidly increase the number of chromosomally localized genes in that species. Combinations of cytological and biochemical techniques are being used to localize human genes in hybrid cell cultures and also to establish linkage groups in other domestic species. Linkage of genes can be used in a practical way in the design of experiments.

Marker genes that have easily observed phenotypes can be used as indicators of the presence of closely linked genes. For example a gene that prevents the development of retinal pigment such as *p* (pink eye) or *c* (albino) could be used to identify fetuses on day 12 of gestation because pigment develops in the retina then. If the action of a gene such as *pu* (pudgy), a recessive that causes malformations of the spine, is to be studied *in utero* it could be recognized at day 12 in selected litters by using the *c* or *p* gene effect. The *c* and *p* genes are both on the same chromosome as *pu*. LA VAIL and SIDMAN (1974) have used this technique to study *rd* (retinal degeneration) using the marker *W* (dominant spotting). Electrophoretic variations of enzymes would be easy to use in this type of experiment.

In most species genetic linkage and chromosome identification are not far enough advanced to be of much use as proof of major gene action and so the occurrence of regular genetic proportions and constant phenotypes in different background genomes must be sufficient evidence for major gene action. There are, however, some disadvantages in these tests. They will permit false positive conclusions to be drawn and also the falsley negative rejection of a trait which is in fact due to major gene action. However, if backcrosses to several different backgrounds are carried out the chance of false positive conclusions can be minimized.

Phenotypic similarity of hereditary traits does not provide an assurance that the genes involved are the same, or even allelic, unless the phenotype is examined at the primary gene product level. Morphological similarity can arise from a common primary defect, as in the case of identical or allelic genes, but this need not be so. In long developmental pathways subsequent pathological events based on normal repair mechanisms so modify the phenotype prior to birth that the primary defect is obscured. Only by examining embryos at or near the time of primary insult can the obscuring effects of healing, repair and scar formation be avoided.

Genetic evidence of difference or similarity in primary insult can be obtained by demonstration of allelism or lack of allelism in the genes causing the defects. Following the basic rule that each locus effects synthesis of a particular polypeptide, evidence of allelism of two genes can be taken as strong evidence that the same peptide is being modified. The converse is also true: that two traits controlled by genes which are not alleles are unlikely to have the same primary peptide defect as a basis.

Phenotypically identical traits can result from either polygenic or major gene effects. A well worked out example of this phenomenon is in the control of the number of toes in the guinea pig. This often quoted example of a trait inherited by polygenic pattern with a threshold is inherited in an autosomal single locus pattern in some guinea pig strains (WRIGHT, 1968). Similarly, cleft lip with cleft palate is a multifactorial trait in the A/J strain of mice (DAVIDSON *et al.*, 1969) and is also produced by the genes *Tw* or *Dc* when present in homozygous state (GREEN, 1966).

Malformations Related to Errors of Metabolism

Normal development depends on both the genetic instructions for morphogenesis in a specific sense and on the genetically based ability of the tissues to carry out general metabolic processes necessary for cell survival or replication. For example, all developing vertebrate tissues use molecular oxygen but localized malformations may result from reduction of available O_2, in a characteristic pattern involving the occurrence of fluid filled blebs in the tissues (Grabowski, 1970; Petter *et al.*, 1971). These blebs frequently become blood-filled and persist, with resulting defects of differentiation in the area in a pattern similar to that produced by the gene *my* "myelencephalic blebs" in mice (Gruneberg, 1952). One of the most common localizations for blebs is in the digital plate with resulting hypodactylism, polydactylism, or other disturbance of limb morphogenesis. In the case of *my*, blebs and consequent malformations occur widely in development producing a spectrum of malformations.

One of the most extensively studied malformations of this type is in the rabbit where the recessive gene *br* "brachydactyly" results in variable degrees of shortening or even total loss of the digits and metatarsus in one or more feet, associated with a variable degree of shortening or narrowing of one or both ears, usually in an asymmetrical pattern (Greene and Saxton, 1939). In the defective regions of fetuses, epithelium remains intact despite absence of blood supply and in many instances active proliferation is observed even when there is extravasation of blood and necrosis in the underlying mesenchyme. The healing of the underlying tissues is associated with loss of the organization of bone centers in the digits and failure of localized growth in the ear, which produce the phenotype seen in the newborn.

In contrast to *my* in which clear blebs appeared in the tissue and are secondarily filled with blood the *br* defect has a localized enlargement and secondary rupture of vessels between days 18 and 20 of gestation as the earliest observed event in pathogenesis. This is followed by necrosis of local connective tissue, muscle, cartilage and nerve with replacement of the necrotic tissue by loose connective tissue or sloughing of the region which is completed before the 25th day of gestation (Greene and Saxton, 1939). The course of events following the primary defect in the development of local vessels appears to follow a regular pathological sequence such as would follow an abnormal environmental stimulus. Such stimuli as vasopressin. (Jost, 1950) and adrenalin (Jost, 1953) have been found to result in a similar sequence of edema, hemorrhages, necrosis and amputation in the rat.

In these malformations the initial local vascular response appears as the critical abnormality. Prevention or amelioration of this response should therefore prevent the development of the defect in *br/br* rabbits. Heterozygous *br/+* does mated to homozygous *br/br* males were maintained in chambers with increased oxygen concentration during the critical period between days 13 and 20 of gestation (Petter *et al.*, 1971). This treatment resulted in a significant reduction in the number and severity of the defects found in the fetuses of does examined.

As these authors comment, the changes may result from an initial anomaly of circulation pattern, of the hemoglobin carrying the O_2, or of vascular permeability. They have demonstrated that reduction in synthesis of red cells reduces the malformation (Petter *et al.*, 1973). In different genotypes which share a pattern of pathogenesis of malformation in which vascular defect and local necrosis in early development occur, any of these lesions might be primary. Such patterns of pathogenesis are suggested for salicylate induced malformation of A/J mice (Larsson *et al.*, 1964), in thalidomide treated monkeys (Poswillo, 1973) and in diphenylhydantoin treated CL/FR mice (Hetzel and Brown, 1975). Facial clefts and other defects have been reported in human infants after maternal treatment with diphenylhydantoin (SPEIDEL and MEADOW, 1972) and with anticoagulants (PETTIFOR and BENSON, 1975).

Just as regular development may be disturbed by localized responses to reduced O_2, it may be disturbed by any rate limiting change in metabolism that affects localized regions of the body. Since many of the enzymes involved in tissue synthesis require co-factors such as vitamins and trace minerals, deficiencies of these substances might be teratogenic by reducing essential metabolic pathways. Genes that modify the need for such co-factors exist and their role in development interacts with nutritional status (HURLEY, 1969).

One of the best documented and most widely occurring interactions between genetic variation in a trace mineral requirement and nutritional status occurs, in several species, with manganese. In the mouse the recessive gene pallid *pa* is associated with pigment reduction in the fur and increase in the Mn requirements for the normal development of the otoconia of the inner ear (ERWAY *et al.*, 1971; LIM and ERWAY, 1974). After normal diet containing 50 p.p.m. Mn during pregnancy, the calcite crystals of the *pa/pa* fetuses are reduced or absent. Consequently vestibular function is irreversibly abnormal. When the diet during pregnancy is supplemented to 2000 p.p.m., then both defects and behavioral consequences are prevented. In the normal genotype of several species, manganese deficiency has consequences similar to those of normal Mn in *pa/pa* genotype of mice (ERWAY *et al.*, 1970). Normal mice show differences in malformation rates between strains (HURLEY and BELL, 1974). This indicates that there are other strain specific factors controlling the requirements for Mn.

The gene *pastel* in mink is apparently homologous to *pa* and causes vestibular defects of behavior which can be prevented by manganese supplementation of the diet during gestation (ERWAY and MITCHELL, 1973).

An example of genetic control of the action of a vitamin in the embryonic single comb white leghorn chicken has been described (CLEGETT, 1971). The gene controls the production of the riboflavin carrier protein. The abnormal homozygote has no carrier protein so the egg has no riboflavin and the embryo dies between day 11 and 14 unless supplemented by injected vitamin. The heterozygote has reduced carrier which might make it differentially responsive to vitamin deficiency.

Hereditary Cell Surface Antigens and Malformation

A possible insight into the problem of the localized organ or tissue defects that result in malformation without any generalized deficiency may be supplied by the recognition of the role of the histocompatibility antigens on cell surfaces. These antigens are the basis of the recognition of cells as being foreign or "self". They are thus important in organ transplantation and much has been learned about them in the last decade. This information has implications for their role in control of normal and abnormal development (Committee for the Conference on Biological significance of Histocompatibility antigens, 1972).

The most highly investigated and potent of over thirty different histocompatibility genes scattered throughout the mouse genome is the *H-2*. Variation at this locus is complex and widely distributed among strains. There are many genetic determinants, each coding for several antigens on the cell surface. Some of these antigens vary from organ to organ and some are capable of transient phenotypic modification or modulation by the presence of antibody. Thus this system of surface antigens has several properties that would be useful in controlling morphogenesis.

Two recent demonstrations of the effects of the H-2 system on hereditary malformation use the technique of the *congenic strain comparison* (MICKOVÁ and IVÁNI, 1974; BONNER and SLAVKIN, 1975). Two lines of mice "congenic" at all loci except H-2 are produced by selective backcrossing of a cross between two strains of different types with testing of the H-2 type and selection for the type not usually found in the backcross parent strain. This results in the isolation of the H-2 allele in question on the background of its congenic partner. The congenic partners can then be compared for any characteristic of interest with confidence that H-2 locus has the only genetic difference between them.

The expression of the gene *T* "Brachyury" was demonstrated to be strongly modified by H-2 type in crosses among three different congenic mouse lines with different *H-2* haplotypes (C57BL/10, $H\text{-}2^b$; C3H, $H\text{-}2^k$; A, $H\text{-}2^a$) (MICKOVA and IVANI, 1974). The expression of Brachyury in the animals with $H\text{-}2^b$ was the most extreme with complete absence of tail occurring in 58% of $T/+$ animals of C57BL/10-T and a modal tail to body length of 50% for the animals having tails. This contrasted with no tailless animals and tail to body length of 76 ± 0.6% and 72 ± 0.8% for the A-T and C3H-T stocks. These differences are the result of the differences of the entire genome between these strains. When 120 $T/+$ offspring of a cross between (C3H × B10) F_1 and B-10-T were classified by H-2 type, 58 $H\text{-}2^b/H\text{-}2^b$ had mean tail body ratio of 38.5 ± 3.3% while the 62 $H\text{-}2^b/H\text{-}2^k$ heterozygotes had ratios of 46.8 ± 3.2%. Since all these animals had their *T* and t^+ alleles from the same sources and the rest of the genome showed no evidence of abnormal assortment, the effects on tail length were attributed to the differential effects of the $H\text{-}2^b/H\text{-}2^b$ and $H\text{-}2^b/H\text{-}2^k$ genotypes.

One of the most interesting aspects of the $H\text{-}2^b$ effect on $T/+$ expression is its sexual dimorphism. MICKOVÁ and IVÁNI report that the majority of the tailless animals in the C57BL/10-T strain were male and the mean tail-body ratio for males was 11.7 ± 2.8% compared to 25.0 ± 3.9% for females. Similarly in the backcross data only the males differed significantly in tail length when grouped by H-2 type. They speculate that, since the time of *T* gene action coincides with the beginning of androgen synthesis in the mouse embryo, this action may be one of the earliest indications of sexual dimorphism. This interpretation also suggests that hormones and hormone synthesis can have many different effects on morphogenesis.

Susceptibility to cleft palate in the mouse has also been linked to H-2 type (BONNER and SLAVKIN, 1975). Congenic strains C57BL/10 and C57BL/10.A which differ in homozygosity for the histocompatibility haplotypes $H\text{-}2^b$ and $H\text{-}2^a$ but are otherwise genetically similar have 27% and 81% isolated cleft of the secondary palate (CP) respectively in fetuses when given 2.5 mg of cortisone intramuscularly on days 11 to 14 of pregnancy. The C57BL/6 gave 25% CP and A/J mice 99% in the same experiment. They have the same H-2 relationship as the congenic strains.

These results suggest that the largest part of the difference in response to cortisone between these congenic strains and also the parent strains is the result of their differences in H-2 type. Since the cell surface glycoprotein of the H-2 antigen may also have differential binding for other molecules such as steroids, this differential binding may be a cause of the difference between types. Androgen binding may also account for the differences in response to different H-2 types by *T*/+ embryos due to the proteins controlled by the *Ss* and *Slp* parts of the H-2 region.

The close linkage of H-2 and *T* locus in mice means that very careful controls must be done to separate the effects of the two loci. In the case of the steroid response in the congenic pair C57BL/10 and C57BL/10·A it may be possible that their differences are related to recessive *T* locus alleles which accompany the H-2 alleles. Some recessive *T* locus alleles are known to modify the anterior development of the neural tube (GLUECKSOHN-WAELSCH and ERICKSON, 1970).

Genetic Control of Response to Hormones during Development

Developing embryos respond to a variety of hormones such as thyroxine, glucagon and glucocorticoids by the synthesis of specific groups of enzymes (GREENGARD, 1973). A striking illustration of the control of the response to a specific hormone by a gene occurs with *Tfm* (testicular feminization), an X-linked gene in mouse and in apparently homologous mutations in cattle, rats, dogs and man (OHNO, 1974). When this gene is present, the embryonic responses associated with masculinization of XY individuals do not occur and they do not occur in response to the administration of androgen. The embryonic wolfian ducts regress, as in females, the embryonic urogenital sinus is not masculinized (GOLDSTEIN and WILSON, 1972) so the animal is externally female but is sterile with internal testes. In later development the connections between the nipple and the mammary glands are not severed (LYON and HAWKES, 1970), and the submaxillary salivary glands do not hypertrophy or produce specific proteins (LYON *et al.*, 1973). In these animals androgens have none of the normal negative feedback effect on pituitary release of luteinizing hormone (ITAKURA and OHNO, 1973) nor do they cause kidney hypertrophy and induction of enzymes in the kidney proximal tubules (DOFUKU *et al.*, 1971). These effects all appear to result from the reduced binding affinity of the androgen receptor protein on the cell surface of *Tfm* cells. The simple genetic behavior of this trait suggests that *Tfm* in the mouse is a primary regulatory locus controlling sexual phenotypes.

The pleotropic effects of *Tfm* illustrate the wide spectrum of tissues which respond to testosterone as a direct stimulus to normal morphological and biochemical development. The sharp characterization of the target tissues for this hormone has been possible by the study of these animals. The analysis of the *Tfm* mouse has facilitated the understanding of several similar hereditary traits in man (GOLDSTEIN and WILSON, 1974).

An autosomal gene *Sxr* (sex-reversed) in the mouse causes genetic females to develop as males in all respects except sperm formation which stops soon after birth (CATTANACH *et al.*, 1971). This gene apparently acts solely on the primary determination of the gonad. The developmental endocrine aspects of sex differentiation are normal and there are no associated malformations, but sterility results from the action of the genes, in contrast to those that affect the receptors for the hormones.

A recessive gene linked to "Polled" (Hornless) in the goat also causes sex reversal as complete as that of the mouse while in the pig a gene giving incomplete sex reversal with ovotestes or even retention of ovaries has been observed (Cattanach, 1974). The reproductive tracts and the gonads are relatively clear examples of gene-hormone interaction because the structures and functions involved are relatively well understood and have been well studied. Other hormones also effect development; for example, the action of insulin on chick limb development (Hinchliffe, 1974). A well documented association between thyroid hormone synthetic defects and defects of the inner ear, Pendred's syndrome, occurs as a recessive trait in man (Fraser, 1965). The basis of the association between defects of innner ear and thyroid is unknown. It is unknown whether hypothyroidism during gestation is teratogenic for the inner ear or whether the two defects are the pleotrophic results of a gene and are not related as cause and effect. Some suggestion that the relation is that of cause and effect is found in the discovery that "Pendred's" cases have a variety of different metabolic errors in thyroid synthesis (Hollander *et al.*, 1964). End organ insensitivity to thyroxine occurred in one family (Refetoff *et al.*, 1972).

An experimental model of this syndrome has been produced in the mouse (Deol, 1973). Treatment of C57BL/G1 females with 0.1% propylthiouracil (PTU) in drinking water during the first ten days of gestation produced a characteristic inner ear defect and deafness in the offspring. When thyroxine was added along with PTU, no effect was observed. This demonstrated the causal relation between deafness and maternal thyroid deficiency. The effect was strain specific (Deol, personal communication). The same dose of PTU was not compatible with pregnancy or was ineffective in other strains tested. The genetics of this response to PTU have not yet been described but the critical period of sensitivity is in the first 10 days of gestation.

Hereditary Differences in Programmed Cell Death

The changes in form of limbs and toes and of many other organs involves selective cell death in localized areas. The cells in such areas are said to undergo "programmed cell death" because of the exact localization and timing of the process. Such cell death occurs in the morphogenesis of the chicken limbs in which it has been studied extensively (Saunders, 1966). An anterior necrotic zone appears along the anterior mesenchyme of the limb bud as it separates from the body wall and extends distally while a posterior necrotic zone occupies a similar position on the posterior margin of the limb bud. In later stages a deep necrotic zone "the opaque patch" separates the mesenchymal condensation of the limb into femur, tibia and fibula or humerus, radius and ulna. Still later the interdigital necrotic zones appear, separating and forming the digits.

Mutants in chickens demonstrating abnormally increased necrosis in areas where "programmed cell death" occurs include *Rumplessness* (Zwilling, 1942) and *ws* "wingless" (Hinchliffe and Ede, 1967). Deficiency malformations characterized by their names, following enlarged areas of programmed death that remove instead of remodel the developing tissues, result from these two genes.

The reduction of normal programmed cell death in the chicken limb due to ta^3 "$talpid^3$" gene appears to result in the failure of normal long bone and digit organization in the ta^3/ta^3 embryos. The elongation and separation of the long bones is restricted and there is polysyndactyly due to suppression of cell death in all of the four regions of the limb that normally show programmed cell death (HINCHLIFFE and THOROGOOD, 1974).

In mice the *Os* "Oligosyndactylous" gene results in a phenotype in which fusion and abnormality of the tarsals and digits suggests a similar process to ta^3 of chickens. MILAIRE (1967) has described abnormal localized cell death in the mesoderm of the foot plate of day 11 and 12 *Os*/+ embryos, while a recessive mutant *sm*/*sm* "syndactylous" showed clear cut hyperplasia of the preaxial apical ectodermal ridge on early day eleven.

The mouse genes *Hm* "Hammertoe" and *Hx* "Hemimelic extra toes" are allelic or very closely linked (MNL ≠ 52 GREEN, M. personal communication, 1975). Preliminary examination of Hammertoe demonstrates reduced cell deaton day 13 in the interdigital spaces. If homology is a guide and the two genes are alleles, then it might be expected that *Hx* will be similar in phenotype to $talpid^3$ in the chicken.

Genes such as *Os*, *sm*, *Hm*, and *Hx* may play a role in characterizing morphological development of the limb similar to that played by alkaptonuria, cystinuria, albinism and pentosuria in characterizing the metabolic processes. Inborn errors of metabolism include, in the broad sense, inborn errors of development. The methods of analysis and even some of the techniques that have resulted in the advances of biochemical genetics during the last two decades will provide much of the foundation for the future progress of developmental genetics and teratology.

Recognition by teratologists of the help that specific genes can give in the analysis of responses to teratogens will increase the pace of teratological research. Conversely, the recognition of the intrinsic variability among individuals of particular species including man, will require continuous reevaluation of the environmental changes introduced by civilization. In particular, their effect on malformation rates and fetal death in generations to come must be assessed. Animal model systems can provide an effective warning system, if genetically defined laboratory animals are used.

References

BERGSMA, D. R., BROWN, K. S.: White fur, blue eyes and deafness in the domestic cat. J. Hered. **62**, 171 (1971).

BEVERIDGE, W. I. B.: Bibliography on congenital defects in animals. Geneva: World Health Organization 1974.

BONNER, J. J., SLAVKIN, H. C.: Cleft palate susceptibility linked to histocompatability-2 (H-2) in the mouse. J. Immunogenet. (in press 1975).

BREWBAKER, J. L.: Agricultural Genetics. Englewood Cliffs: Prentice-Hall 1964. Chapters three and nine.

CATTANACH, B. M.: Genetic disorders of sex determination in mice and other mammals, p. 129. Birth Defects, A. MOTULSKY, W. LENZ, Eds. Amsterdam: Excerpta Medica 1974.

CATTANACH, B. M., POLLARD, C. E., HAWKES, S. G.: Sex-reversed mice: XX and XO males. Cytogenet. **10**, 318 (1971).

CLEGETT, C. O.: Genetic control of the riboflavin carrier protein. Fed. Proc. **30**, 127 (1971).

Committee for the Conference on Biological significance of Histocompatibility antigens. Fed. Proc. **31**, 1087 (1972).

DAVIDSON, J. G., FRASER, F. C., SCHLAGER, G.: A maternal effect on the frequency of spontaneous cleft lip in the A/J mouse. Teratology **2,** 371 (1969).

DEOL, M. S.: An experimental approach to the understanding and treatment of hereditary syndromes with congenital deafness and hypothyroidism. J. med. Genet. **10,** 235 (1973).

DOFUKU, R., TETTENBORN, U., OHNO, S.: Testosterone-"Regulon" in the mouse kidney. Nature (Lond.) New Biol. **232,** 5 (1971).

ERWAY, L. C., FRASER, A. S., HURLEY, L. C.: Prevention of congenital otolith defect in pallid mutant mice by manganese supplementation. Genet. **67,** 97 (1971).

ERWAY, L., HURLEY, L. S., FRASER, A. S.: Congenital ataxia and otolith defects due to manganese deficiency in mice. J. Nutr. **100,** 643 (1970).

ERWAY, L. C., MITCHELL, S. E.: Prevention of otolith defect in pastel mink by manganese supplementation. J. Hered. **64,** 111 (1973).

Excerpta Medica, Section 21, Human Developmental Biology (Cont. as Developmental Biology and Teratology). Amsterdam: Excerpta Medica.

FRASER, G. R.: Association of congenital deafness with goitre (Pendred's syndrome). Ann. Hum. Genet. **28,** 201 (1965).

GLUECKSOHN-WAELSCH, S., ERICKSON, R. P.: The T-locus of the mouse: implications for mechanisms of development. Chapter 8, current topics in developmental biology, vol. 5, A. A. MOSCONA, A. MONROY, Eds. New York-London: Academic Press 1970.

GOLDSTEIN, J. L., WILSON, J. D.: Studies on the pathogenesis of the pseudohermaphroditism in the mouse with testicular feminization. J. clin. Invest. **51,** 1647 (1972).

GOLDSTEIN, J. L., WILSON, J. D.: Hereditary disorders of sexual development in man, p. 165. Birth Defects, A. MOTULSKY, W. LENZ, Eds. Amsterdam: Excerpta Medica 1974.

GRABOWSKI, C. T.: Embryonic oxygen deficiency — a physiological approach to analysis of teratological mechanisms. Advances in teratology, vol. 4, D. H. M. WOOLLAM, Ed. New York-London: Academic Press 1970.

GREEN, E. L., Ed.: Biology of the laboratory mouse, second edition. New York-Toronto-Sydney-London: McGraw-Hill 1966.

GREENE, H. S. N., SAXTON, J. A., Jr.: Hereditary brachydactylia and allied abnormalities in the rabbit. J. exp. Med. **69,** 301 (1939).

GREENGARD, O.: Effects of hormones on development of fetal enzymes. Clin. Pharmacol. Ther. **14,** 721 (1973).

GRÜNEBERG, H.: The genetics of the mouse, second ed. The Hague: Nijhoff 1952.

HETZEL, S., BROWN, K. S.: Facial clefts and lip hematoma in mouse fetuses given diphenylhydantoin. J. dent. Res. **54 A,** 83 (1975).

HINCHLIFFE, J. R.: Experimental modification of cell death and chondrogenesis in insulin-induced micromelia of the developing chick limb. Teratology **9,** 263 (1974).

HINCHLIFFE, J. R., EDE, D. A.: Limb development in the polydactylous talpid^3 mutant of the fowl. J. Embryol. exp. Morph. **17,** 385 (1967).

HINCHLIFFE, J. R., THOROGOOD, P. V.: Genetic inhibition of mesenchymal cell death and the development of form and skeletal pattern in the limbs of talpid^3 (ta^3) mutant chick embryos. J. Embryol. exp. Morph. **31,** 747 (1974).

HOLLANDER, C. S., PROUT, T. E., RIENHOFF, M. C., RUBEN, R. J., ASPER, S. P.: Congenital deafness and goiter. Amer. J. Med. **37,** 630 (1964).

HURLEY, L. S.: Nutrients and genes: interactions in development. Nutr. Rev. **27,** 3 (1969).

HURLEY, L. S., BELL, L. T.: Genetic influences on response to dietary manganese deficiency in mice. J. Nutr. **104,** 133 (1974).

HUTT, F. B.: Animal Genetics. New York: Ronald Press 1964. p. 380.

ITAKURA, H., OHNO, S.: The effect of the mouse x-linked testicular feminization mutation on the hypothalamus-pituitary axis. Clin. Genet. **4,** 91 (1973).

JOST, A.: Dégénérescence des extrémités du foetus de rat sous l'action de certaines preparations hypophysaires. C. R. Soc. Biol. **144,** 1324 (1950).

JOST, A.: Dégénérescence des extrémités du foetus de rat provoquéé par l'adrenaline. C. R. Soc. Biol. **236,** 1510 (1953).

LARSSON, K. S., ERICKSON, B., BOSTROM, H.: Salicylate-induced skeletal and vessel malformations in mouse embryos. Acta Morphol. Neerl. Scand. **6,** 34 (1964).

LA VAIL, M. M., SIDMAN, R. L.: C57BL/6J mice with inherited retinal degeneration. Arch. Ophthalmol. **91**, 394 (1974).
LIM, D. J., ERWAY, L. C.: Influence of manganese on genetically defective otolith. Ann. Otol. (St. Louis) **83**, 565 (1974).
LYON, M. F., HAWKES, S. G.: X-linked gene for testicular feminization in the mouse. Nature (Lond.) **225**, 1217 (1970).
LYON, M. F., HENDRY, I., SHORT, R. V.: The submaxillary salivary glands as test organs for response to androgen in mice with testicular feminization. J. Endocr. **58**, 357 (1973).
MCKUSICK, V. A.: Heritable disorders of connective tissue, 3rd edition. St. Louis: Mosby 1966.
MCKUSICK, V. A.: Human Genetics, 2nd edition. Englewood Cliffs: Prentice-Hall 1969. Chapter 5.
MICKOVÁ, M., IVÁNI, P.: Sex-dependent and H-2 linked influence on expressivity of the brachyury gene in mice. J. Hered. **65**, 369 (1974).
MILAIRE, J.: Histochemical observations on the developing foot of normal, oligosyndactylous (*Os*/+) and syndactylous (SM/SM) mouse embryos. Arch. Biol. (Liège) **78**, 223 (1967).
MOTULSKY, A. G., LENZ, W.: Birth Defects. Amsterdam: Excerpta Medica 1974.
MULVIHILL, J. J.: Congenital and genetic disease in domestic animals. Science **176**, 132 (1972).
NISHIMURA, H., TAKANO, K., TANIMURA, T., YASUDA, M.: Normal and abnormal development of human embryos: first report of the analysis of 1213 intact embryos. Teratology **1**, 281 (1968).
OHNO, S.: Regulatory genetics of sex differentiation. Birth Defects, p. 148, A. MOTULSKY, W. LENZ, Eds. Amsterdam: Excerpta Medica 1974.
PATTERSON, D. F.: Comparative medical genetics: studies in domestic animals. Birth Defects: Original Article Series, vol. X, no. 10, 263, D. BERGSMA, Ed. White Plains, New York: The National Foundation-March of Dimes 1974.
PETTER, C., BOURBON, J., MALTIER, J. P., JOST, A.: Prevention des amputations congenitales hereditaires du lapin par une hyperoxie maternelle. C. R. Acad. Sci. (Paris) **273**, 2639 (1971).
PETTER, C., BOURBON, J., MALTIER, J. P., JOST, A.: Production d'hemorragies des extremites chez le foetus de rat soumis a une hypoxie in utero. C. R. Acad. Sci. (Paris) **272**, 2488 (1971 A).
PETTER, C., BOURBON, J., MALTIER, J. P., JOST, A.: Hematies primordiales et amputations congenitales chez les foetus de lapin porteurs du gene *br*. C. R. Acad. Sci. (Paris) **277**, 801 (1973).
PETTIFOR, J. M., BENSON, R.: Congenital malformations associated with the administration of oral anticoagulants during pregnancy. J. Pediat. **86**, 459 (1975).
POSWILLO, D.: The pathogenesis of the first and second branchial arch syndrome. Oral Surg. **35**, 302 (1973).
REFETOFF, S., DE GROOT, L. J., BERNARD, B., DE WIND, L. T.: Studies of a sibship with apparent hereditary resistance to the intracellular action of thyroid hormone. Metabolism **21**, 723 (1972).
SAUNDERS, J. W., Jr.: Death in embryonic systems. Science **154**, 604 (1966).
SAXÉN, L., RAPOLA, J.: Congenital Defects. New York-Toronto-London: Holt, Reinhart and Winston 1969. Chapter 3.
SEARLE, A. G., Ed.: Mouse News Letter, No. 52, 1975. A private communication. M. R. C. Laboratory animals centre Carshalton Surrey, England.
SPEIDEL, B. D., MEADOW, S. R.: Maternal epilepsy and abnormalities of the fetus and newborn. Lancet **1972 II**, 839.
STAATS, J.: Subject-Strain bibliography listing. Supplement to Mouse News Letter, No. 51, A. G. SEARLE, Ed., the Jackson Laboratory, Bar Harbor, Maine 1975.
STANBURY, J. B., WYNGAARDEN, J. B., FREDRICKSON, D. S., Eds.: The Metabolic Basis of Inherited Disease, 2nd edition, New York-London: McGraw-Hill 1966.
STERN, C.: Principles of Human Genetics, 3rd edition. San Francisco: Freeman 1973. Chapter 13.
WIESNER, E.: Die Erbschäden der landwirtschaftlichen Nutztiere. Jena: Gustav Fischer 1960.
WILSON, J. G.: Environment and Birth Defects. New York-London: Academic Press 1973. Chapter 4.

Witkop, C. J., White, J. G., King, R. A.: Oculocutaneous albinism, chapter 11. Heritable Disorders of Amino Acid Metabolism, W. C. Nyhan, Ed. New York: John Wiley and Sons 1974.
Wright, S.: Evolution and the Genetics of Populations, vol. 1, p. 95. Chicago: University of Chicago Press 1968.
Zwilling, E.: The development of dominant rumplessness in chick embryos. Genet. 27, 641 (1942).

4. Cytotoxic Agents in Teratogenic Research

T. A. Connors

With 3 Figures

The term cytotoxic agent was initially used to describe a number of chemically unrelated agents which had in common only the ability to inhibit the growth of animal tumours. A detailed investigation of their effects in a variety of experimental models showed that, at physiological dose levels, they acted specifically on cells in cycle. Thus, the most sensitive vegetable cells were growing root tips and shoots of plants and germinating seedlings, while bacteria in exponential growth were more affected than when growing slowly in minimal media. Similar observations have been made on a variety of systems ranging from bacteria, yeast, higher plants and invertebrates, to vertebrates including primates. In most cases, acutely toxic doses cause death by damaging proliferating tissues, such as bone marrow and intestinal mucosa. Survivors may show symptoms of damage to epithelial surfaces, to ovarian and testicular tissues, growing hair follicles and indeed to any organ which contains cells in cycle and with a short cycle time. On chronic administration of low doses, cellular abnormalities and nuclear gigantism eventually occur and deaths may result from cirrhosis or pulmonary fibrosis, for example, or from induction of some form of cancer.
Because of their broad spectrum of action, the cytotoxic agents have been used not only in the treatment of cancer but also as immunosuppressants to prevent rejection of tissue homografts, in the treatment of psoriasis and of auto-immune diseases, as sheep epilating agents and as insect chemosterilants. They are also used in the laboratory for studying mechanisms of carcinogenesis, mutagenesis and teratogenesis.
The actual mechanisms by which these chemicals cause cell death is not clear but has been loosely ascribed to some form of unbalanced growth, RNA and protein synthesis being out of phase with DNA synthesis. This phenomenon of unbalanced growth has been described in detail for a number of cytotoxic agents (Kim and Eidinoff, 1965) and is very similar to 'thymine-less' death seen in bacteria (Cohen and Barner, 1954).
Although broadly similar in their biological properties, cytotoxic agents can vary widely in their effects depending on the experimental systems used. A dimethyltriazene, for example, when injected into pregnant rats at day 10 post coitum has little teratogenic action, but is extremely effective if administered on day 14 (Table 1, Druckrey, 1974). Conversely, a closely related diethyltriazene is teratogenic at day 10 but not at day 14. It can also be seen from the table that there is no correlation between LD_{50}, teratogenicity and carcinogenicity. Thus, although a compound may be classed as a cytotoxic agent, its biological effects will vary from system to system.

Table 1. Differential cytotoxicity of two related dialkyltriazenes. (From data of DRUCKREY, 1973)

Compound	Route of Administration	LD_{50} on fetus mg/kg		Teratogenicity		Carcinogenicity	
		Day 10	Day 14	Day 10	Day 14	Day 15	Day 22
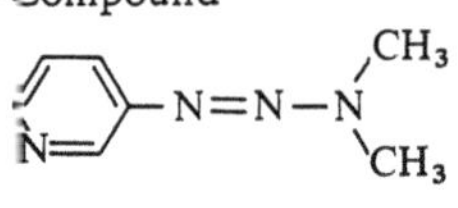 1-(3-Pyridyl)3,3-dimethyltriazene	Subcutaneous	10	100	0	+++	0	+
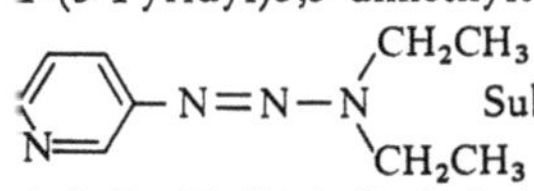 1-(3-Pyridyl)3,3-diethyltriazene	Subcutaneous	60	170	+++	0	++	++

These differences in biological properties between cytotoxic agents do not imply any major differences in their mechanism of action but reflect differences in their physico-chemical properties and in their physiological disposition. For instance, there may be differences in chemical half-life, in their tissue distribution, in their metabolism and excretion and in the ability of target cells to repair the damage they cause. When these agents are being studied as teratogens, the degree and nature of the lesions they cause will depend on a large number of variables, the most important of which are:

1. The age of the embryo when the drug is administered (and hence the organs that are most rapidly proliferating at that time).
2. The total amount of drug administered, the route of administration and the dose schedule used.
3. The ability of the drug to pass the placenta and to penetrate embryonic tissues.
4. The ability of maternal tissues (especially liver) to either detoxify the drug or convert it to an active teratogenic metabolite.
5. The biological and chemical half-life of the agent, especially if it is one that requires activation by maternal liver.
6. The ability of embryonic tissues to detoxify or activate the drug.
7. The status of the target cells, that is whether or not they are in a sensitive stage of the cell cycle during the period when the drug is present at a cytotoxic concentration.
8. The ability of the damaged cells to repair or recover from the cytotoxic lesion.

These variables explain why an agent may be found to be highly teratogenic under one set of experimental conditions and inactive in another.
The means by which the cytotoxic agents destroy dividing cells and exert their characteristic biological properties, can vary from one class of compound to another and cytotoxic agents are usually classified according to their site of action in the cell. Table 2 lists the agents that have been shown to be teratogenic in laboratory animals or which are suspected of being so in man. Tables 3—9 summarise the teratogenic lesions that have been induced by cytotoxic agents and the species used.

Table 2. Mechanism of action of cytotoxic agents with teratogenic activity

Agent	Site of action
Bifunctional alkylating agents	
Nitrogen mustard Uracil mustard Cyclophosphamide Chlorambucil Tretamine ThioTEPA MeTEPA Busulphan	Inter or intrastrand cross-linking of DNA (many other molecules are alkylated but DNA is probably the most important target molecule).
Electrophilic reactants	
Aflatoxin Aminoazobenzenes Benzpyrenes Carbon tetrachloride Cycasin 1,2-Diethylhydrazine Benzanthracenes Alkyltriazenes Ethionine Acetylaminofluorene Pyrollizidine alkaloids Methyl cholanthrene Nitrosourea 6	Usually require metabolism in the host, most frequently by liver microsomes to produce a variety of electrophilic reactants which, like the alkylating agents, can combine co-valently with many molecules. Metabolism may also, in some cases, be extra-microsomal or by gut bacteria. Some agents can break down spontaneously to the active species.
Antimetabolites	
Methotrexate Aminopterin Primethamine Mercaptopurine Azathioprine Thioguanine Azaguanine Halogenated pyrimidines Cytosine arabinoside Aza uracils Diaminopurine	Inhibition of pathways of purine or pyrimidine biosynthesis. Inhibition of formation of thymidylic acid. Inhibition of nucleic acid replication and function by incorporation into nucleic acids as base analogues.
Amino acid antagonists	
Asparaginase Azaserine DON Ethionine Hadacidine Mimosine p-Fluorophenylalanine	Inhibition of protein and nucleic acid synthesis by interfering with specific amino acids required for either protein or nucleic acid synthesis. Specific inhibition of utilisation of asparagine, glutamine, methionine, aspartic acid, tyrosine and phenylalanine.
Intercalating agents	
Acriflavin Actinomycin D Chloroquine Daunomycin (Rubidomycin) Mithramycin Quinacrine	Insertion between stacked base pairs of DNA double helix interfering with transcription and replication.

Table 2 (Continued)

Agent	Site of action
Spindle poisons	
Griseofulvin Podophyllotoxin Vinblastine Vincristine Colchicine	Condensation with microtubular protein so interfering with the formation of cellular organelles especially the spindle apparatus.
Other agents	
Caffeine Formaldehyde Procarbazine Urethane Hydroxyurea	Co-valent reaction with DNA, inhibition of DNA synthesis or inhibition of DNA repair.

Table 3. Bifunctional alkylating agents

Chemical	Type of abnormality	Species studied	References
Nitrogen mustard (HN2, Mustine)	Skeletal Cleft palate CNS Limb defects	Rat Mouse Chick	MURPHY *et al.*, 1958; JURAND, 1961; CHAUBE and MURPHY, 1968; MULLER, 1966; KALTER, 1968
Uracil mustard	CNS Skeletal	Rat	CHAUBE and MURPHY, 1968
Cyclophosphamide (Cytoxan, Endoxan)	Skeletal Cleft palate CNS Limb defects	Rat Mouse Man	CHAUBE and MURPHY, 1968; CHAUBE *et al.*, 1967; GREENBERG and TANAKA, 1964
Chlorambucil	CNS Palate Skeletal Urogenital Chromosomes	Rat Man	CHAUBE and MURPHY, 1968; MONIE, 1961; SHOTTON and MONIE, 1963; SOUKUP *et al.*, 1967
Mitomycin C	Skeletal Palate CNS	Mouse Rat (inactive)	CHAUBE and MURPHY, 1968; TANIMURA, 1968 b
Triethylenemelamine (Tretamine, TEM)	Embryolethal CNS Palate Skeletal	Rat Mouse	THIERSCH, 1957; JURAND, 1961; CHAUBE and MURPHY, 1968; KAGEYAMA and NISHIMURA, 1961
ThioTEPA	Growth inhibition Limbs Skeletal CNS Resorptions	Rat Chick (inactive)	MURPHY *et al.*, 1958; THIERSCH, 1957; TANIMURA, 1968

Table 3 (Continued)

Chemical	Type of abnormality	Species studied	References
MeTEPA	Resorptions Limbs CNS	Rat	GAINES and KIMBROUGH, 1966
Busulphan (Myleran)	Palate Stunting Limbs Ocular Cytomegaly	Rat Man	MURPHY *et al.*, 1958; DIAMOND *et al.*, 1960

Some references given in this table and in Tables 4—9 have been abstracted from 'A Catalog of Teratogenic Agents' by T. H. SHEPARD. John Hopkins University Press, Baltimore and London, 1973.

Table 4. Other electrophilic reactants

Chemical	Type of abnormality	Species studied	References
Aflatoxin	CNS Umbilical hernia Palate Liver necrosis	Guinea pigs	ELIS and DIPAOLO, 1967
Aminoazobenzenes (Azo dyes)	Skeletal Palate	Mouse	SUGIYAMA *et al.*, 1960
Benzopyrene (Poly-nuclear hydrocarbons)	Resorptions Embryotoxicity	Rat	RIGDON and RENNELS, 1964
Carbon tetrachloride	Blastocysts	Rat Rabbit (inactive)	WILSON, 1954; ADAMS *et al.*, 1961
Cycasin (Methyl-azoxy methanol)	CNS Limbs	Guinea pigs	SPATZ *et al.*, 1967
1,2-Diethylhydrazine	Limbs CNS	Rat	DRUCKREY *et al.*, 1968
Dimethylbenzanthracene	CNS Palate Ocular Kidney	Rat	CURRIE *et al.*, 1970
3,3-Dimethyl-phenyltriazene	Skeletal Palate Jaw bone	Chick Rat	MURPHY *et al.*, 1957
Ethionine	CNS	Chick Rat (inactive)	FELDMAN and WADDINGTON, 1955; PROFFIT and EDWARDS, 1962
Ethylnitrosourea	Limbs CNS Ocular	Rat	DRUCKREY *et al.*, 1966; ALEXANDROV and JANISCH, 1970

Table 4 (Continued)

Chemical	Type of abnormality	Species studied	References
N-2-Fluorenylacetamide (AAF)	Skeletal CNS Palate Lips	Mouse	IZUMI, 1966
Heliotrine	Skeletal Palate	Rat	GREEN and CHRISTIE, 1961
Methylcholanthrene	Limb Lymphomas Lung tumours	Mouse	SAVKUR *et al.*, 1961; TOMATIS *et al.*, 1971
Methyl nitrosourea	CNS	Rat	KOYAMA *et al.*, 1970

Table 5. Anti-purines, -pyrimidines and -folates

Chemical	Type of abnormality	Species studied	References
Aminopterin	CNS Abortive Palate Skeletal Ocular Limbs Mitotic block	Rat Man Chick	BARANOV, 1966; PUCHKOV, 1967; THIERSCH and PHILLIPS, 1950; MELTZER, 1956
8-Azaguanine	CNS Embryotoxicity	Rat Chick	WADDINGTON and PERRY, 1958
Azathioprine (Ismuran)	Limb	Mouse (inactive) Rat (inactive) Rabbit	TUCHMANN-DUPLESSIS and MERCIER-PAROT, 1968
5-Azauracil	Embryotoxicity Ocular	Chick	KOSMACHEVSKAYA, 1968
6-Azauracil	Embryotoxicity Ocular	Chick	KOSMACHEVSKAYA, 1968
6-Azauridine	Abortive Skeletal Palate Kidney	Mouse Monkey Man	SANDERS *et al.*, 1961; VAN WAGENEN *et al.*, 1970; VOJTA and JIRASEK, 1966
5-BUdR (5-bromouracil-deoxyriboside)	Limbs CNS Palate Skeletal	Mouse Rat Hamster Rabbit (inactive)	CHAUBE and MURPHY, 1968; ADAMS *et al.*, 1961; DIPAOLO, 1964; RUFFOLO and FERM, 1965
5-ClUdR (deoxyriboside of 5-chlorouracil)	CNS Palate Skeletal	Rat	CHAUBE and MURPHY, 1964

Table 5 (Continued)

Chemical	Type of abnormality	Species studied	References
6-Chloropurine	Palate Skeletal	Rat	MURPHY and CHAUBE, 1962; THIERSCH, 1957 b; TUCHMANN-DUPLESSIS and MERCIER-PAROT, 1959
Cytosine arabinoside	Facial Skeletal Palate CNS	Chick Rat Hamster Mouse	CHAUBE and MURPHY, 1965; CHAUBE and MURPHY, 1968; FISCHER and JONES, 1965; KARNOFSKY and LACON, 1966
2,6-Diaminopurine	Resorption Stunted foetus	Rat	CHAUBE and MURPHY, 1968; THIERSCH, 1957 b
5-Fluorocytosine (5-FC)	Palate Lip Skeletal	Rat	CHAUBE and MURPHY, 1969
5-FCdR (deoxyriboside of 5-FC)	CNS Palate Skeletal	Rat	CHAUBE and MURPHY, 1968; DEGENHARDT *et al.*, 1968
5-Fluorouracil (5-FU)	CNS Skeletal	Mouse Rat Chick	CHAUBE and MURPHY, 1968; PUCHKOV, 1967; DAGG, 1960
5-Fluorouridine	CNS Palate Skeletal	Rat	CHAUBE and MURPHY, 1968
5-FUdR (deoxyriboside of 5-FU)	CNS Palate Skeletal Embryonic haemorrhage	Mouse Rat Chick	CHAUBE and MURPHY, 1968; BRO-RASMUSSEN *et al.*, 1971
5-Fluoroorotic acid	Skeletal	Rat	CHAUBE and MURPHY, 1968
Methotrexate	Skeletal Limbs DNA inhibition	Rat Rabbit (inactive) Man	ADAMS *et al.*, 1961; BERRY, 1971; MILUNSKY, GRAEF and GAYNOR, 1968
6-Mercaptopurine (and riboside)	Limbs Palate	Mouse Rat Rabbit Chick Man (inactive)	CHAUBE and MURPHY, 1968; ADAMS *et al.*, 1961; KARNOFSKY, 1960; SOKAL and LESSMANN, 1960
Primethamine	Palate Skeletal Limb Chromosomal	Rat Guinea pig Chick	ANDERSON and MORSE, 1966; STANZHEUSKAYA, 1966; SULLIVAN and TAKACS, 1971; THIERSCH, 1954
Thioguanine (and riboside)	Skeletal Resorption Runting	Rat	CHAUBE and MURPHY, 1968; THIERSCH, 1957 b
5-Trifluoromethyl UdR	Palate Skeletal Kidney	Chick	KURY and CROSBY, 1967

Table 6. Amino acid antagonists

Chemical	Type of abnormality	Species studied	References
Asparaginase	Intestinal Skeletal Lung Kidney	Rabbit Rat (inactive)	Adamson *et al.*, 1970
Azaserine	Skeletal Palate	Chick Rat	Blattner *et al.*, 1958; Dagg and Karnofsky, 1955; Murphy and Karnofsky, 1956
DON (Diazo-oxo-norleucine)	Lip Palate	Rat Dog	Chaube and Murphy, 1968; Murphy, 1960
Hadacidin (Formylhydroxy-glycine)	CNS Palate Skeletal	Rat	Chaube and Murphy, 1963; Lejour-Jeanty, 1966
Mimosine	Resorption Uterus	Rat	Dewreede and Wayman, 1970
p-Fluorophenylalanine	Growth inhibition (*in vitro*)	Chick	Waddington and Perry, 1958

Table 7. Intercalating agents

Chemical	Type of abnormality	Species studied	References
Acriflavin	Skeletal	Chick	Ancel, 1946
Actinomycin D	CNS Optic nerve Rumplessness	Rat Rabbit Chick	Takaya, 1963; Dyban and Akimova, 1967; Pierro, 1961; Tuchmann-Duplessis and Mercier-Parot, 1960; Wilson, 1966
Chloroquine	Ototoxicity Ocular Wilm's tumour Embryotoxicity	Rat Man	Smith, 1966; Udalova, 1967; Hart and Naunton, 1964
Daunomycin (Rubidomycin, Daunorubicin)	None found	Rat	Chaube and Murphy, 1968
Mithramycin	None found	Rat	Chaube and Murphy, 1968
Quinacrine	Embryotoxicity	Rat	Rothschild and Levy, 1950
Rubidomycin (Daunomycin, Daunorubicin)	Ocular Heart Kidney CNS	Rat Chick (inactive) Mouse (inactive) Rabbit (inactive)	Julou *et al.*, 1967; Roux and Taillemite, 1969

Table 8. Spindle poisons

Chemical	Type of abnormality	Species studied	References
Griseofulvin	Ocular Skeletal Urogenital CNS	Rat	KLEIN and BEALL, 1972
Podophyllotoxin	Resorption	Mouse Rat (inactive)	CHAUBE and MURPHY, 1968; THIERSCH, 1963; WIESNER and YUDKIN, 1955
Vinblastine and Vincristine	CNS Skeletal Ocular Metaphase arrest Limb	Rat Hamster Rabbit Monkey Man (inactive)	ARMSTRONG *et al.*, 1964; COHLAN and KITAY, 1965; FERM, 1963; MORRIS *et al.*, 1967
Colchicine	Embryotoxicity Neural	Rabbit Monkey Rat Sperm	ADAMS *et al.*, 1961

Table 9. Other cytotoxic agents

Chemical	Type of abnormality	Species studied	References
Caffeine	Limb Palate	Mouse Rat Rabbit (inactive)	NISHIMURA and NAKAI, 1960
Formaldehyde	Reduced DNA content	Rat	PUSHKINA *et al.*, 1968
Procarbazine	Ocular Limb	Rat	CHAUBE and MURPHY, 1968; TUCHMANN-DUPLESSIS and MERCIER-PAROT, 1967
Urethane	CNS Palate Skeletal Ocular	Mouse Rat	HALL, 1953; SINCLAIR, 1950; TAKAORI *et al.*, 1966; NISHIMURA and KUGINUKI, 1958
Hydroxyurea	CNS Palate Skeletal DNA inhibition Limb Beak	Rat Chick	SOUKUP *et al.*, 1967; CHAUBE and MURPHY, 1966; MURPHY and CHAUBE, 1964; SCOTT *et al.*, 1971

Alkylating Agents

The biological properties of certain alkylating agents have been known for more than 50 years, but they began to be studied in detail only in the 1940s when it was shown that aliphatic nitrogen mustards (originally synthesised as potential chemical warfare agents) had good effects in the treatment of lymphomas (CONNORS, 1975). From the many thousands of chemicals investigated since that time, it is now apparent that different classes of alkylating agent can have good anti-cancer activity but that with very few exceptions they must be polyfunctional, i. e. have at least two alkylating arms per molecule. In order to be effective anti-cancer agents they must also have an optimum level of chemical reactivity (ROSS, 1962).
The alkylating agents in polar solvents are very reactive towards molecules which have negative charges (nucleophiles) such as ionised carboxylic and phosphoric acids and thiols, or which have negative areas due to presence of amine groups. Thus these agents react with many biological constituents including nucleic acids, proteins, nucleotides and amino acids. At least four chemical classes of alkylating agent have cytotoxic properties, the nitrogen mustards, ethyleneimines (aziridines), sulphonoxy-alkanes and epoxides (oxiranes). As shown in Fig. 1, they react after formation of a positively charged species, although in practice this species may not exist in free form, reaction with a negatively charged molecule taking place through a transition complex. All the derivatives shown in Fig. 1 are bifunctional containing two alkylating arms, the corresponding monofunctional analogues being usually less toxic and without anti-tumour activity. However, the latter are sometimes just as potent carcinogens as the corresponding bifunctional compound and it is likely that they will also be teratogenic, although to date relatively few alkylating agents have been investigated, all of which are difunctional (Table 3). Like anti-cancer activity, terato-

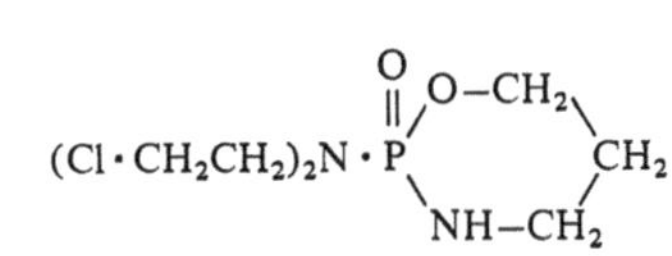

(I)

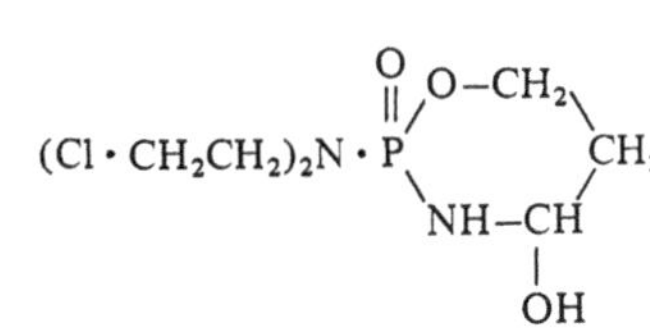

(II)

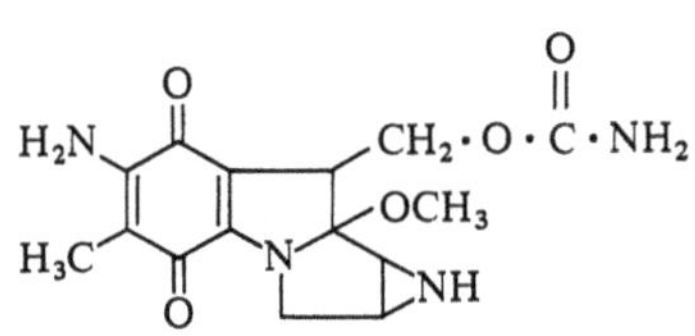

(III)

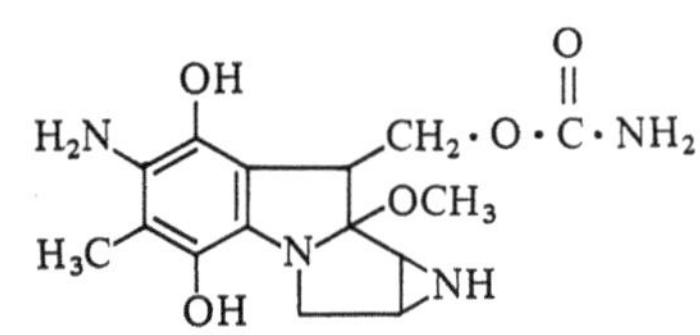

(IV)

genicity also depends on the chemical reactivity of the alkylating agent which will have an optimal value. An alkylating agent that reacts too rapidly may never reach embryonic tissues in active form and one which reacts only slowly may be excreted before effective cellular alkylation has occurred. Alkylating agents can kill dividing cells at any stage of the cell cycle and, unlike many anti-metabolites, it is not likely

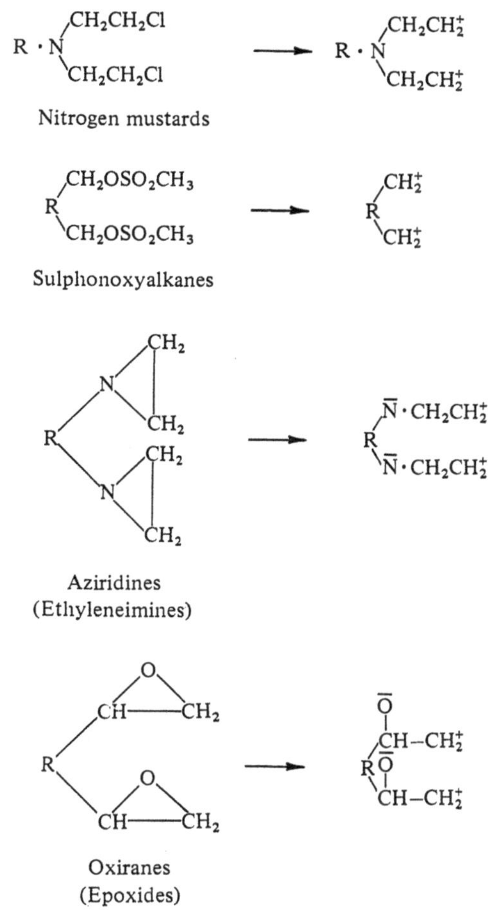

Fig. 1

that there will be any great difference in teratogenicity between a single injection of an agent and the same amount given over a period of hours. The day of gestation on which alkylating agent is given can of course greatly influence the severity and type of teratogenic effect observed, due to differences in organ proliferation rates on various days. Thus, for both chlorambucil and cyclophosphamide, the defects found and their severity are dependent on the day of gestation on which the compound is administered (Chaube *et al.*, 1967). Alkylating agents are known which are not active *per se* but which must be metabolised *in vivo* to an active species and thus factors which influence this metabolism, e. g. hormonal, nutritional, may alter the teratogenic properties of the compound. Cyclophosphamide (I), for instance, requires to be hydroxylated by the liver to the corresponding 4-hydroxy derivative (II; Connors *et al.*, 1974) and any factor which influences the liver microsomes which carry out this reaction will affect the teratogenicity of this compound. Similarly, Mitomycin C (III) probably requires activation by initial reduction of its quinone ring (IV). The ability of embryonic tissues to reduce mitomycin may be the main factor which determines its teratogenicity, since the active metabolite probably has a very short half-life and would not reach the embryo if it were generated only in maternal liver.

At the molecular level, difunctional alkylating agents have been claimed to act by their effects on cell membranes, on nucleoprotein, glycolytic enzymes or on cyclic AMP levels. However, the alkylating agents are quite similar in their biological properties, despite their varied chemical structure, and usually a cell with acquired or natural resistance to one alkylating agent is cross resistant to all others. This implies that they share a common pathway in exerting their effects, if not a common mechanism of action. The majority of the evidence favours DNA as the principle target site for all alkylating agents since it is known that low levels of alkylation of this molecule can cause considerable toxicity. The requirement for bifunctionality is explained by a cross-linking reaction which links together two areas of the DNA molecule and which is more toxic than a monofunctional alkylation. Whether cross-linking is more toxic when it is between the complementary strands of DNA, between two regions of the same strand or between nucleic acid and protein is not known. Although at one time it was considered that the cross-linking of two guanine moieties in adjacent strands was the important cytotoxic event, this view has been modified. New methods to isolate alkylated DNA have now shown that reaction takes place with many different groups in the molecule. To explain the special sensitivity of dividing cells, it is postulated that resting cells may repair their DNA by known enzymatic processes, while dividing cells are forced into mitosis before this repair is completed.

Many monofunctional alkylating agents are often as mutagenic and carcinogenic as their corresponding difunctional analogues and one theory is that DNA is again the most sensitive molecule. At sub-lethal doses repair is attempted but if this is faulty, changes in the function of DNA occurs which lead to the malignant change or some other form of mutation.

Other Electrophilic Reactants

It is now becoming increasingly clear that many synthetic and natural carcinogens must be converted *in vivo* to an alkylating agent or some other form of electrophilic reactant before they have this property. Characteristically, these compounds are acutely toxic if given in a single high dose and carcinogenic on chronic administration. Thus ingestion of large amounts of aflatoxin contaminated foodstuffs is known to cause acute hepatotoxicity, while injection of small amounts can cause hepatocellular carcinoma in a wide range of animal species. Any carcinogen which acts by an intermediate electrophilic reactant will have the general properties of cytotoxic agents and under the appropriate conditions will probably be a carcinogen. Already a number of organic chemicals, highly carcinogenic in animals and suspected of causing cancer in man, are known to be powerful teratogens (Table 4).

Many variables are involved in determining whether a chemical can be transformed *in vivo* to an electrophilic reactant and one of the most comprehensive studies has been carried out on 2-acetylaminofluorene (V; Fig. 2; MILLER and MILLER, 1969). This compound is a potent liver carcinogen in a variety of species, although the

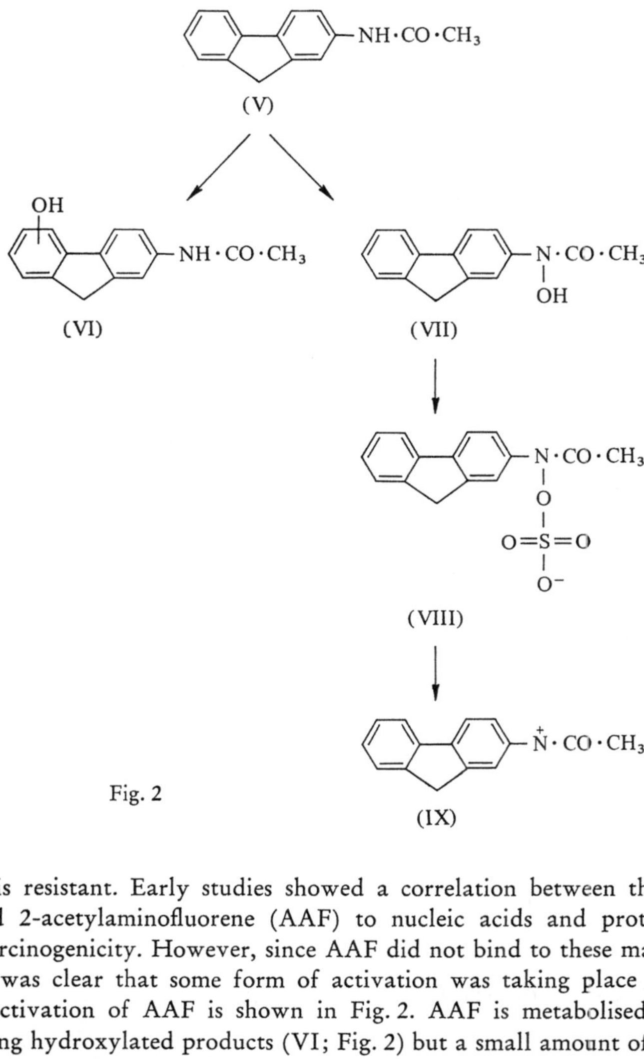

Fig. 2

guinea pig is resistant. Early studies showed a correlation between the binding of administered 2-acetylaminofluorene (AAF) to nucleic acids and proteins and the degree of carcinogenicity. However, since AAF did not bind to these macromolecules *in vitro*, it was clear that some form of activation was taking place *in vivo*. The scheme of activation of AAF is shown in Fig. 2. AAF is metabolised in the liver mainly to ring hydroxylated products (VI; Fig. 2) but a small amount of N-hydroxylation (VII; Fig. 2) also takes place. The latter compound is a more potent carcinogen than AAF and can induce tumours at sites of application (e. g. subcutaneous) where AAF has no activity. The N-hydroxy derivative thus lies on the activation pathway, but is not the ultimate carcinogen because it is still not very reactive to nucleic acids and proteins *in vitro*. The finding that synthetic esters of VII reacted powerfully with macromolecules, suggested that the final activation step *in vivo* was the formation of a sulphate ester (VIII; Fig. 2) and its subsequent breakdown to an electrophilic reactant (IX). This pathway neatly explains the difference in carcinogenicity between species. Part of the resistance of the guinea pig to this compound is that it is not very efficient in converting AAF to its N-hydroxy derivative and the guinea pig and mouse are resistant because they only have low levels of the sulphotransferase enzyme (MILLER and MILLER, 1969). The electrophilic reactant formed now attacks

Table 10

Teratogen	Active metabolite
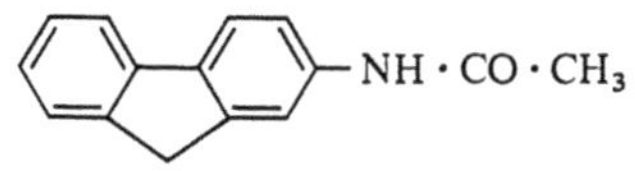 Acetylaminofluorene	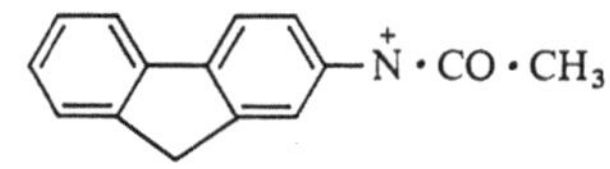
CCl_4 Carbon tetrachloride	$CCl_3^{\bullet}$
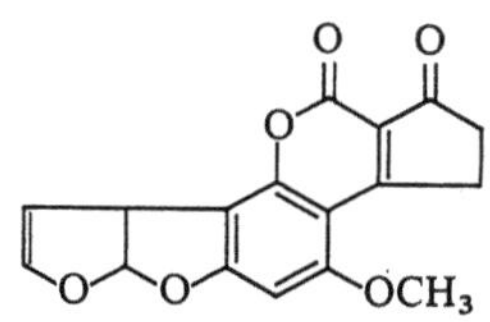 Aflatoxin B_1	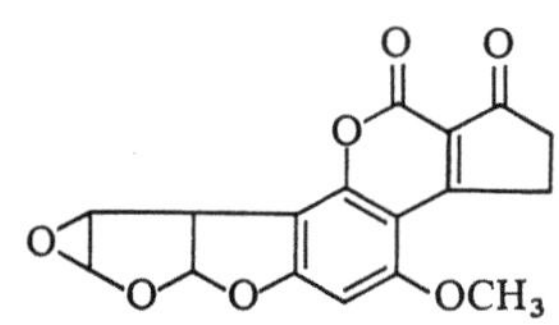
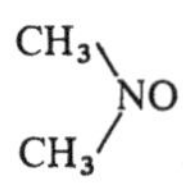 Dimethylnitrosamine	CH_3^+
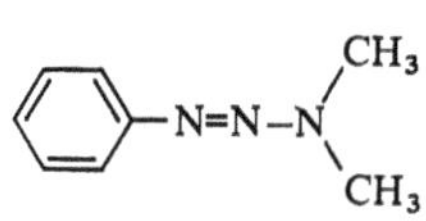 3,3-Dimethyl-1-phenyltriazene	CH_3^+
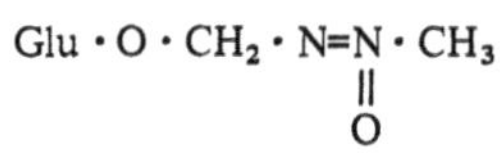 Cycasin	CH_3^+
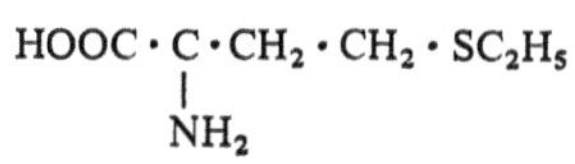 Ethionine	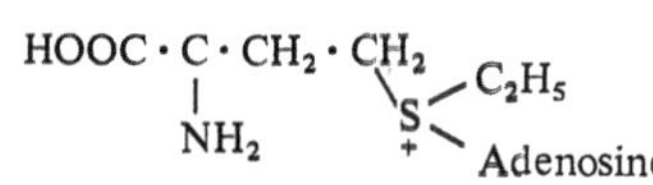
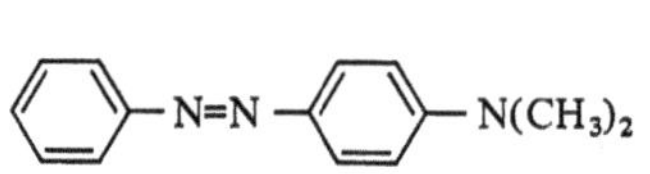 Dimethylamino azobene	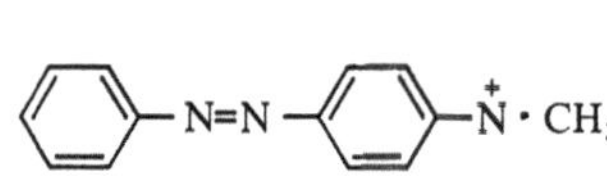

any cellular molecule in its vicinity which has a negatively charged region (nucleophile) and if the appropriate level of reaction takes place with the essential target molecule, then the malignant transformation occurs. It is apparent from the scheme of Fig. 2 that whether or not a critical level of the electrophilic reactant is formed is determined by a large number of variables. Metabolism by liver microsomes is an

Table 10 (Continued)

Teratogen	Active metabolite
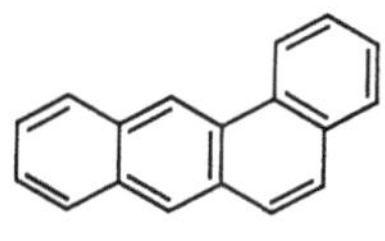 Benz(a)anthracene	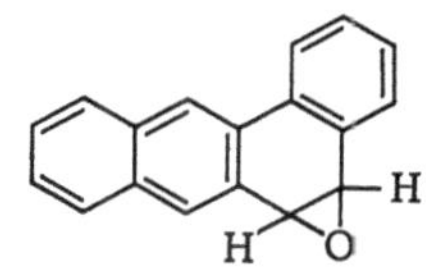
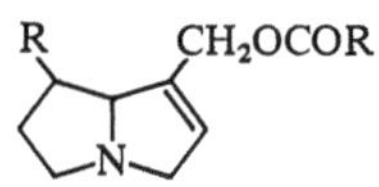 Pyrollizidine alkaloids	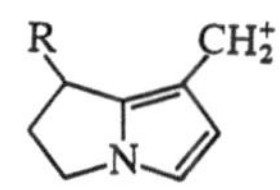
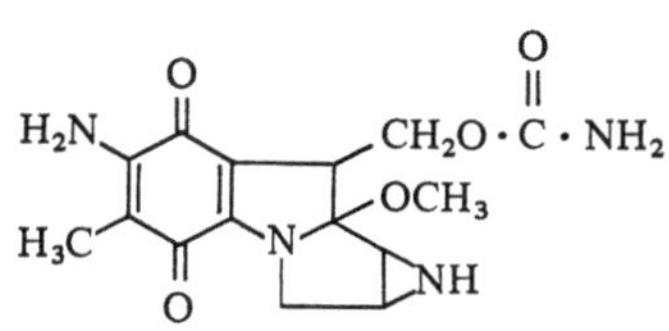 Mitomycin C	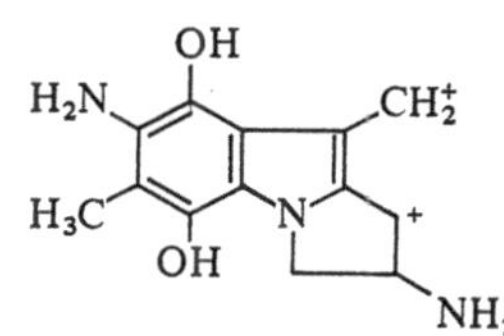

essential first step in activation and microsomal activity is dependent on a number of factors, including the hormonal and nutritional status of the animal. The major metabolites of microsomal metabolism are ring hydroxylated detoxification products, and if the carcinogen is given to an animal whose microsomes have been 'induced' by, for example, phenobarbitone, there may be lowered carcinogenicity although increased metabolism. The degree of carcinogenicity will depend on the balance between detoxification and activation reactions and this balance may vary depending on the microsomal inducer used.

AAF is predominantly a liver carcinogen, presumably because the active sulphate is such a reactive chemical that it cannot travel far from its site of formation in the liver. However, AAF does induce tumours in sebaceous ear duct gland, mammary gland and epithelium of the small intestine, implying that either these tissues can also activate AAF or that another, as yet unidentified, carcinogenic metabolite is formed in the liver which is stable enough to diffuse from the liver and reach distant tissues.

When AAF was given to mice between the 8th and 15th gestational days, skeletal defects were the main abnormality observed (Izumi, 1966). The implication of this finding is that foetal liver does not metabolise AAF since no hepatotoxicity was observed, but that some form of cytotoxic agent is being produced by maternal tissues which reaches the embryo in active form.

All of the electrophilic reactants in Table 4 are highly carcinogenic as well as teratogenic. Since a number of these are naturally occurring, it is clear that some of the teratogenicity seen in man could be due to accidental ingestion of these compounds. The metabolism of most of them has been studied, and without exception it has been found that the ultimate carcinogen is an electrophilic reactant (Table 10). Thus, if a compound is known to be an electrophilic reactant in its own right (for example, an alkylating agent) it must be considered to be a potential teratogen, the most important feature of the compound being its chemical half-life which determines whether it can travel from the site of injection to sensitive embryonic tissues. Other compounds with no reactivity to nucleophiles *per se* must also be considered as potential teratogens if they are related in structure to the chemical classes listed in Table 10 or to any other known carcinogen. Many of these agents require liver microsomal metabolism and the half-life of the active metabolite will be an important factor. Thus, if it is very reactive, such as the $CCl_3^{\cdot}$ radical formed from carbon tetrachloride, it will be unstable and react at the site of formation. Hence, carbon tetrachloride is very toxic to adult liver where it is generated (providing the microsomal system has not been inhibited by, for instance, protein deprivation) but not very toxic in new born rats whose metabolic enzymes are not fully developed (REYNOLDS, 1967). This is in agreement with the weak teratogenic action of carbon tetrachloride which caused no congenital defects in the offspring of rats (WILSON, 1954) and only slight effects on the embryonic discs of rabbit blastocysts (ADAMS *et al.*, 1961). The aflatoxins are again metabolised, principally by the liver, to an epoxide which has a very short half-life and hence the predominant action of these derivatives is on the liver (GARNER, 1974). However, despite the short half-life of the metabolite, the aflatoxins are teratogenic and cause fetal liver cell necrosis (ELIS and DIPAOLO, 1967). This implies that fetal liver has the ability to metabolise the aflatoxins, which is a little surprising since this reaction is thought to be mediated by microsomes.

The nitrosamines are similarly activated in the liver to highly reactive carbonium ions which act mainly at the site of formation, thus causing hepatotoxicity or liver cancer. Despite their high carcinogenicity in adult rats, they are not powerful inducers of transplacental cancer because the active metabolite is too unstable to reach the fetus, which is itself unable to activate the nitosamines until shortly before birth (DRUCKREY, 1973). The related nitrosoureas, on the other hand, are teratogenic because they are stable enough to cross the placenta and to be demonstrable in the embryo (WUNDERLICH and TETZLAFF, 1970). Dialkyltriazenes are potent both as antitumour agents and as carcinogens. They are activated by microsomal demethylation to monoalkyltriazenes which then break down spontaneously to form alkylating metabolites. The monoalkyltriazenes formed in the liver from phenyltriazenes are relatively stable, having half-lives of the order of ten minutes. They thus have adequate time to diffuse from maternal liver and penetrate embryonic tissue and their teratogenic properties are not unexpected (MURPHY *et al.*, 1957).

Cycasin, a naturally occurring constituent of certain plants which are used as a source of edible starch in some countries, is the β-glycoside of methylazoxymethanol. This compound is only an electrophilic reactant after the sugar residue has been removed and *in vivo* this is carried out enzymatically by the β-glucosidase of gut bacteria. Thus, the presence of enterobacteria will determine whether an active agent is formed, but once this has occurred it is stable enough to be distributed systematically and to be carcinogenic and teratogenic. The β-glucosidase content of the intestinal bacteria of laboratory animals can vary considerably depending on the species, age and condition of the animals, and thus the teratogenicity of this compound is widely variable.

Ethionine is converted by the methionine activation enzyme in the liver to S-adenosyl-L-ethionine and in this form can ethylate macromolecules, especially nucleic acids, causing cell abnormalities. Adenosylethionine is stable and can penetrate embryonic tissues and cause teratogenic effects. However, the rate at which it ethylates macromolecules is slow compared with the rate of (normal)methylation by S-adenosylmethionine and the adverse effects of ethionine can easily be reversed by methionine. It is known, for instance, that the defective neurulation in chicks induced by ethionine can be prevented by concomitant administration of methionine (FELDMAN and WADDINGTON, 1955). Obviously the availability of methionine in the embryo must play a role in determining whether or not ethionine is teratogenic. The inability of ethionine to cause defects in rats during the second week of gestation (PROFFIT and EDWARDS, 1962) may indicate that during this period there is a plentiful supply of methionine.

The teratogenic and carcinogenic 4-dimethylaminoazobenzene is metabolised by N-hydroxylation followed by esterification in a manner analogous to that previously described for acetylaminofluorene. Substitution of either of the aromatic rings can greatly alter the carcinogenicity of the compound (and presumably its teratogenicity). Certain substitutions in the aromatic ring make the molecule much more sensitive to reduction, this cleavage of the azo linkage representing a detoxification reaction. At high dose levels, at least three aminoazobenzenes are teratogenic (SUGIYAMA *et al.*, 1960) and if, as is likely, activation takes place in maternal liver, then the active metabolite must be stable enough to reach embryonic tissue. In view of the close similarity of activation pathways of acetylaminofluorenes and aminoazobenzenes, it is of interest that in both cases the predominant teratogenic defects were skeletal abnormalities.

The polycyclic hydrocarbons are converted by microsomal enzymes to epoxides which are very reactive to nucleophiles. The strong mutagenicity of this class of compounds is thought to be due to their planar structure which enables them to fit between the base pairs of the DNA double helix (intercalation). The intercalated metabolite containing a reactive epoxide group can thus react with specific centres of DNA. As a consequence of this reaction, an abnormal 'base' is inserted in the DNA strand and the following faulty transcription of the triplet sequence can cause mutations. Not all the hydrocarbons are alike in their teratogenic properties however, for while benzpyrene is not a particularly effective teratogen at tolerated doses (RIGDON and RENNELS, 1964), 7,12-dimethylbenzanthracene produces a high incidence of defects of various types (CURRIE *et al.*, 1970). For this latter compound, there is an interesting correlation between adrenolytic activity and teratogenicity.

The pyrollizidine alkaloids, such as heliotrine, are hepatotoxic agents isolated from various plants. They have the same basic structure as mitomycin C and are probably only active after conversion to the corresponding pyrrole analogue.

Antimetabolites

The anti-metabolites are a particularly important class of anti-tumour agent and are divided into purine and pyrimidine antagonists and anti-folates. Amino acid antagonists rarely have cytotoxic properties and are not effective as anti-tumour agents, although a few have teratogenic properties (Table 6).

An antimetabolite is generally defined as an analogue of an essential metabolite which prevents its further utilisation by competing with it for an enzyme. As might be expected, analogues acting in this way are very similar in chemical structure to the metabolite they inhibit.

Anti-Purines

Anti-purines with teratogenic activity are the 6-substituted purines such as azathioprine, mercaptopurine, thioguanine and chloropurine and heterocyclic ring analogues such as 8-azaguanine. In every case it can be seen that the alteration to the molecule is a slight one (Fig. 3). Thus 6-mercaptopurine (XIII) is an analogue of hypoxanthine, the base of the nucleotide inosinic acid (X), an essential precursor of nucleic acid biosynthesis, where the only modification has been substitution of an SH group for an OH group. This slight change is sufficient to prevent the formation of the nucleic acid bases, adenylic (XI) and guanylic acids (XII) from inosinic acid. 6-Chloropurine (XIV) acts in the same way and azathioprine (XV), which is used widely as an immunosuppressant, is hydrolysed to 6-mercaptopurine soon after injection and probably acts *in vivo* as this compound. 6-Thioguanine (XVI) is an analogue of guanylic acid (XII) obtained similarly to 6-mercaptopurine by substitution of the 6-hydroxy group for a thiol. In this case, although it inhibits a number of pathways of purine biosynthesis, its predominant toxic action is a result of its incorporation into nucleic acids. 2,6-Diaminopurine (XVII) is a further analogue obtained by the substitution of a hydroxyl group by an amino group. Since its cytotoxic effects are reversed by adenine, it is likely that it acts by preventing the synthesis of adenylic acid (XI). Analogues can also be formed by isosteric replacement of the imidazole ring of the purine to form, for example, 8-azaguanine (XVIII).

These base analogues are not active *per se,* since all the important pathways they interfere with operate at the nucleotide di- and triphosphate levels, which means that they must be converted to the appropriate ribotide or deoxyribotide before they act as antagonists. Thus many bases which resemble a natural metabolite, e. g. 8-azaxanthine (XIX), have no cytotoxic properties in mammals because they are not converted to their nucleotides. Similarly, resistance to these compounds can occur by the cell losing the enzyme necessary to convert the base analogue to its active nucleotide. Activation of bases is either by a two-stage process involving enzymatic attachment of first the ribose and then the phosphate moiety or a single stage reaction where the base is converted directly to its nucleotide by a phosphoribosyl transferase enzyme. Thus the level of the appropriate activating enzyme in a cell will be one factor determining its sensitivity to the anti-metabolite. Many of the purine antagonists can also be catabolised by the enzymes that break down the normal metabolite and thus the activity of an anti-metabolite may depend on the balance between activating and deactivating enzymes. Most of the teratogenic anti-metabolites are reversible antagonists acting specifically at one stage of the cell cycle, usually the DNA synthetic phase. Because of these properties they are dose schedule dependent (unlike electrophilic reactants which react irreversibly at all stages of the cell cycle). A single high dose of an anti-metabolite may be ineffective while a much smaller total dose administered over a period of time may be much more effective. For cytotoxicity to

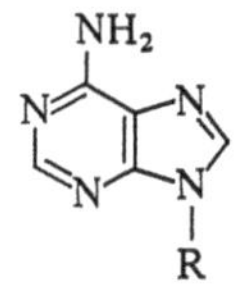
(XI)

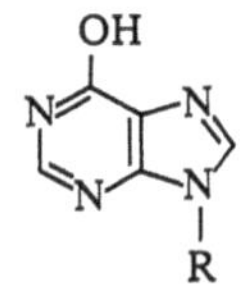
(X)

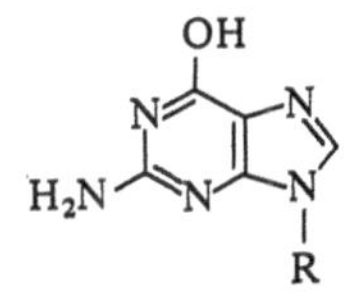
(XII)

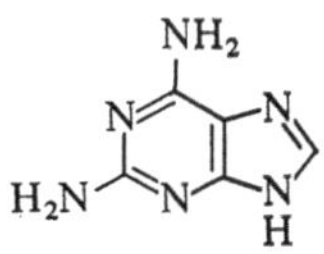
(XVII)

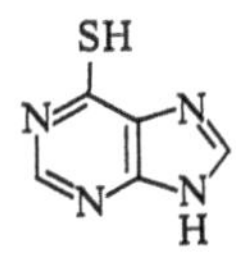
(XIII)

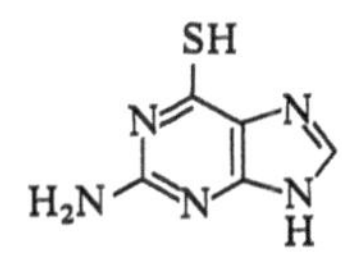
(XVI)

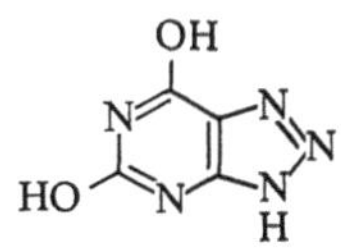
(XIX)

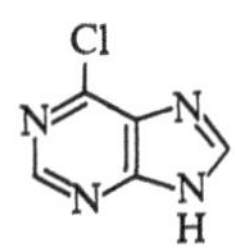
(XIV)

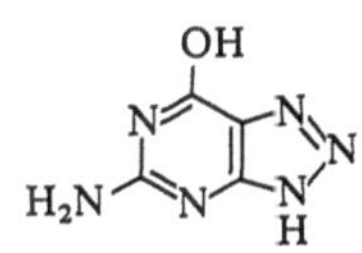
(XVIII)

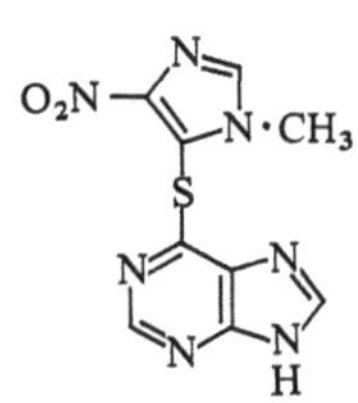
(XV)

Fig. 3

occur, the drug must be present in the body for the period of time that it takes all target cells to enter and pass through the sensitive phase of the cycle. In a tumour comprising a population of asynchronously dividing cells, for example, a single dose of an anti-metabolite may have little effect, especially if it is rapidly broken down or excreted, because only a proportion of the cells are exposed to the drug when they are in a sensitive phase. On the other hand a small minimum effective dose of the compound maintained for at least one cell cycle time, may be completely lethal to a rapidly-growing tumour. If fetal tissues contain cells growing almost synchronously and of a very short cycle time, then given at the right time, a single dose of an anti-metabolite can be teratogenic (WADDINGTON and PERRY, 1958; TUCHMANN-DUPLESSIS and MERCIER-PAROT, 1968; THIERSCH, 1957b; CHAUBE and MURPHY, 1968; SOKAL and LESSMANN, 1960) but even in this case an agent would be a more powerful teratogen if it were infused over a period of time.

Anti-Pyrimidines

Anti-pyrimidines have been made by the same sort of chemical alterations that led to anti-purines and like the latter must be converted to nucleotides before having activity. They can also be catabolised by intracellular enzymes and since they act on specific phases of the cell cycle they are dose schedule dependent.

At least nine 5-substituted halogenated pyrimidines have been tested for their teratogenicity in laboratory animals (Table 5), the most potent member being the deoxyribotide of 5-fluorocytosine (XX) which causes embryonic defects at doses of 0.15 mg/kg given on the 11th or 12th day of gestation (CHAUBE and MURPHY, 1969). It is some 200-times more toxic to the rat fetus than to the mother. The base, 5-fluorocytosine is itself a teratogen (CHAUBE and MURPHY, 1969) although to be effective, doses of as high as 1000 mg/kg are required. The lack of cytotoxic activity

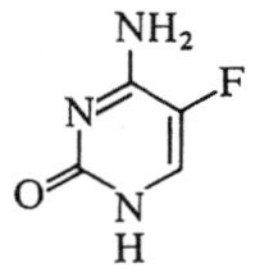

(XX)

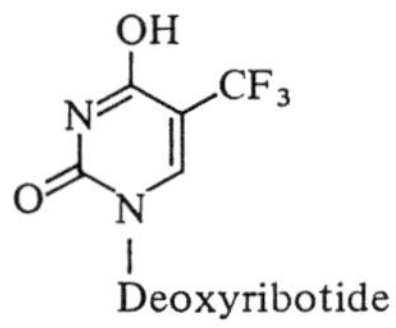

(XXI)

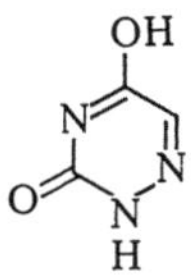

(XXII)

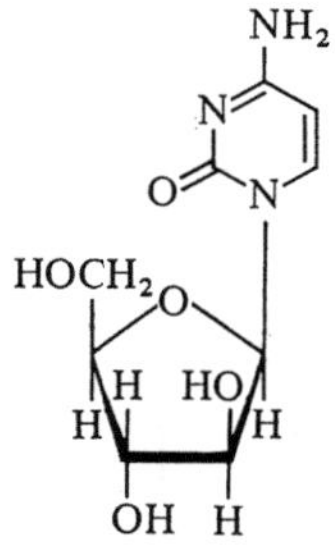

(XXIII)

of 5-fluorocytosine in mammalian cells is thought to be due to the inability of these cells to deaminate the compound to 5-fluorouracil under the action of a cytidine deaminase enzyme. The deoxyriboside of 5-fluorocytosine is a substrate for mammalian cytidine deaminase and is readily converted to the cytotoxic 5-fluorodeoxyuridine (TATTERSALL *et al.*, 1974). 5-Fluorocytosine is a good anti-fungal agent, presumably because fungi can either convert it to its ribotide (which mammalian cells cannot) or because it is a good substrate for fungal cytidine deaminase. The finding of teratogenicity with 5-fluorocytosine, albeit at very high dose levels, may mean that there is some activation of this agent in embryonic tissues.

The fluorinated pyrimidines inhibit various stages of pyrimidine biosynthesis, particularly the formation of thymidylic acid from deoxyuridylic acid. In most cases they act reversibly but one of them, 5-trifluoromethyldeoxyuridine (XXI) is an irreversible inhibitor of thymidylate synthetase. After binding to the enzyme, a covalent bond is formed between inhibitor and enzyme so that the inhibitor cannot be displaced from the enzyme surface even by large amounts of deoxyuridylic acid. Thus, although, with most pyrimidine anti-metabolites the inhibited pathways gradually recover (in surviving cells), due to a build up of precursors, the inhibition caused by the trifluoro derivative is much more prolonged. Although 5-fluorouracil is a powerful anti-metabolite, the corresponding halogeno derivatives, 5-iodo- and 5-bromouracil have no anti-metabolite activity in mammalian cells. This is due to their inability to anabolise these agents to their ribosides and ribotides, because the corresponding ribosides are cytotoxic and act on many pyrimidine biosynthetic pathways. One notable property of 5-bromo- and 5-iododeoxyuridine is their ability to replace the thymidine residues of DNA by as much as 50% of the total thymidine content. It is the consequences of their incorporation as base analogues into DNA that lead to many of the toxic effects of these agents.

Other types of pyrimidine antagonist have been synthesised by making isomers of the heterocyclic ring, for example 5- and 6-azauracil (XXII) and their ribosides, which prevent the decarboxylation of orotidylic acid to uridylic acid. A further type of modification is to replace the ribose sugar of the nucleoside by an isomeric pentose. A powerful anti-metabolite made in this way is cytosine arabinoside (XXIII) which affects DNA synthesis specifically, by inhibiting DNA polymerase. This compound, like other anti-metabolites, is dose schedule dependent, is rapidly excreted *in vivo* and can also be deactivated by the cytidine deaminase enzyme. Its cytotoxicity will depend on the balance between the activating enzymes which convert it to its triphosphate, and the deactivating enzyme which deaminates it to arabinosyl uridine. Since it is excreted so quickly, multiple injections or infusion of the agent give much greater anti-tumour effects than single injections and although relatively large dose levels are needed to produce teratogenic effects in rats or mice (Chaube and Murphy, 1968), it is likely that the same effects could be produced by infusions of much smaller doses over a period of a few hours. Like other reversible anti-metabolites, the teratogenicity of cytosine arabinoside can be reversed by high concentrations of the natural metabolite it inhibits. In this case, injections of deoxycytidine (which is converted to the natural metabolite deoxycytidylic acid intracellularly) given simultaneously, can prevent the teratogenicity of cytosine arabinoside (Chaube and Murphy, 1968).

Anti-Folates

Folic acid (XXIV) is a precursor of a number of co-enzymes vital for the synthesis of many important molecules. These derivatives of folic acid referred to collectively as 'active formate' and 'active formaldehyde' are responsible for the addition of a one carbon containing group to molecules during the enzymatic synthesis of essential compounds such as in the formation of thymidylic acid from deoxyuridylic acid. Before folic acid can act as an acceptor of one carbon fragments it has to be reduced by a folate reductase enzyme to tetrahydrofolic acid (XXV). Anti-folates such as methotrexate (XXVI) bind to the folate reductase enzyme, inhibiting the production of tetrahydrofolate which eventually results in inhibition of nucleic acid and protein synthesis. In methotrexate the slight change in structure, substitution of a hydroxyl group by an amino group and a hydrogen by a methyl, is sufficient to increase its affinity for the reductase enzyme by some 10^4—10^5 fold with the result that the inhibition is essentially irreversible. The cytotoxicity of methotrexate may be reversed but only by by-passing the block by administering folinic acid as a source of tetra-

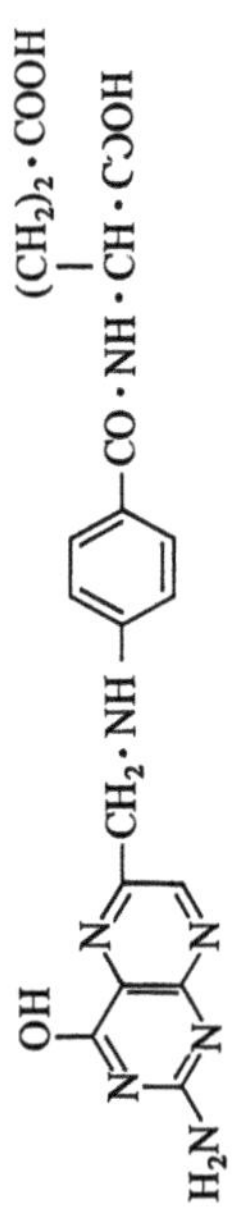

(XXIV)

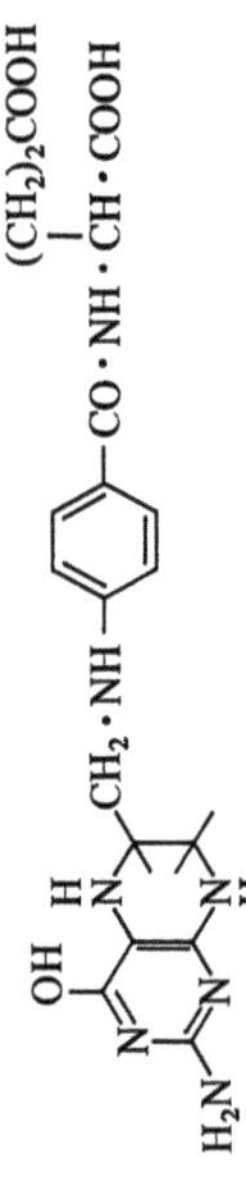

(XXV)

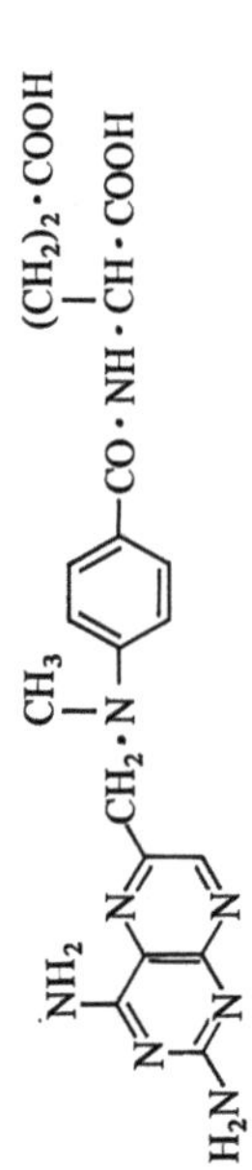

(XXVI)

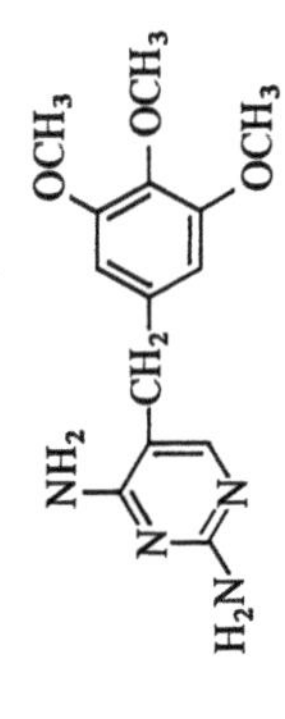

(XXVII)

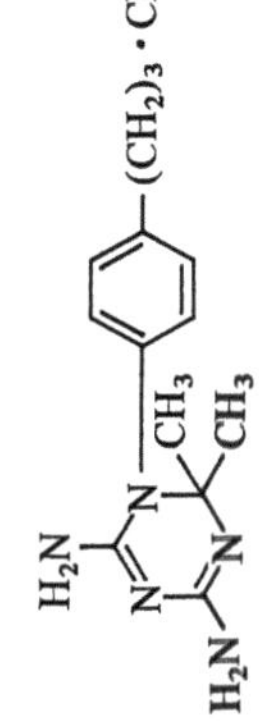

(XXVIII)

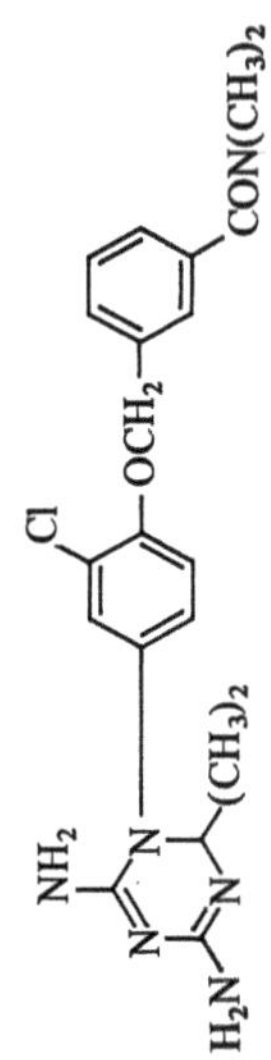

(XXIX)

hydrofolate. Obviously, whether or not a cell has a reserve of reduced folates and its requirement for folate co-enzyme will be important factors in determining whether cytotoxicity will occur. Although methotrexate is the only anti-folate in general use as an anti-cancer agent, it is now realised that the potency of an anti-folate very much depends on the test system used to investigate it. Pyrimethamine (XXVII) for instance, is an anti-folate inhibiting the folate reductases of many different sources. However, the reductase of Proteus vulgaris is 100 000 times more sensitive to inhibition by pyrimethamine than the reductase of rat liver. Conversely, rat liver folate reductase is 100 times more sensitive to p-butylphenyltriazine (XXVIII), a related anti-folate, than the reductase of Proteus vulgaris. Differences in response to anti-folates even occur between mammalian cells. Methotrexate is very active against the L1210 leukaemia but has only slight effects against the Walker carcinoma. On the other hand, a triazine anti-folate (XXIX) is very active against the Walker tumour causing tumour regression at doses as low as 1/100 of the LD_{50} but has no effect on the L1210 leukaemia (SKEEL *et al.*, 1973). In this case the differences are due to drug transport. Only three anti-folates have been shown to be teratogens — aminopterin, methotrexate and pyrimethamine — but in view of the possibly large differences in tissue specificity, it may be that compounds judged to be only weak anti-folates by their action on a single transplanted tumour system may turn out to be very powerful and specific teratogens. Many of the teratogenic effects of the anti-folates can be simulated by folic acid deficiency (KALTER and WARKANY, 1959) while their teratogenicity can be reversed by administration of folinic acid (SULLIVAN and TAKACS, 1971).

Amino Acid Antagonists

In contrast to the highly cytotoxic properties of many purine and pyrimidine analogues, the majority of amino acid analogues investigated have proved to be much less toxic, although some have anti-bacterial properties such as p-fluorophenylalanine and others are carcinogenic, e. g. ethionine (SELS, 1970). It is apparently much more difficult for an amino acid antagonist to inhibit protein synthesis, because the activation step which would enable the antagonist to be incorporated into protein, the formation of the transfer RNA-amino acid complex, is much more specific than the corresponding phosphorylation of bases to their active nucleotides.
A few amino acid antagonists have teratogenic activity. *p*-Fluorophenylalanine, for example, causes growth inhibition of chick embryo explants, but this can be reversed by equimolar concentrations of L-phenylalanine (WADDINGTON and PERRY, 1958). Hadacidin (XXX) is a derivative of glycine and probably acts as an antagonist of aspartic acid. It causes defects in rat embryos, but whether this was due to a direct competition with glycine or aspartic acid was not clear since no reversal experiment with the natural amino acids was attempted (CHAUBE and MURPHY, 1963; LEJOUR-JEANTY, 1966). Mimosine (XXXI), an amino acid extracted from plants, is an antagonist of tyrosine and can cause severe weight loss in animals and specific anti-tumour effects at relatively low dose levels (DE WYS and HALL, 1973). In pregnant rats fed mimosine in the diet, there was an increased resorption rate at a level of 0.7% and some fetal deformation associated with uterine perforations (DEWREEDE and WAYMAN, 1970). More cytotoxic are two glutamine antagonists, azaserine (XXXII) and DON (XXXIII). These compounds are structurally similar to glutamine but also contain an alkylating moiety which enables them to inhibit the appropriate enzyme irreversibly by formation of a covalent bond. Unlike many other antagonists where the block is soon reversed by the build-up of precursors immedi-

ately prior to the site of the inhibition, these antagonists are irreversible and very toxic. When added to cells, it can be shown that the inhibition is reversible for a short period but soon becomes irreversible as a result of the inhibitor alkylating the enzyme, probably through a sulphhydryl group of a cysteine residue. The major sites of action of these two glutamine antagonists are on the enzymes which use glutamine in purine biosynthesis and thus in many of their biological properties they resemble purine anti-metabolites. Not surprisingly, they are powerful teratogens in a number of species (CHAUBE and MURPHY, 1968; BLATTNER *et al.*, 1958; DAGG and KARNOFSKY, 1955; MURPHY and KARNOFSKY, 1956; MURPHY, 1960).

$HOOC \cdot CH_2 \cdot N(OH) \cdot CHO$

(XXX)

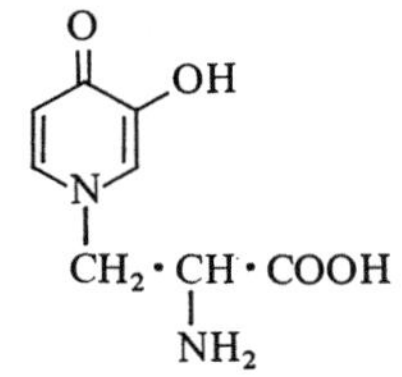

(XXXI)

$\bar{N}{=}\overset{+}{N}{=}CH \cdot COO \cdot CH_2 \cdot CH(NH_2) \cdot COOH$

(XXXII)

$\bar{N}{=}\overset{+}{N}{=}CH \cdot CO \cdot CH_2CH_2CH(NH_2) \cdot COOH$

(XXXIII)

Asparaginase enzymes, isolated from a variety of sources, when injected into animals are confined to the extracellular fluids where they hydrolyse circulating asparagine to aspartic acid. These enzymes are relatively non-toxic provided they are not administered over a long period, but are highly effective against tumour cells which have lost the asparagine synthetase enzyme and thus rely on the extracellular fluid for their supply of this amino acid. Rapidly-growing embryonic tissues may not be able to synthesise sufficient asparagine from aspartic acid to meet all their requirements and may depend on the extracellular fluids to supplement their asparagine. This is probably the reason why asparaginase at relatively low doses (50 I.U./kg) causes a variety of fetal defects in rabbits (ADAMSON *et al.*, 1970). The absence of teratogenicity in rats must imply that all cells can synthesise adequate amounts of asparagine. The enzyme is of a high molecular weight but since it acts by hydrolysing material in extracellular fluids, it does not necessarily need to cross the placenta to produce an asparagine deficient fetal concentration.

Intercalating Agents

A number of compounds are known to form very stable complexes with DNA. These complexes are of a precise structure, but unlike alkylating agent — DNA complexes, they do not involve co-valent linkages since both compounds may be dissociated in unaltered form by modification of the ionic environment. The effect of complexing is to modify the configuration of the DNA double helix and to interfere with its template activity. Agents most efficient in binding to DNA are usually planar molecules containing a number of conjugated aromatic rings. Binding to DNA (which is dependent on an intact helical structure) is by a process of intercalation. The intercalating agent reacts with the double helix (presumably causing it to unwind) and single molecules are inserted between the stacked base pairs. The molecules intercalated in this way are held firmly in position by electronic interaction with the base pairs immediately above and below it. Besides the strict requirement of a double helix and planar structure for calation, the agent must also be of a precise size and small alterations in the structure of intercalating agents can lead to complete loss of activity. An intercalating agent should bind to the DNA of all cells on administration, but selectivity does occur, for example the anti-tumour effects of actinomycin D or the anti-malarial properties of quinacrine. Intercalating agents would be expected to be teratogenic and this has proved to be the case for a number of such compounds (Table 7), although in some cases the day of administration is an important factor (TUCHMANN-DUPLESSIS and MERCIER-PAROT, 1960) and in others no congenital effects have been obtained even with high doses (CHAUBE and MURPHY, 1968). In the case of quinacrine, this failure to cause fetal malformation may be due to poor penetration since it has been reported that rats receiving quinacrine by subcutaneous injection of 122 mg/kg accumulated 549 μg in maternal liver but only 9 μg in fetal liver (ROTHSCHILD and LEVY, 1950).

Daunomycin and adriamycin are effective agents in the treatment of certain forms of cancer, but are rapidly excreted and have severe side effects, especially on bone marrow and cardiac muscle. In attempts to overcome these side effects, the compounds have been administered as complexes with fragments of DNA. In this form the intercalating agent is non-toxic but can be released from the macromolecule in unchanged form by the action of DNA-ase. DNA-daunomycin complexes are more selective anti-tumour agents than daunomycin alone (TROUET *et al.*, 1972) probably because the high molecular weight complex is selectively endocytosed by tumour cells. Once ingested, the complex is incorporated into a lysosome, where it is broken down by the action of DNA-ase. This releases daunomycin in unchanged form and this can diffuse to the nucleus and intercalate nuclear DNA. Complexes of this sort have not yet been tested for their teratogenicity but they may well have a quite different spectrum of action compared with the intercalating agents themselves.

Spindle Poisons

A number of organic materials of natural origin have the ability to inhibit growth by arresting cells at mitosis. At low dose levels, all these compounds inhibit cells in metaphase by interfering with the formation of the mitotic spindle apparatus. Collectively they are referred to as the spindle poisons and at least four have been shown to be teratogenic (Table 8). Although they all act by similar pathways, there are differences in their biological properties. Podophyllotoxin and colchicine have only marginal anti-tumour activity while the vinca alkaloids are routinely used in the clinic in the treatment of certain forms of cancer. Furthermore, while two of the vinca alkaloids, vinblastine and vincristine are closely related in chemical structure, they differ in some biological properties, the dose-limiting toxicity of the former, for instance, being bone marrow toxicity and of the latter, neural toxicity. It is of interest in this respect that vinblastine causes neural toxicity in the embryo. It is believed that all spindle poisons act basically in the same manner by condensing with microtubular protein and preventing the formation of essential cell structures. Cells are arrested in mitosis because the fan-shaped structure of the mitotic apparatus which requires microtubular proteins does not form properly in the presence of spindle poisons. Microtubular proteins form the basis of many intracellular organelles and in order to explain this highly selective effect on the spindles, it is claimed that the permeability of cells to these agents increases just prior to mitosis. If dividing cells of different organs had different permeabilities for the spindle poisons, this would for instance explain the different toxicity of, for example, vincristine and vinblastine. That embryotoxicity is also due to metaphase arrest is indicated by the finding that the embryos of pregnant rats and hamsters treated with the vinca alkaloids show an increase in the number of mitotic figures (FERM, 1963; COHLAN and KITAY, 1965).

Miscellaneous Agents

A number of other agents with cytotoxic properties are teratogenic in laboratory animals. These include hydroxyurea and urethane which have both been used in the treatment of cancer and which act by inhibition of nucleic acid synthesis, the former by preventing reduction of ribonucleotides and the latter by reacting directly with nucleic acid bases. Procarbazine (natulan) probably breaks down *in vivo* to a number of products which can combine co-valently with DNA. Formaldehyde is mutagenic as well as causing slight effects in embryos and probably acts by reacting with the amino groups of the purines of nucleic acids. Caffeine is a known inhibitor of DNA repair and its teratogenicity may possibly reflect natural damage to DNA which would normally be repaired by enzymatic pathways known to exist in cells.

References

ADAMS, C. E., HAY, M. F., LUTWAK-MANN, C.: The action of various agents upon the rabbit embryo. J. Embryol. exp. Morph. **9,** 468 (1961).

ADAMSON, R. H., FABRO, S., HAHN, M. A., CREECH, C. E., WHANGPENG, J.: Evaluation of the embryotoxic activity of L-asparaginase. Arch. int. Pharmacodyn. Ther. **186,** 310 (1970).

ALEXANDROV, V. A., JANISCH, W.: Die teratogene Wirkung von Äthylharnstoff und Nitrit bei Ratten. Experientia (Basel) **27,** 538 (1970).

ANCEL, P.: Recherche experimentale sur le spina bifida. Arch. Anat. micr. Morph. exp. **36,** 45 (1946).

ARMSTRONG, J. G., DYKE, R. W., FONTS, P. J.: Vinblastine sulfate treatment of Hodgkin's disease during pregnancy. Science **143,** 703 (1964).

BARANOV, V. S.: Mechanism of aminopterin pathogenic effect upon embryogenesis in the albino rat. Arch. Anat. **51,** 17 (1966).

BERRY, C. L.: Transient inhibition of DNA synthesis by methotrexate in the rat embryo and fetus. J. Embryol. exp. Morph. **26,** 469 (1971).

BLATTNER, R. J., WILLIAMSON, A. P., SIMONSEN, L.: Teratogenic changes in early chick embryos following administration of anti-tumor agent (azaserine). Proc. Soc. exp. Biol. (N.Y.) **97,** 560 (1958).

BRO-RASMUSSEN, F., JENSEN, B., HANSEN, O. M., OSTERGAARD, A. H.: Fluorodeoxyuridine-induced malformations in mice. Studies of early embryogenesis. Acta path. microbiol. scand. (A) **79**, 55 (1971).

CHAUBE, S., KURY, G., MURPHY, M. L.: Teratogenic effects of cyclophosphamide (NCA 26271) in the rat. Cancer Chemother. Rep. **51**, 363 (1967).

CHAUBE, S., MURPHY, M. L.: Teratogenic effect of Hadacidin (a new growth inhibitory chemical) on the rat fetus. J. exp. Zool. **152**, 67 (1963).

CHAUBE, S., MURPHY, M. L.: Teratogenic effects of 5-chlorodeoxyuridine on the rat fetus: protection by physiological pyrimidines. Cancer Res. **24**, 1986 (1964).

CHAUBE, S., MURPHY, M. L.: Teratogenic effects of cytosine arabinoside (CA) in the rat fetus. Proc. Amer. Ass. Cancer Res. **6**, 11 (1965).

CHAUBE, S., MURPHY, M. L.: The effects of hydroxyurea and related compounds on rat fetus. Cancer Res. **26**, 1448 (1966).

CHAUBE, S., MURPHY, M. L.: The teratogenic effects of the recent drugs active in cancer chemotherapy. Advanc. Teratology **3**, 181 (1968).

CHAUBE, S., MURPHY, M. L.: The teratogenic effects of 5-fluorocytosine in the rat. Cancer Res. **29**, 554 (1969).

COHEN, S. S., BARNER, H. D.: Studies on unbalanced growth in Escherichia coli. Proc. Nat. Acad. Sci. (Wash.) **40**, 885 (1954).

COHLAN, S. Q., KITAY, D.: The teratogenic action of vincaleukoblastine in the pregnant rat. J. Pediat. **66**, 541 (1965).

CONNORS, T. A.: 'Mechanism of action of 2-chloroethylamine derivatives, sulfur mustard, epoxides and aziridines' *in* 'Antineoplastic and Immunosuppressive Agents. Part II.' Handb. Exp. Pharm. XXXVIII. SARTORELLI, A. C. and JOHNS, D. G. Eds. Berlin, Heidelberg, New York: Springer 1975.

CONNORS, T. A., COX, P. J., FARMER, P. B., FOSTER, A. B., JARMAN, M.: Some studies of the active intermediates formed in the microsomal metabolism of cyclophosphamide and iposphamide. Biochem. Pharmacol. **23**, 115 (1974).

CURRIE, A. R., BIRD, C. C., CRAWFORD, A. M., SIMS, P.: Embryopathic effects of 7,12-dimethylbenz (A) anthracene and its hydroxymethyl derivatives in the Sprague Dawley rat. Nature (Lond.) **226**, 911 (1970).

DAGG, C. P.: Sensitive stages for the production of developmental abnormalities in mice with 5-fluorouracil. Amer. J. Anat. **106**, 89 (1960).

DAGG, C. P., KARNOFSKY, D. A.: Teratogenic effects of azaserine on the chick embryo. J. exp. Zool. **130**, 555 (1955).

DEGENHARDT, K. H., FRANZ, J., YAMAMURA, H.: A model in comparative teratogenesis. Dose responses to 5-fluoro-2-deoxycytidine in organogenesis of mouse strains. Teratology **1**, 311 (1968).

DEWREEDE, S., WAYMAN, O.: Effect of mimosine on the rat fetus. Teratology **3**, 21 (1970).

DE WYS, W. D., HALL, T. C.: Anti-tumor effect of the amino acid mimosine. Europ. J. Cancer **9**, 281 (1973).

DIAMOND, I., ANDERSON, M. M., MCCREADIE, S. P.: Transplacental transmission of busulfan (myleran) in a mother with leukaemia. Production of fetal transformation and cytomegaly. Pediatrics **25**, 85 (1960).

DIPAOLO, J. A.: Polydactylism in the offspring of mice injected with 5-bromodeoxyuridine. Science **145**, 501 (1964).

DRUCKREY, H.: 'Chemical structure and action in transplacental carcinogenesis and teratogenesis' *in* Transplacental carcinogenesis. Ed. L. TOMATIS and U. MOHR, IACR Scientific Publications No. 4, Lyon, pp. 45—58 (1973).

DRUCKREY, H., IVANKOVIC, S., PREUSSMANN, R.: Teratogenic and carcinogenic effects in the offspring after a single injection of ethylnitrosourea to pregnant rats. Nature (Lond.) **210**, 1378 (1966).

DRUCKREY, H., IVANKOVIC, S., PREUSSMANN, R., LANDSCHUTZ, C., STEKAR, J., BRUNNER, U., SCHAGEN, B.: Transplacental induction of neurogenic malignomas by 1,2-diethyl-hydrazine and azoxyethane in rats. Experientia (Basel) **24**, 561 (1968).

DYBAN, A. P., AKIMOVA, I. M.: Some pecularities of embryogenesis. Disturbances caused by blockade of RNA synthesis in mammals. Experiments with actinomycin D in rats. Arch. Anat. **52,** 36 (1967).

ELIS, J., DIPAOLO, J. A.: Aflatoxin B1. Induction of malformations. Arch. Path. **83,** 53 (1967).

FELDMAN, M., WADDINGTON, C. H.: The uptake of methionine S(35) by the chick embryo and its inhibition by ethionine. J. Embryol. exp. Morph. **3,** 44 (1955).

FERM, V. H.: Congenital malformations in hamster embryos after treatment with vinblastine and vincristine. Science **141,** 426 (1963).

FISCHER, D. S., JONES, A. M.: Cerebellar hypoplasia resulting from cytosine arabinoside treatment in the neonatal hamster. Clin. Res. **13,** 540 (1965).

GAINES, T. B., KIMBROUGH, R. D.: The sterilising carcinogenic and teratogenic effects of MeTepa on rats. Bull. W.H.O. **34,** 317 (1966).

GARNER, C.: Moulds, bacteria and cancer. New Scientist **63,** 325 (1974).

GREEN, C. R., CHRISTIE, G. S.: Malformations on foetal rats induced by the pyrrolizidine alkaloid heliotrine. Brit. J. exp. Path. **42,** 369 (1961).

GREENBERG, L. H., TANAKA, K. R.: Congenital abnormalities probably induced by cyclophosphamide. J. Amer. med. Ass. **188,** 423 (1964).

HALL, E. K.: Developmental anomalies in the eye of the rat after various experimental procedures. Anat. Rec. **116,** 383 (1953).

HART, C. W., NAUNTON, R. F.: The ototoxicity of chloroquine phosphate. Arch. Otolaryngol. **80,** 407 (1964).

IZUMI, T.: Developmental anomalies in offspring of mice induced by administration of 2-acetylaminofluorene during pregnancy. Acta anat. Nippon **37,** 239 (1966).

JULOU, L., DUCROT, R., FOURNEL, J., GANTER, P., MARAL, R., POPULAIRE, P., KOENIG, F., MYON, J., PASCAL, S., PASQUET, J.: Un novel antibiotique doue d'activité anti-tumorale. Arzneimittel-Forsch. **17,** 948 (1967).

JURAND, A.: Further investigation on the cytotoxic and morphogenetic effects of some nitrogen mustard derivatives. J. Embryol. exp. Morph. **9,** 492 (1961).

KAGEYAMA, M., NISHIMURA, H.: Developmental anomalies in mouse embryos induced by triethylene melamine (T.E.M.). Acta Med. Univ. Kyoto **37,** 318 (1961).

KALTER, H.: Teratology of the central nervous system. Chicago: University of Chicago Press, pp. 139—140 (1968).

KALTER, H., WARKANY, J.: Experimental production of congenital malformations in mammals by metabolic procedures. Physiol. Rev. **39,** 69 (1959).

KARNOFSKY, D. A.: Influences of antimetabolites inhibiting nucleic acid metabolism on embryonic development. Trans. Ass. Amer. Phycns **73,** 334 (1960).

KARNOFSKY, D. A., LACON, C. R.: The effects of 1-β-D-arabinofuranosylcytosine on the developing chick embryo. Biochem. Pharmacol. **15,** 1435 (1966).

KIM, J. H., EIDINOFF, M. L.: Action of 1-β-D-arabinofuranosylcytosine on the nucleic acid metabolism and viability of HeLa cells. Cancer Res. **25,** 698 (1965).

KLEIN, M. F., BEALL, J. R.: Griseofulvin: a teratogenic study. Science **115,** 1483 (1972).

KOSMACHEVSKAYA, E. A.: Comparison of pathogenic activity of 5- and 6-azauracil. Arch. Anat. **3,** 85 (1968).

KOYAMA, T., HANDA, J., HANDA, H., MATSUMOTO, S.: Methylnitrosourea-induced malformations of brain in SD-JCL rat. Arch. Neurol. (Chic.) **22,** 342 (1970).

KURY, G., CROSBY, R. J.: The teratogenic effect of 5-trifluoromethyl-2-deoxyuridine in chicken embryos. Toxicol. appl. Pharmacol. **11,** 72 (1967).

LEJOUR-JEANTY, M.: Becs-de-lievre provoques chez le rat par un derive de penicilline, l'hadacidine. J. Embryol. exp. Morph. **15,** 193 (1966).

MELTZER, H. J.: Congenital anomalies due to attempted abortion with 4-aminopteroylglutamic acid. J. Amer. med. Ass. **161,** 1253 (1956).

MILLER, E. C., MILLER, J. A.: Studies on the mechanism of activation of aromatic amine and amide carcinogens to ultimate carcinogenic electrophilic reactants. Ann. N.Y. Acad. Sci. **163,** 731—750 (1969).

MILUNSKY, A., GRAEF, J. W., GAYNOR, M. F.: Methotrexate induced congenital malformations with a review of the literature. J. Pediat. **72,** 790 (1968).

Monie, I. W.: Chlorambucil-induced abnormalities of the urogenital system of rat fetuses. Anat. Rec. **139**, 145 (1961).

Morris, J. M., van Wagenen, G., Hurteau, G. D., Johnstone, D. W., Carlsen, R. A.: Compounds interfering with ovum implantation and development. Fertility, Sterility **18**, 7 (1967).

Muller, M.: Does nitrogen mustard affect the foetus directly or secondarily by its effect on the mother? Experientia (Basel) **22**, 247 (1966).

Murphy, M. L.: Teratogenic effects of tumor inhibitory chemicals in the rat in Wolstenholme, G. E. W. and O'Connor, C. M. (eds.). A CIBA Foundation Symposium on Congenital Malformations. London: J. and A. Churchill Ltd., pp. 92—95, 1960.

Murphy, M. L., Chaube, S.: Teratogenic effects of abnormal purines and their ribosides in the rat. Proc. Amer. Ass. Cancer Res. **3**, 347 (1962).

Murphy, M. L., Chaube, S.: Hydroxyurea (NSC 32065) as a teratogen. Cancer Chemother. Rep. **40**, 1 (1964).

Murphy, M. L., Dagg, C. P., Karnofsky, D. A.: Comparison of teratogenic chemicals in the rat and chick embryos. Pediatrics **19**, 701 (1957).

Murphy, M. L., Karnofsky, D. A.: Effect of azaserine and other growth inhibiting agents on fetal development of the rat. Cancer **9**, 955 (1956).

Murphy, M. L., Moro, A. D., Lacon, C. R.: The comparative effects of five polyfunctional alkylating agents with additional notes on the chick embryo. Ann. N.Y. Acad. Sci. **68**, 762 (1958).

Nishimura, H., Kuginuki, M.: Congenital malformations induced by ethyl-urethane in mouse embryos. Okajimas Folia anat. jap. **31**, 1 (1958).

Nishimura, H., Nakai, K.: Congenital malformations in offspring treated with caffeine. Proc. Soc. exp. Biol. (N.Y.) **104**, 140 (1960).

Pierro, L. J.: Teratogenic action of actinomycin D in the embryonic chick. J. exp. Zool. **147**, 203 (1961).

Proffit, W. R., Edwards, L. E.: Effects of ethionine administration during pregnancy in the rat. J. exp. Zool. **150**, 135 (1962).

Puchkov, V. F.: Teratogenic action of aminopterin and 5-fluorouracil on 4 to 23 somite chick embryos after application in ovo. Bull. exp. Biol. Med. **7**, 99 (1967).

Pushkina, N. N., Gofmekler, V. A., Klertsova, G. N.: Changes in content of ascorbic acid and nucleic acids produced by benzene and formaldehyde. Bull. exp. Biol. Med. **66**, 868 (1968).

Reynolds, E. S.: Liver parenchymal cell injury IV. J. Pharmacol. exp. Ther. **155**, 117 (1967).

Rigdon, R. H., Rennels, E. G.: Effect of feeding benz(a)pyrene on reproduction in the rat. Experientia (Basel) **20**, 224 (1964).

Ross, W. C. J.: Biological Alkylating Agents. London: Butterworths, 1962.

Rothschild, B., Levy, G.: Action de la quinacrine sur la gestation chez le rat. C. R. Soc. Biol. (Paris) **144**, 1350 (1950).

Roux, C., Taillemite, J. L.: Action teratogene de la rubidomycine chez le rat. C. R. Soc. Biol. (Paris) **163**, 1299 (1969).

Ruffolo, P. R., Ferm, V. H.: The embryocidal and teratogenic effects of 5-bromodeoxyuridine in the pregnant hamster. Lab. Invest. **14**, 1547 (1965).

Sanders, M. A., Wiesner, B. P., Yudkin, J.: Control of fertility by 6-azauridine. Nature (Lond.) **189**, 1015 (1961).

Savkur, L. D., Batra, B. K., Sridharan, B. N.: Effect of 20-methylcholanthrene on mouse embryos. J. Reprod. Fertil. **2**, 374 (1961).

Scott, W. J., Ritter, E. J., Wilson, J. G.: DNA synthesis inhibition and cell death associated with hydroxyurea teratogenesis in rat embryos. Dev. Biol. **26**, 306 (1971).

Sels, A.: 'Analogues of Amino Acids' in 'Fundamentals of Biochemical Pharmacology'. Z. M. Bacq, ed. Oxford and New York: Pergamon Press, pp. 505—514, 1970.

Shotton, D., Monie, I. W.: Possible teratogenic effect of chlorambucil on a human fetus. J. Amer. med. Ass. **186**, 74 (1963).

Sinclair, J. G.: A specific transplacental effect of urethane in mice. Tex. Rep. Biol. Med. **8**, 623 (1950).

Skeel, R. T., Sawicki, W. L., Cashmore, A. R., Bertino, J. R.: The basis for the disparate sensitivity of L1210 leukaemia and Walker 256 carcinoma to a new triazine folate antagonist. Cancer Res. **33**, 2972 (1973).

Smith, D. W.: Dysmorphology (Teratology). J. Pediat. **69**, 1150 (1966).

Sokal, J. E., Lessmann, E. M.: Effects of cancer chemotherapeutic agents on the human fetus. J. Amer. med. Ass. **172**, 1765 (1960).

Soukup, S., Takacs, E., Warkany, J.: Chromosome changes in embryos treated with various teratogens. J. Embryol. exp. Morph. **18**, 215 (1967).

Spatz, M., Dougherty, W. J., Smith, D. W. E.: Teratogenic effects of methylazoxymethanol. Proc. Soc. exp. Biol. (N.Y.) **124**, 467 (1967).

Stanzheuskaya, T. L.: Effect of chloridin on chick embryogenesis. Bull. exp. Biol. Med. **61**, 427 (1966).

Sugiyama, T., Nishimura, H., Fukui, K.: Abnormalities in mouse embryos induced by several aminoazobenzene derivatives. Okajimas Folia anat. jap. **36**, 195 (1960).

Sullivan, G. E., Takacs, E.: Comparative teratogenicity of pyrimethamine in rats and hamsters. Teratology **4**, 205 (1971).

Takaori, S., Tanabe, K., Shimamoto, K.: Developmental abnormalities of skeletal system induced by ethylurethan in the rat. Jap. J. Pharmacol. **16**, 63 (1966).

Takaya, M.: Teratogenic effects of the anti-tumour anti-biotics. Proceedings of the Congenital Abnormalities Research Association of Japan **3**, 47 (1963).

Tanimura, T.: Relationship of dosage and time of administration to teratogenic effects of thiotepa in mice. Sonderabdruck Okajimas Folia Anatomica Japonica **44**, 203 (1968).

Tanimura, T.: Effects of mitomycin C administered at various stages of pregnancy upon mouse fetuses. Okajimas Folia anat. jap. **44**, 337 (1968 b).

Tattersall, M. H. N., Ganeshaguru, K., Hoffbrand, A. V.: The mechanisms of action of three fluorine substituted cytosine analogues. Implications for Cancer Chemotherapy. Biochem. Pharmacol. **23**, 2533 (1974).

Thiersch, J. B.: The effect of substituted 2,4-diamino pyrimidines on the rat fetus in utero. Proc. Int. Cong. on Chemotherapy **3**, 367 (1954).

Thiersch, J. B.: Effect of 2,4,6-Triamin-S-Triazin (TR), 2,4,6-Tris(ethyleneimino)-S-triazine (TEM) and N,N,N,-Triethyleneiminophosphoramide (TEPA) on rat litter in utero. Proc. Soc. exp. Biol. (N.Y.) **94**, 36 (1957).

Thiersch, J. B.: Effect of 2,6-diaminopurine (2,6-DP), 6-chloropurine (CLP) and thioguanine (THG) on rat litter in utero. Proc. Soc. exp. Biol. (N.Y.) **94**, 40 (1957 b).

Thiersch, J. B.: Effect of podophyllin and podophyllotoxin on the rat litter in utero. Proc. Soc. exp. Biol. (N.Y.) **113**, 124 (1963).

Thiersch, J. B., Phillips, F. S.: Effect of 4-aminopteroylglutamic acid (aminopterin) on early pregnancy. Proc. Soc. exp. Biol. (N.Y.) **74**, 204 (1950).

Tomatis, L., Turosov, V., Guibbert, D., Duperray, B., Malaveille, C., Pachelo, H.: Transplacental carcinogenic effect of 3-methylcholanthrene in mice and its quantitation in fetal tissues. J. nat. Cancer Inst. **47**, 645 (1971).

Trouet, A., Deprez de Campeneere, D., de Duve, C.: Chemotherapy through lysosomes with a DNA-daunorubicin complex. Nature (Lond.) New Biol. **239**, 110 (1972).

Tuchmann-Duplessis, H., Mercier-Parot, L.: The teratogenic action of the anti-biotic actinomycin D in Wolstenholme, G. E. W. and O'Connor, C. M. Eds. CIBA Foundation Symposium on Congenital Malformations. Boston: Little Brown and Co. 1960. pp. 115—128.

Tuchmann-Duplessis, H., Mercier-Parot, L.: Sur l'action abortive et teratogene de la 6-chloropurine. C. R. Soc. Biol. (Paris) **153**, 1133 (1959).

Tuchmann-Duplessis, H., Mercier-Parot, L.: Production chez le rat de malformations oculaires et squalettiques par administration d'un methyl hydrazine. C. R. Soc. Biol. (Paris) **161**, 2127 (1967).

Tuchmann-Duplessis, H., Mercier-Parot, L.: Foetopathes therapeutiques. Production experimentale de malformations des membres. Union Med. Can. **97**, 283 (1968).

Udalova, L. D.: The effect of chloroquine on the embryonal development of rats. Pharmacol. Toxicol. **2**, 226 (1967).

VAN WAGENEN, G., DECONTI, R. C., HANDSCHUMACHER, R. E., WADE, M. E.: Abortifacient and teratogenic effects of triacetyl-6-azauridine in the monkey. Amer. J. Obstet. Gynec. **108**, 272 (1970).

VOJTA, M., JIRASEK, J.: 6-Azauridine induced changes of the trophoblast in early human pregnancy. Clin. Pharmacol. Ther. **7**, 162 (1966).

WADDINGTON, C. H., PERRY, M. M.: Effects of some amino acid and purine antagonists on chick embryos. J. Embryol. exp. Morph. **6**, 365 (1958).

WIESNER, B. P., YUDKIN, J.: Control of fertility by anti-mitotic agents. Nature (Lond.) **176**, 249 (1955).

WILSON, J. G.: Influence on the offspring of altered physiologic states during pregnancy in the rat. Ann. N.Y. Acad. Sci. **57**, 517 (1954).

WILSON, J. G.: Effects of acute and chronic treatment with actinomycin D on pregnancy and the fetus in the rat. Harper Hospital Bulletin **24**, 109 (1966).

WUNDERLICH, V., TETZLAFF, J.: Alkylierung der Kern-DNS verschiedener Organe der Ratte durch Nitrosomethylharnstoff in vivo. Arch. Geschwulstforsch. **35**, 251 (1970).

Problems of Predictive Teratology

The chapters in this section describe current approaches to the development of a structured teratological programme for screening environmental hazards of small or large effect, at widely different stages of development. The problems of interpretation of the results of this type of study are often underemphasised. The shortcomings of existing methods are described and suggestions for more suitable statistical techniques are made.

Man is constantly exposed to chemical agents which may be teratogenic, including drugs, food additives, cosmetics and pesticides. Extensive reproductive and teratological studies have been introduced to screen these agents, but there is considerable doubt, in scientific circles, about their effectiveness. Perhaps the greatest difficulty in designing appropriate tests is the lack of knowledge of the fundamental mechanism of the vast majority of malformations. If these were known, the choice of species, drug administration procedures and interpretation of results would be easier.

In recent years its has been suggested that structured tests should be used in teratological testing. For example, Wilson and Layton have both suggested that the information obtained from pharmacological and toxicological tests, including details of metabolic pathways and pharmacokinetics, should be combined with knowledge of animal physiology and pharmacology in determining the choice of test animals. The results of particular tests should then be interpreted in order to determine the next step. From discussions with industrial toxicologists it is apparent that this pragmatic approach is often followed; what is lacking in this method is a scientific basis for predictive teratology.

References

LAYTON, W. B.: Congenital defects, new directions in research. JANERICH, D. J., SKALKO, R. G., and PORTER, I. H., Eds. New York and London: Academic Press, Inc. 1974.

WILSON, J. G.: Environment and birth defects. New York and London: Academic Press 1973.

5. Polygenic Models in Teratological Testing

C. L. Berry and J. P. Germain

With 7 Figures

Most of the malformations that occur in man develop as a result of the combined effects of many genes; these provide a background of predisposition to a particular defect against which environmental agents exert their influence. This concept, often referred to as polygenic or multifactorial inheritance, has been described in detail by Carter (1965, 1969) and modified by Falconer (1967) and Edwards (1969).
In its simplest form the hypothesis requires that the genetic predisposition to a particular malformation is distributed Normally in a population, and that at some point a "threshold" of predisposition exists above which there is a risk of malformation. The position of the threshold may be shifted by environmental factors, and the whole Normal curve representing genetic predisposition may be moved up or down the x axis by factors such as closeness of relationship. Malformations determined in this way have well defined characteristics; the abnormality is common, there are familial aggregates, the recurrence rate in siblings is 1—5%, in twin studies the recurrence rate in non-identical pairs is that of siblings (1—5%), but in identical twins it is between 20 and 50%. Evidence for the influence of non-genetic factors is seen in the effects of parental age, socio-economic class, birth rank, variation in seasonal incidence and geographical variation. Such characteristics have been found in epidemiological studies of malformations of the central nervous system, cardiovascular system and musculoskeletal tissues in man (Carter, 1970; Woolf, 1971) which collectively form the bulk of major abnormalities. As Leck (1972) has pointed out, in a population in which the predisposition to any malformation is Normally distributed the mean would only have to be reduced slightly, by tackling one factor in this predisposition, to cause a valuable decline in incidence. How may one discover the factors which are susceptible to modification? Epidemiological studies have yielded most of the valuable information obtained in studies of human malformation to date but, by their nature, tend to stop short of identification of specific factors in the diet, water supply, or social background of a group. Additional applied studies are necessary to establish causal connections and mechanisms.

Possible Testing Systems

The search for alternative testing systems in animals is always complicated by the difficulty of interpretation of results, with possible "transfer of the argument" between species.

This problem arises from a fundamental lack of knowledge of the pathogenesis of most malformations. The reasoned view of the World Health Authority (W.H.O., 1967) concerning animal testing programmes is that "there is no absolute assurance that negative results obtained by testing drugs in these species can be used to predict that an agent will lack teratogenic effects in man". It seems unlikely that a single, directly transferable testing system of general application will be devised. Specific problems may have specific solutions, which focus our attention on areas in which further study in man is indicated. Such models exist in, for example, the work of POSWILLO (1973) on the genesis of first arch anomalies. Perhaps the best example of this type is that of FRASER, TRASLER and their colleagues on cleft lip in the mouse (FRASER, 1971 for review). In considering the genesis of this malformation it should be remembered that the palatal shelves must meet above the tongue before the lateral growth of the face has carried them too far appart to reach each other. TRASLER (1968) examined the effects of aspirin on the expression of cleft lip in A/J and C57BL mice. She found that face shape differed markedly in the two groups, and that this influenced the frequency of the defect. FRASER and PASHAYAN (1970) explored the hypothesis further. If face shape is at least in part genetically determined, and if it is indeed related to the predisposition to cleft lip, it follows that the parents of children with congenital cleft lip should have faces that are, on the average, of a different shape to those of the general population. They found that the parents of individuals with cleft lip with or without cleft palate had less prominent maxillae than controls, and that in general there were more rectangular and trapezoid face shapes and fewer ovoid, than in controls. Broad flat faces would seem to predispose to cleft lip, and FRASER and PASHAYAN pointed out that the Japanese have a relatively high incidence of this defect.

If studies of this type are to be employed in the search for environmental teratogens it is possible to describe an ideal system. It would involve a defect, readily recognised, the expression of which is affected by several genes and by environmental factors. It should show threshold characteristics, offer the possibility for agents under test to interfere with the principle components of embryogenesis (growth, differentiation and morphogenesis) and have metric characteristics so that sub-threshold effects could be recognised.

Relevant Previous Work

The examination of large numbers of animals to comply with current testing regulations has led to the accumulation of a great deal of normal data on the frequency of malformations (GIBSON *et al.*, 1966; PALMER, 1968, 1972). PALMER has pointed out that in most teratological testing programmes low rates of malformations are the rule and it is often difficult to decide whether they are related to treatment or not. He divides spontaneous anomalies into four main classes, examples of which are given below:

1. *Common variations.* Supernumary ribs at the thoraco-lumbar border, variations in sternebral ossification etc., in rodents.

2. *Minor skeletal anomalies.* In rabbits — Bipartate sternebrae, reduced skull ossification, unossified odontoid phalanges or astragali. In mice — retarded ossification at various sites. In rats — Similar changes and the presence of vertebral and rib anomalies.
3. *Minor visceral anomalies.* Lung and gall bladder anomalies (rabbit) rotation of the heart (rat) anterior displacement of the gonads (rat and mouse).
4. *Major malformations.*

From an examination of tens thousands of animals, he finds that the incidence of anomalies in categories 2, 3 and 4 are as shown in Table 1.

Table 1. Incidence of spontaneous malformations in laboratory animals (%) (PALMER, 1972)

	Rabbits	Rats	Mice
No. of foetuses examined	36,508	51,349	22,389
Minor skeletal anomalies	8.60	2.35	5.32
Minor visceral anomalies	2.53	2.02	3.68
Major malformations	0.74	0.41	0.84

Table 2. Aspirin and extra ribs (CD rat)

Dosage (mg/kg b. wt/day)	Percentage of pups with extra ribs
0	10
150	58
300	98

The incidence of common variations may differ widely and for this reason they are often ignored in teratological studies. Their frequency may be affected by teratogens, as PALMER himself has shown (Table 2), and it is our contention that such anomalies may be excellent testing systems in which to look for agents of small effect.

What possible variations of this kind exist in animals? There have been a number of genetic studies over a period of time which have established both polygenic determination and the influence of the environment in particular defects. The studies of WRIGHT (1934 a, b) on polydactyly in guinea pigs were perhaps the first to demonstrate polygenic inheritance in animals. Since that time many papers have described other systems, and a few examples will be given. In 1954, SEARLE (1954 a) described the variations in twenty skeletal characteristics in pure line mice and found that "residual intangible non-genetic factors" accounted for 80% of the variance in three-quarters of the characters studied. In a further paper, published in the same year SEARLE (1954 b) showed that in the variation within pure lines most of the non-genetic variation was due to "intangible factors" acting independently on individuals. There was evidence of a maternal effect in some variations, revealed by trends with maternal age, parity, litter size, or length of gestation. Correlations were also found between litter mates for a particular character, due to factors acting on the litter as a whole.

Further studies by McLAREN and MICHIE (1958) demonstrated that uterine environment influenced sacralisation of the lumbar vertebrae in mice, an effect that was not related to birth weight. They suggested that specific deficiencies might be responsible for the changes found since, at the stage at which the eventual morphology was determined the total fetal demand was insufficient to account for a general deficiency producing growth inhibition. Later GREEN (1962) demonstrated that within inbred stains of mice, the differences in skeletal variation were almost exclusively non-genetic although differences from strain to strain were genetic. The underlying distribution which represented the combinations of genetic and non-genetic factors that affect the number of presacral vertebrae might be regarded as Normal or nearly Normal in form. Changes in the environment of developing mice might be expected to change the relative percentage of the various numbers of presacral vertebrae, but not to bring about an abrupt conversion of the treated mice to a new number of presacral vertebrae.

In a number of papers, polygenic inheritance has been considered to be the basis of variability of response to particular teratogens with variable genetic and environmental contributions. DAGG (1963, 1966) has demonstrated that polydactyly in mice induced by 5-fluorouracil is controlled by a minimum of four genes, and that 80% of the response is genetically determined. More recently YASUDA and MAEDA (1972) have demonstrated that there is a dose-related increase in the incidence of lumbar ribs in rats after exposure to a herbicide and a tetracycline derivative. Vitamin A in massive doses had a similar effect. KIMMEL and WILSON (1973) found changes in the frequency of supernumerary ribs after sodium salicylate.

These examples indicate that minor variations are often polygenically determined and may be susceptible to the effects of environmental agents and various drugs. We shall now discuss the use of a specific variation, absence of the third molar tooth in the mouse, as a screening system.

Absence of the Mouse Third Molar

The normal mouse dentition consists of an incisor and three molars in each quadrant which develop and erupt in sequence from anterior to posterior. The various stages of development are shown diagrammatically in Fig. 1 a—c. The changes occur between day 1 and day 18 for the mouse third molar i. e., they are entirely post-natal. Initially undifferentiated mesenchyme condenses at specific sites under the dental lamina, associated with collections of capillaries. The dental lamina thickens, and the resultant epithelial-mesodermal complex is known as the "bud" stage (Fig. 1 a). The epithelium proliferates and the mesoderm is partly surrounded by it, producing a dental cap (Fig. 1 b). The epithelial cells differentiate to form an inner and outer dental epithelium separated by the stellate reticulum. The inner layer of cells (pre-ameloblasts) invaginates to make a bell like structure enclosing the dental papilla, within which the odontoblasts and pulp of the tooth develop. Subsequent stages will not be con-

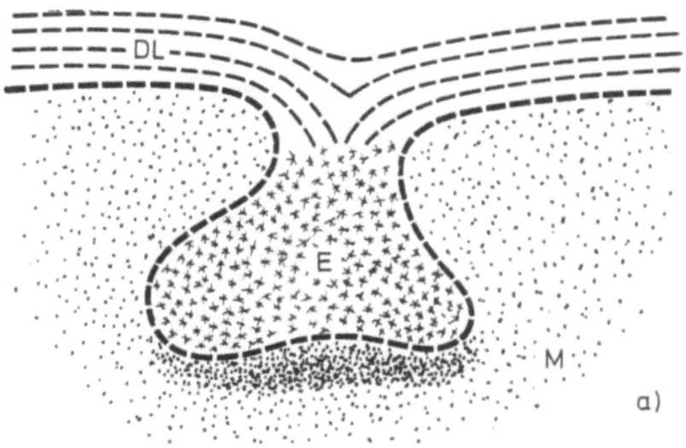

Fig. 1. (a) *Bud stage*. A thickening of the epithelium is seen at the site of mesodermal condensation. (b) *Cap stage*. Epithelial proliferation surrounds the area of mesodermal condensation. (c) *Bell stage*. The epithelial cells have differentiated to form an inner and outer dental epithelium, separated by the stellate reticulum. *Key:* DL. Dental lamina, E. Epithelial proliferation, M. Mesoderm, IDE. Inner dental epithelium, SR. Stellate reticulum

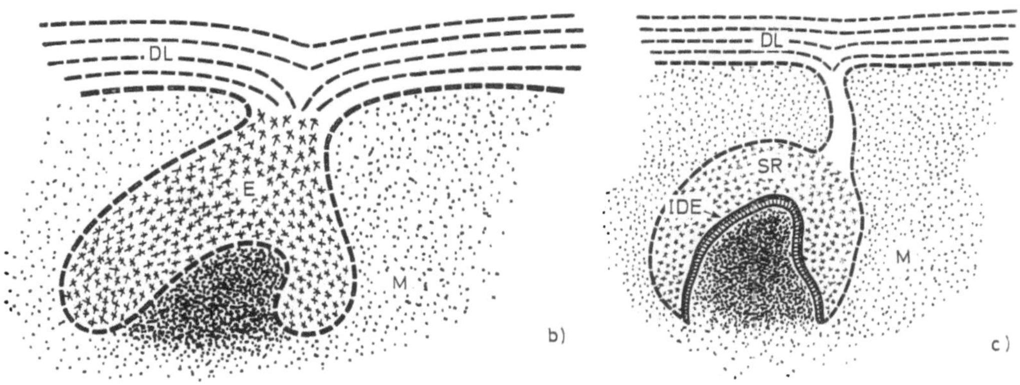

sidered in detail here; tooth form and size is probably determined by the pattern of epithelial growth by the time the degree of development indicated by Fig. 1 c has been reached. Fig. 2 shows the developing second and third molars at day 6 in the CBA mouse; the second molar is now well differentiated and the third is in the late "bell" stage. Grewal (1962) considered that it was before this stage that the event, or events, which determined whether a tooth will be present or not took place. Our own histological studies confirm this (Berry and Germain, 1972).

The third molar is the smallest tooth in both jaws, and may be absent in wild mice (Deol, 1958; Harold and Zimmermann, 1960), where the upper tooth is most often missing. In contrast the lower third molar is most frequently missing from the jaws of inbred strains at a frequency which varies from 1.5 to 18% in AGr and CBA mice respectively (Gruneberg, 1951; Searle, 1954). Gruneberg, examining the CBA mouse, has shown that there is no parent-offspring correlation as regards the absence of third molars; normal and affected animals are therefore genetically similar and the presence or absence of the tooth is determined in part by non-genetic factors. From crosses with C57BL animals it is evident that several genes are involved. His work has indicated that underlying the discontinuous variant "absence of third molars" is a continuous variation involving the size of the third molars. He suggested that what

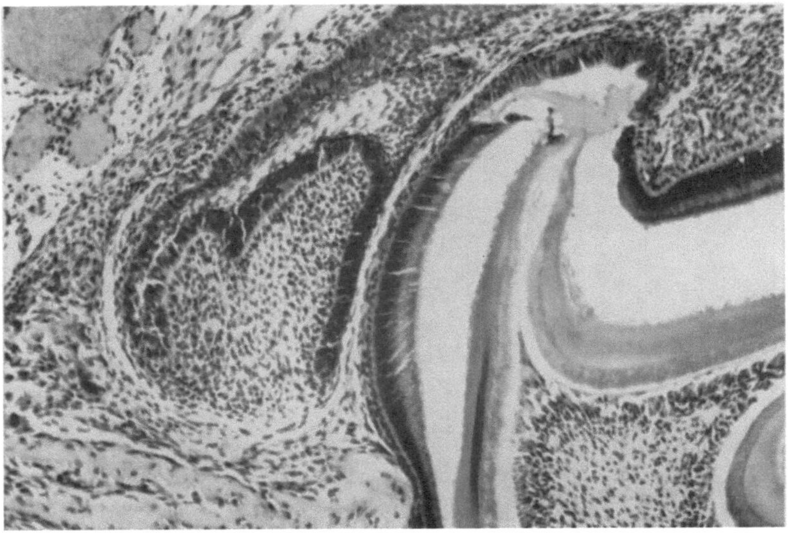

Fig. 2. CBA mouse. 6 day. Section through second and third molar. The third molar is in the "bell" stage, with formation of inner and outer enamel epithelium and stellate reticulum. (HE X 240)

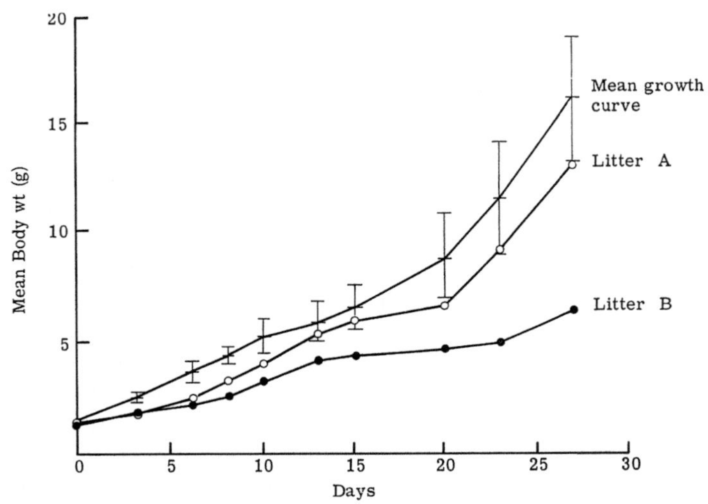

Fig. 3. Growth curves for normal litter of ICI mice (mean size 10, range 8—11) and two litters with missing teeth. Litter B numbered 14 at birth; 8 at 1 week; litter A 11 at birth; 9 at 1 week. This emphasises the importance of the first week of post-natal growth in this system

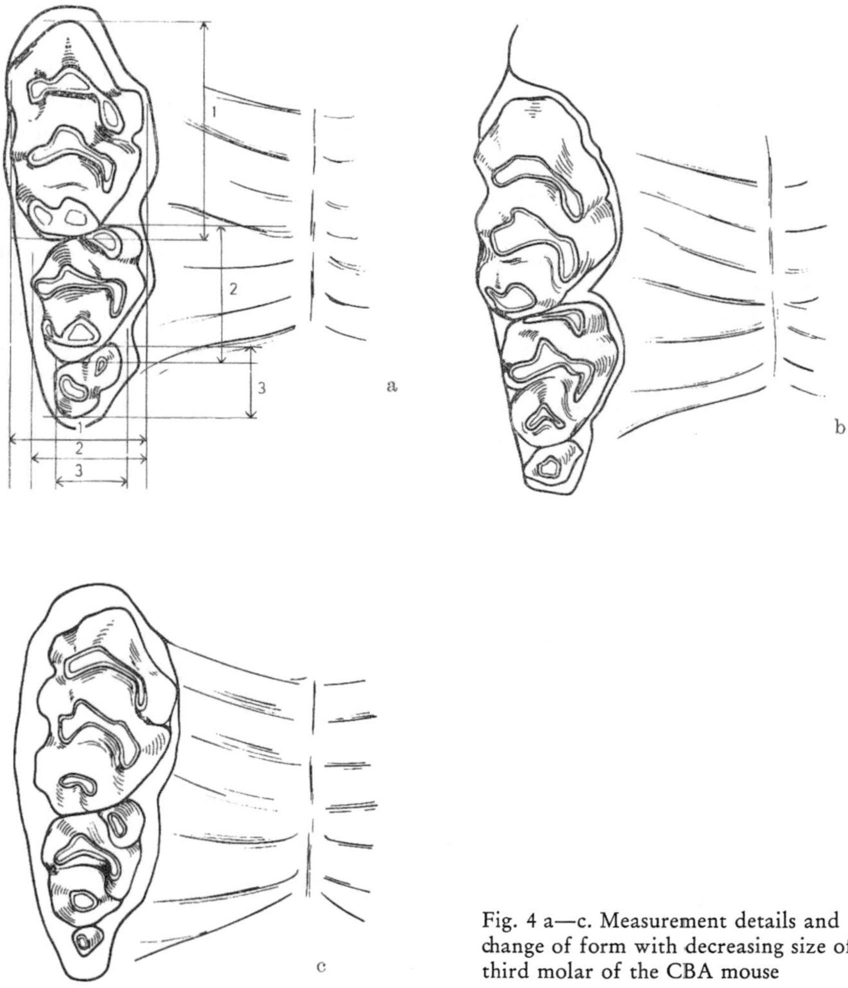

Fig. 4 a—c. Measurement details and change of form with decreasing size of the third molar of the CBA mouse

was really inherited was the size of the tooth, and when that fell below a certain critical point the tooth was absent. One further point is of importance, the tendency for teeth to be missing from animals from larger litters. Maternal lactational capacity is probably important here (Fig. 3 shows growth curves from normal and affected litters in ICI derived white mice bred at GUY's).

Absence of the third molar is thus considered to be a polygenically determined anomaly, susceptible to the influence of environmental factors, with metric characteristics and a readily observed "threshold". We have examined the frequency of occurrence of the defect in the CBA mouse, and have attempted to modify both size, form, and number of missing teeth in a series of experiments.

Experimental Details

In each experiment, control litters were studied concurrently with test animals to exclude the effects of unsuspected environmental changes (e. g. noise levels etc.). In practice alternate litters were allocated to control and test groups. In an unscheduled investigation a faulty window led to cold injury of many animals with considerable influence on tooth size and the frequency of missing teeth, emphasising the possible effects of less obvious events of this type. In the work described below the animals have been maintained on a standard diet, in a temperature and light controlled environment.

One observer made control and test measurements of tooth size in each study. Fig. 4 a illustrates the normal mouse upper dentition, and indicates how antero-posterior and bucco-lingual measurements are made. Fig. 4 b and 4 c indicate a progressive alteration in form as the third molar becomes smaller, with loss of a cusp. All measurements and observations were carried out at five weeks of age — shortly after the third molar had erupted.

Control Data

The initial examination of control animals gave frequencies of missing teeth as 11.8% in males and 4.3% in females in our strain (Table 3). This study confirmed GRUNEBERG's observations that animals with one or more teeth missing had smaller remain-

Table 3. Incidence of missing teeth in CBA mice (controls)

	Males	Females
No. of mice	160	137
No. with missing teeth	19 (11.8%)	6 (4.3%)
	s. e. of %: 2.55	s. e. of %: 1.70

Table 4. Mean size of third molar teeth in normal CBA mice with a full complement of teeth and in those with one or more teeth absent

	Mean tooth size ± SE (mm²) with range in brackets			
Third molar tooth	CBA male mice		CBA female mice	
	with all teeth present	with one or more teeth absent	with all teeth present	with one or more teeth absent
Upper	0.318 ± 0.004 (0.187—0.418)	0.297 ± 0.008 (0.187—0.360)	0.303 ± 0.005 (0.187—0.425)	0.312 ± 0.061 (0.160—0.360)
Lower	0.257 ± 0.004 (0.160—0.360)	0.237 ± 0.013 (0.160—0.284)	0.263 ± 0.008 (0.173—0.320)	0.269 ± 0.122 (0.249—0.300)

ing third molars (Table 4), and showed that there was no change in size of the first or second molars in the two groups (missing/normal), and no significant differencies between left and right sided teeth; in all subsequent experiments measurements of the two sides have been pooled in compiling the results.

Table 5. Effect of 8 hrs treatment with methotrexate on the frequency of the absence of third molar teeth in mice

Treatment	Sex of mice examined	Number of mice examined	Mice with one or more teeth missing	
			Number	Percentage ± SE
None (controls)	M	169	19	11.2 ± 2.43
	F	143	6	4.1 ± 1.66
Methotrexate on:				
3rd day	M	22	4	18
	F	27	2	7.4
4th day	M	24	5	20.8
	F	21	4	19
5th day	M	22	0	0
	F	22	2	9

Table 6. Size of third molar teeth in methotrexate-treated CBA mice with a full complement of teeth and in those with one or more teeth absent

Third molar tooth	Day of methotrexate treatment	Size (mm²) of third molar tooth in methotrexate-treated male CBA mice		female CBA mice	
		with all teeth present	with one or more teeth absent	with all teeth present	with one or more teeth absent
Upper	3	0.237 ± 0.004 [a] (0.202—0.284)	0.173 [8] [b] (0.047 [c]—0.284)	0.236 ± 0.004 (0.160—0.340)	0.111, 0.267, 0.320
Lower	3	0.199 ± 0.004 (0.166—0.249)	0.217, 0.217, 0.217	0.198 ± 0.004 (0.133—0.267)	0.187, 0.218, 0.249
Upper	4	0.225 ± 0.005 (0.187—0.284)	0.251 [7] (0.213—0.320)	0.225 ± 0.005 (0.160—0.281)	0.144, 0.178, 0.213, 0.213
Lower	4	0.187 ± 0.005 (0.111—0.250)	0.173 [7] (0.071 [c]—0.284)	0.195 ± 0.005 (0.111—0.267)	0.202, 0.213, 0.268
Upper	5	0.246 ± 0.004 (0.817—0.320)	—	0.238 ± 0.005 (0.160—0.320)	0.160, 0.160, 0.202
Lower	5	0.203 ± 0.004 (0.089—0.284)	Peg teeth present in animals with 4 teeth	0.219 ± 0.005 (0.160—0.284)	0.018 [c], 0.06 [c], 0.160

[a] Mean ± SE, with range in round brackets below.
[b] Number of third molars measured.
[c] "Peg" tooth.

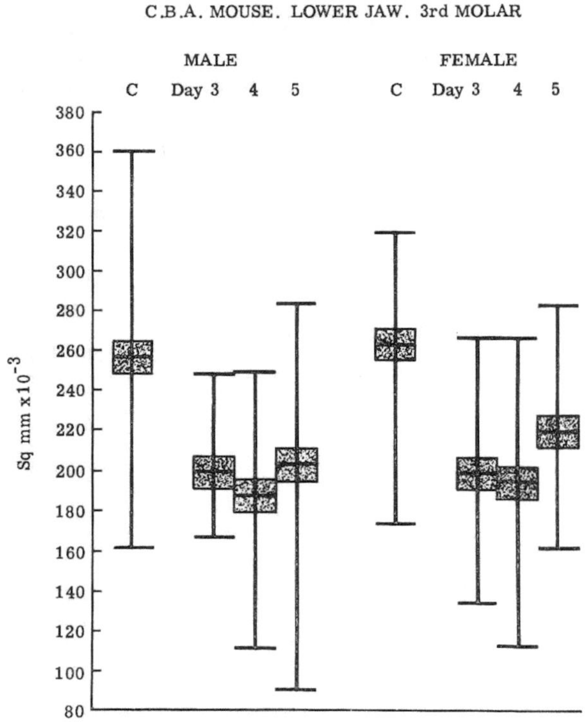

Fig. 5. Tooth size in lower join after methotrexate

Growth Inhibition Studies

The critical stages of tooth development that control size, form or absence of the tooth take place on days 3—6, before the tooth reaches the bell stage (Fig. 2). The effects of a finite period of growth inhibition on days 3—5 were therefore examined. Massive doses of methotrexate were given, inhibiting the action of the enzyme dihydrofolate reductase. This prevents the formation of tetrahydrofolate, a coenzyme in the conversion of deoxyuridylate to thyuridylate, and the *de novo* synthesis of the purine moiety of inosinic acid, the precursor for adenylic and guanylic acid synthesis. Since folinic acid will counteract this effect this is an effective means of inhibiting and restarting thymidine and hence DNA synthesis (Berry *et al.*, 1972). Treatment of this type causes growth retardation and has been shown to affect the size of vertebral body anlage in the rat (Berry, 1971). From Tables 5 and 6 and Figs. 5 and 6 it is evident that the treatment was effective in reducing the size of the tooth and increasing the frequency of expression of the defect. In addition simple peg-like teeth were found (Fig. 7). This suggests that a simple threshold explanation for the absence of the tooth is an inadequate one, since form may be altered to a pattern not seen in control animals before "disappearance" occurs. This is not surprising since a tooth of normal size and form is a result of co-ordinated mesodermal and epithelial interaction

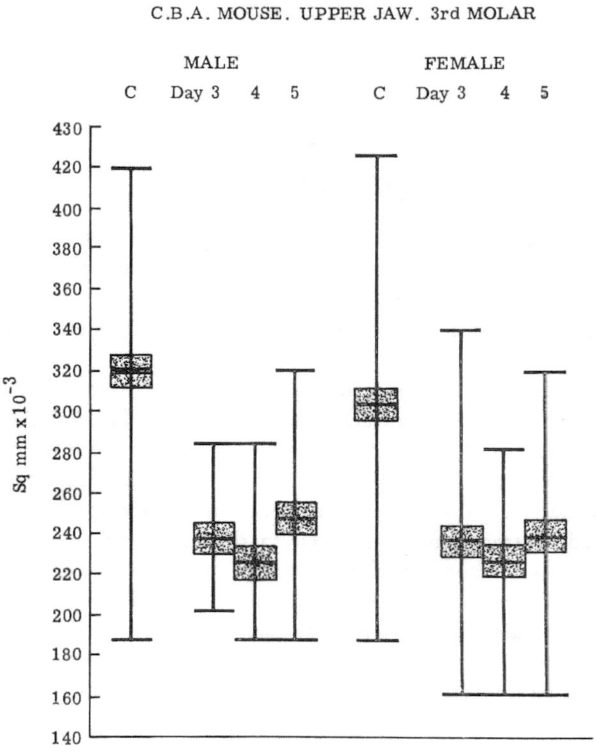

Fig. 6. Tooth size in upper join after methotrexate

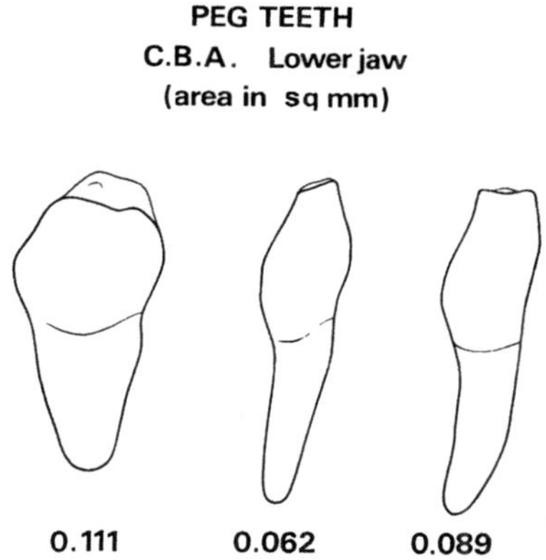

Fig. 7. Line drawing of peg teeth found in growth inhibition experiment

(a well developed vascular papilla is necessary for the growth of a tooth of normal size, and epithelial development probably controls the development of tooth form, RAMADAN SADEK, 1972).

Factors Affecting Late Tooth Development

Following these experiments, demonstrating sub-threshold metric changes, tetracycline and Vitamin A were studied as examples of compounds that might affect tooth morphology directly. In general, such compounds act late in development and theoretically should not affect the expression of the defect, although tooth size might be affected.

Vitamin A was given to mothers on day 3 post-partum as 2,500 I.U. by stomach tube. Mean blood level in control animals was found to be 16 I.U./100 mls. Treated animals had values of 1,790 I.U./100 ml 24 hrs after administration, falling to 40 I.U./100 ml at 48 hrs. MOORE (1971) has shown that Vitamin A transfer occurs freely during lactation and so it was considered that blood levels in the suckling mice would be raised. Tetracycline was given in drinking water (25 mg/100 mls) from day 0—14, and was demonstrated in suckling mouse tooth dentine of the first and second molars and incisors by fluorescence microscopy. In both experimental groups the mortality of treated litters was increased (controls 4.6%, tetracycline 11.8%, Vitamin A 28.5%). There was no significant change in the frequency of missing teeth (Table 7). It will be noticed that in this, as in subsequent experiments, the frequency

Table 7. Number and per cent third molars missing

		Maximum possible number of 3rd molars	Number missing 3rd molars	Percentage 3rd molars missing
Control	M	200	8	4.0
	F	228	6	2.6
Vitamin A	M	124	3	2.4
	F	107	2	1.8
Tetracycline	M	87	6	6.8
	F	94	4	4.2

of missing teeth is recorded as a percentage of the theoretical maximum of teeth present in order to permit the animal with a more severe defect i. e., 3 or 4 teeth missing, to weight the results in what was felt to be an appropriate manner. This problem will be discussed later (see page 100).

Table 8 shows the relevant data for the tooth area. There was a slight increase in size of Vitamin A treated animals, which subsequent events have suggested might be due to dietary deficiency in controls; mean tooth size was diminished, but not significantly, in tetracycline treated animals. Thus the early stages of tooth morphogenesis do not seem unduly sensitive to agents which affect the later stages of mineralization and

Table 8. Mean tooth area of the third molar tooth

	Male	n	Range of observations	Female	n	Range of observations
Controls						
Upper	0.193 (0.004)	58	0.133—0.249	0.195 (0.004)	62	0.130—0.280
Lower	0.144 (0.004)	55	0.100—0.267	0.145 (0.003)	56	0.089—0.213
Vitamin A						
Upper	0.215 (0.005)	62	0.106—0.311	0.215 (0.007)	52	0.111—0.302
Lower	0.160 (0.007)	59	0.044—0.320	0.191 (0.007)	53	0.035—0.284
Tetracycline						
Upper	0.176 (0.004)	45	0.073—0.249	0.187 (0.006)	47	0.089—0.320
Lower	0.145 (0.005)	38	0.038—0.187	0.150 (0.004)	43	0.044—0.249

The figures in parentheses denote the standard error of the mean, and n the number of teeth examined.

tooth formation. The choice of Vitamin A and tetracycline, and the results of these experiments are discussed in more detail elsewhere (GERMAIN and BERRY, 1973). It is of interest to note that as in previous experiments, teeth smaller than the smallest in control animals were found in the experimental groups.

Trace Elements

In order to examine the effects of trace minerals on the expression of this anomaly we have administered zinc, fluoride and selenium at various dose levels to CBA mice. In all experiments the additive was given in "Analar" water from 1—14 days post-partum. Zinc was given at 1,000 parts per million (p.p.m.) zinc carbonate, fluoride as 2 p.p.m. sodium fluoride and selenium as 5 p.p.m. sodium selenate. Each group of animals was weighed to confirm that their growth rate was normal. The results are shown in Tables 9—14.

From these preliminary experiments it can be seen that a large amount of zinc in drinking water appears to affect the frequency of absent teeth considerably. Tooth size in upper teeth is significantly reduced. A small amount of fluoride has a similar effect although the difference in tooth size is significant at a lower level of probability. Selenium has a greater effect on tooth size. The effects of fluoride support the observations of COOPER and LUDWIG (1965) in man, and of PAYNTER and GRAINGER (1956, 1961) in the rat. These authors have found reduction of tooth size in populations to which fluoride had been administered. It should be noticed that the frequency of

Table 9. % Teeth missing after fluoride administration

CONTROLS

	Possible No. teeth	No. absent teeth	% age missing teeth
Male			
Upper	62	0	0
Lower	62	1	1.6
Female			
Upper	40	0	0
Lower	40	1	2.5

FLUORIDE

	Possible No. teeth	No. absent teeth	% age missing teeth
Male			
Upper	74	4	5.4
Lower	76	36	47.3
Female			
Upper	52	3	5.7
Lower	52	17	32.6

TOTALS

	Male	Female
Controls	0.82	1.25
Fluoride (2 ppm)	26.7 [a]	19.2 [a]

[a] Indicates significant difference.
$P = < 0.001$ for males and females.

missing teeth increases in both sexes although the change is more common in males. Tooth size is reduced in both sexes although significant changes are often seen in females. It is possible that this is due to a closer approximation of normal tooth size to the threshold in males; thus teeth may disappear more readily.

These pilot studies indicate that minerals affect the expression of the defect, and since a number have been incriminated as teratogens (lithium, selenium, lead, cadmium, tellurium, arsenic and mercury in excess, and manganese, calcium and zinc in deficiency, Germain, 1975 for bibliography) these results are given as evidence to suggest that the molar tooth model may provide an appropriate system in which to examine their potential effects.

Table 10. Tooth size

	Male Mean ± SE	n (Teeth)	Female Mean ± SE	n (Teeth)
Controls				
Upper	0.232 ± 0.004 (0.156—0.292)	62	0.231 ± 0.005 (0.140—0.294)	40
Lower	0.159 ± 0.002 (0.113—0.192)	61	0.164 ± 0.004 (0.113—0.229)	39
Fluoride (2 ppm)				
Upper	0.221 [a] ± 0.004 (0.112—0.295)	70	0.214 [a] ± 0.005 (0.141—0.278)	49
Lower	0.161 ± 0.002 (0.122—0.186)	40	0.168 ± 0.002 (0.141—0.200)	35

[a] Indicates significant difference.
Males P = < 0.05 > 0.02.
Females P = <0.02 >0.01.
Figures in parentheses denote range of tooth sizes.

Table 11. % Missing teeth after selenium administration

CONTROLS

	Possible No. teeth	No. absent teeth	% age missing teeth
Male			
Upper	44	0	0
Lower	44	0	0
Female			
Upper	30	0	0
Lower	30	1	3.4

SELENIUM

	Possible No. teeth	No. absent teeth	% age missing teeth
Male			
Upper	74	4	5.4
Lower	74	24	32.4
Female			
Upper	70	1	1.4
Lower	70	9	12.8

Table 11 (Continued)

TOTALS

	Male	Female
Controls	0	1.7
Selenium (5 ppm)	18 [a]	14 [a]

[a] Indicates significant difference.
Male $p = < 0.001$.
Female $p = < 0.001$.

Table 12. Tooth size

	Male mean ± SE	n (Teeth)	Female mean ± SE	n (Teeth)
Controls	0.230 ± 0.005	(44)	0.231 ± 0.005	(30)
Upper	(0.156—0.292)		(0.140—0.276)	
Lower	0.155 ± 0.004	(43)	0.158 ± 0.004	(29)
	(0.113—0.192)		(0.113—0.209)	
Selenium	0.203 [b] ± 0.004	(70)	0.205 [b] ± 0.005	(69)
Upper	(0.087—0.269)		(0.031 [a]—0.313)	
Lower	0.138 [b] ± 0.003	(50)	0.143 [b] ± 0.002	(61)
	(0.028 [a]—0.179)		(0.102—0.176)	

[a] Peg shaped tooth.
[b] Indicates significant difference $p = < 0.001$ male, $p = < 0.01$ female.
Figures in parentheses denote range of tooth sizes.

Table 13. % Missing teeth after zinc administration

CONTROLS

	Possible No. teeth	No. absent teeth	% age missing teeth
Male			
Upper	100	0	0
Lower	100	8	8
Female			
Upper	114	0	0
Lower	114	6	5.2

Table 13 (Continued)
ZINC

	Possible No. teeth	No. absent teeth	% age missing teeth
Male			
Upper	48	4	8.3
Lower	48	26	54.1
Female			
Upper	32	2	6.2
Lower	32	9	28.1

TOTALS

	Male	Female
Controls	4.1	2.7
Zinc	32.2	15.6

Male $p = < 0.001$.
Female $p = < 0.01$.

Table 14. Tooth size

	Male mean ± SE	n (Teeth)	Female mean ± SE	n (Teeth)
Controls	0.193 ± 0.004	(58)	0.195 ± 0.004	(62)
Upper	(0.120—0.249)		(0.130—0.200)	
Lower	0.144 ± 0.004	(55)	0.145 ± 0.003	(56)
	(0.100—0.267)		(0.124—0.199)	
Zinc	0.173 [a] ± 0.003	(43)	0.168 [a] ± 0.007	(30)
Upper	(0.106—0.231)		(0.031 [b]—0.231)	
Lower	0.156 ± 0.007	(22)	0.151 ± 0.007	(23)
	(0.44 [b]—0.202)		(0.035 [b]—0.187)	

[a] Indicates significant difference $p = < 0.01$.
Figures in parentheses denote range of tooth sizes.
[b] Peg shaped tooth.

Inter-Strain Differences

We have recently compared the incidence of missing teeth in the same strain kept in two animal houses with varying degrees of environmental control. In the less controlled situation, marked variation in the frequency of missing teeth was found. This prompted a further study of a number of strains. With the kind permission of Dr. M. FESTING of the Medical Research Council Laboratory Animals Centre one of us (J. P. G.) was able to examine 2,857 mandibles from adult male mice of 16 different strains. The results are shown in Table 15. It is evident that by maintaining a number of strains in a given environment it would be possible to evaluate suspected teratogens in animals with varying degrees of susceptibility to the production of small or missing teeth.

Table 15

Strain	No. of mandibles examined	% Missing teeth
A2G (LAC)	280	7.14
A2G (OLAC)	139	5.75
F/st	58	5.17
CBA (OLAC)	134	1.59
CBA (Harwell)	184	1.19
CBA (LAC)	178	—
C57/BL	128	—
C57/L	126	—
C57/Br	140	—
C3H/Hc	497	—
NZW	194	—
BALB/C	252	—
ICFW	111	—
DBA/I	164	—
LACA	68	—
CBA/Sn Sn	94	—
BIO A	86	—
Bio-LP-*a*	12	—
BIO Br	112	—

Statistical Treatment of Data

In view of the comments of Becker (1974) on the handling of teratological data it is difficult to know exactly how to consider this system. In terms of tooth size, all animals in a group show consistent changes, but threshold effects may be more obvious within litters. Lactational performance can be checked by cross fostering experiments (Germain, 1975) and with reduction of litters to a standard size and careful assessment of growth rates this "within litter" effect can be eliminated. It would then seem reasonable to treat each animal as an individual test; this is obviously true when the compound is administered by injection. This subject is discussed more fully in Chapter 8.

Summary and Conclusions

The process of development of the third molar tooth in the mouse is obviously susceptible to the effects of a number of different types of environmental agent. Gaunt

(1963) has shown that each tooth germ is self-governing in terms of its rate of development and the rapid growth of the third molar in early post-natal life makes it peculiarly vulnerable to environmental factors. There are particular advantages in this system with regard to ease of recognition of end-point, metric characteristics etc. The mechanism of failure of development may be studied in tissue culture, since tooth germs may be grown *in vitro*. With investigation of the nature of the fundamental abnormality and a better understanding of the mechanism, it may well be possible to improve its predictive value. Recent work by GRUNEBERG (1971) has suggested that this system may be an appropriate one in which to examine the early development of any organ which results from an initial downgrowth of solid epithelial buds into mesoderm. In the tabby mouse many organs (including the teeth) which originate in this way may be small or absent.

The development of a battery of tests of this type, based on selective examination of agents likely to affect particular mechanism, offers a scientific basis for the examination of the possible affects of environmental agents in man.

Acknowledgements. This work is supported by the Medical Research Council.

References

BECKER, B. A.: The Statistics of Teratology. Teratology **9**, 261—262 (1974).

BERRY, C. L.: Transient inhibition of DNA synthesis by methotrexate, in the rat embryo and foetus. J. Embryol. exp. Morph. **26**, 469 (1972).

BERRY, C. L., GERMAIN, J. P.: Absence of the third molar tooth in the mouse: its relevances to human malformation. J. Path. 108, 35 (1972).

BERRY, C. L., GERMAIN, J. P., LOOKER, T.: The effect of methotrexate on DNA synthesis and its reversal by folinic acid. J. Embryol. exp. Morph. **28**, 601 (1972).

CARTER, C. O.: The inheritance of common congenital malformations. Prog. Med. Genet. **4**, 59 (1965).

CARTER, C. O.: Genetics of common disorders. Brit. med. Bull. **25**, 52—57 (1969).

CARTER, C. O.: Multifactorial inheritance revisited. In Proc. III Int. Cong. Congenital Malformations, The Hague, 1969, p. 227. Amsterdam: Exerpta Medica (1970).

COOPER, V. K., LUDWIG, T. G.: The effects of fluoride and of soil trace elements on the morphology of the permanent molars in man. N. Z. dent. J. **61**, 33 (1965).

DAGG, C. P.: The interaction of environmental stimuli and inherited susceptibility to congenital deformity. Amer. Zoologist **3**, 223—233 (1963).

DAGG, C. P., SCHLAGER, G., DOERR, A.: Polygenic control of teratogenicity of 5-fluorouracil in mice. Genetics **53**, 1101—1117 (1966).

DEOL, M. S.: Genetical studies on the skeleton of the mouse XXIV. Further data on skeletal variation in wild populations. J. Embryol. exp. Morph. **6**, 569 (1958).

EDWARDS, J. H.: Familial predisposition in Man. Brit. med. Bull. **25**, 58 (1969).

FALCONER, D. S.: The inheritance of liability to diseases with variable age of onset with particular reference to Diabetes mellitus. Ann. Hum. Genet. **31**, 1)1967).

FRASER, F. C.: Etiology of cleft lip and palate. In Cleft Lip and Palate. W. C. GRABB, S. ROSENSTEIN and K. R. BZOCH, Eds. Boston: Little and Brown. p. 54—66 (1971).

FRASER, F. C., PASHAYAN, H.: Relation of face shape to susceptibility to congenital cleft lip. J. med. Genet. **7**, 112—117 (1970).

GAUNT, W. A.: An analysis of the growth of the cheek teeth of the mouse. Acta Anat. **54**, 220 (1962).

GERMAIN, J. P.: A polygenically determined characteristic in the mouse, observations on its pathogenesis, susceptibility to environmental factors, and relevance to human malformation. M. Phil. thesis, University of London (1975).

Germain, J. P., Berry, C. L.: The effects of Vitamin A and tetracycline on a mouse tooth anomaly. Arch. oral. Biol. **18**, 729 (1973).

Gibson, J. P., Staples, R. E., Newberne, J. W.: Use of the Rabbit in Teratogenicity studies. Toxicol. appl. Pharmacol. **9**, 398—408 (1966).

Green, E. L.: Quantitative genetics of skeletal variations in the mouse II Crosses between four inbred strains (C3H, CBS, C57BL, BALB/c). Genetics **47**, 1087—1096 (1962).

Grewal, M. S.: The development of an inherited tooth defect in the mouse. J. Embryol. exp. Morph. **10**, 202 (1962).

Grüneberg, H.: The genetics of a tooth defect in the mouse. Proc. roy. Soc. B. **138**, 437 (1951).

Grüneberc, H.: The tabby syndrome in the mouse. Proc. R. Soc. Lond. B. **179**, 139—153.

Herold, W., Zimmermann, K.: Molaren-Abbau bei der Hausmaus (Mus Musculus L). Z. Säugetierk. **25**, 81 (1960).

Kimmel, C. A., Wilson, J. G.: Skeletal Deviations in Rats: Malformations or Variations. Teratology **8**, 309—315 (1973).

Leck, I.: The Etiology of Human Malformations: Insights from Epidemiology, **5**, 303 (1972).

McLaren, Ann, Michie, D.: Factors affecting Vertebral Variation in Mice. 4 Experimental Proof of the Uterine Basis of a Maternal effect. J. Embryol. exp. Morph. **6**, 645—659 (1958).

Moore, T.: Vitamin A transfer from mother to offspring in mice and rats. Internat. J. Vit. Nutr. Res. **41**, 301 (1971).

Palmer, A. K.: Spontaneous malformations of the New Zealand White Rabbit. The background to safety evaluation tests. Lab. Anim. **2**, 195—206 (1968).

Palmer, A. K.: Sporadic malformations in laboratory animals and their influence on drug testing. In Drugs and Fetal Development. Eds. Klingerg, M., Abramovici, A., and Chemke, J. New York and London: Plenum Press. p. 45—60 (1972).

Paynter, K. J., Grainger, R. M.: The relation of nutrition to the morphology and size of rat molar teeth. J. Canad. dent. Ass. **22**, 519 (1956).

Paynter, K. J., Grainger, R. M.: Influence of nutrition and genetics on morphology and caries susceptibility. J. Amer. med. Ass. **177**, 306 (1961).

Poswillo, D. E.: The pathogenesis of the first and second branchial arch syndrome. Oral Surg. **35**, 302—328 (1973).

Searle, A. G.: Genetical studies on the skeleton of the mouse. IX Causes of skeletal variation in pure lines. J. Genet. **52**, 68 (1954).

Searle, A. G.: IX Causes of skeletal variation with in pure lines. J. Genet. **52**, 68—102 (1954 a).

Searle, A. G.: Genetical studies on the skeleton of the mouse. XI The influence of diet on variation within pure lines. J. Genet. **52**, 413—423 (1954 b).

Trasler, D. G.: Pathogenesis of cleft lip and its relation to embryonic face shape in A/J and C57BL mice. Teratology **1**, 33—50 (1968).

W.H.O.: Principles for the testing of drugs for teratogenicity. Report of a W.H.O. Scientific Group. W.H.O. Tech. Rep. Ser. No. 364. Geneva 1967.

Woolf, C. M.: Congenital Cleft Lip. J. med. Genet. **8**, 65 (1971).

Wright, S.: An analysis of variability in number of digits in an inbred strain of guinea pigs. Genetics **19**, 506—536 (1934 a).

Wright, S.: The results of crosses between inbred strains of guinea pigs, differing in number of digits. Genetics **19**, 537—551 (1934 b).

Yasuda, M., Maeda, H.: Significance of the lumbar rib as an indicator in teratogenicity tests. Teratology **6**, 124—125 (1972).

6. Behavioural Teratology

S. M. Barlow and F. M. Sullivan

With 2 Figures

Following the thalidomide disaster techniques for carrying out reproductive tests (Fitzhugh, 1968) and tests of teratogenicity (Wilson and Warkany, 1965; Robson and Sullivan, 1968) were established. In recent years interest has been aroused in "non-structural" malformations; subtle long term effects on offspring of substances taken during pregnancy. In this way enquiries into the behavioural effects of teratogens have become important factors in the assessment of the influence of drugs on the embryo and fetus.

Although it was known in the 1940's that giving pregnant rats the sedative and anti-epileptic drug sodium bromide could impair the behaviour and learning ability of the offspring (Harned *et al.*, 1940), it was not until the 1960's that the work of Werboff and his collaborators aroused public interest. He showed that the then widely used tranquilliser, meprobamate, if administered to pregnant rats, could affect the learning capacity of the offspring (Werboff, 1962; Werboff and Havlena, 1962). Numerous other studies on psychoactive drugs were instituted at that time. The term "Behavioural Teratology" seems first to have been used by Werboff and Gottlieb (1963) to describe this newly recognised area of teratogenic sensitivity, defined as "the behaviour or functional adaptation of the offspring to its environment".

Behavioural teratology then, is concerned with the identification of agents which may cause behavioural abnormalities in the offspring. It encompasses the study of the subtle anatomical and biochemical disturbances which presumably underlie these functional abnormalities. There is considerable evidence from both human and animal work to suggest that exposure of the developing organism, either prenatally or neonatally, to a wide variety of environmental influences may bring about functional changes, in the absence of any gross structural deformity. Recent work has demonstrated the vulnerability of the developing brain to interference with normal processes of cell growth, differentiation and migration (discussed in Chapter 1) and with normal biochemical maturation. There follows a review of behavioural teratogens and a discussion of some of the practical difficulties which may be encountered in the design, conduct and interpretation of behavioural teratology tests.

Review of Clinical and Animal Studies

The first extensive studies in man were carried out by Pasamanick, Lilienfield, Knobloch *et al.* (reviewed by Joffe, 1969). They observed that a wide spectrum of disorders in children, including cerebral palsy, epilepsy, mental retardation, behavioural, speech and reading difficulties were associated with maternal complications of pregnancy such as toxaemia, vaginal bleeding and premature delivery. These observations have provided a basis for more detailed studies of individual prenatal environmental influences known to be associated with complications of pregnancy, including smoking, stress, poor maternal nutrition and low socio-economic status. The long term effects of smoking in pregnancy include impairment of "general ability", reading and mathematical abilities in children assessed at 7 and 11 years of age (BUTLER and GOLDSTEIN, 1973) though whether these effects are causally related or not is hotly debated (BURCH, 1973). Similarly, maternal psychological stress has been implicated in the aetiology of some behavioural abnormalities in children (STOTT, 1957; FERREIRA, 1965), whilst numerous animal studies demonstrate a variety of effects of prenatal psychological stress on postnatal activity, emotional reactivity, sexual behaviour and learning ability in rats and mice (ARCHER and BLACKMAN, 1971).

Despite the widespread occurrence of protein-calorie malnutrition in developing countries there have been few studies of the adverse effects of malnutrition in infancy on mental development (PAN AMERICAN HEALTH ORGANISATION, 1972) and even fewer studies in man of the effects of maternal malnutrition during pregnancy and lactation. Indirect evidence links maternal malnutrition with those complications of pregnancy (EBBS *et al.*, 1942; BURKE *et al.*, 1943) which are known to cause neuropsychiatric disorders in the offspring. Other studies have shown an association between an unbalanced maternal diet in the first trimester of pregnancy and central nervous system (CNS) malformations of the offspring (RICHARDS, 1969) and demonstrated the beneficial effect on offspring I.Q. of giving vitamin supplements during late pregnancy and lactation to "less well nourished" women (HARREL *et al.*, 1955). In animals the deleterious effects of undernutrition during gestation and the preweaning period include delayed reflex ontogeny, deficits in exploratory behaviour and over-reaction to stress (DOBBING and SMART, 1973).

Not only dietary deficiencies, but specific dietary constituents are of interest to the behavioural teratologist, particularly in view of the increasingly widespread use of processed foods containing many different additives. The flavour enhancer monosodium glutamate, for example, damages hypothalamic neurones when given to fetal and neonatal primates and rodents (OLNEY, 1969; OLNEY and SHARPE, 1969; NAGASAWA *et al.*, 1974). Excessive vitamin A during pregnancy in the rat impairs the learning ability of the offspring (BUTCHER *et al.*, 1970) and in a primate, the marmoset, a maternal diet containing blighted potatoes has been reported to result in abnormal play patterns and excessive clinging behaviour in the offspring (POSWILLO *et al.*, 1973).

Prenatal X-irradiation of the human fetus results in widespread defects of the CNS (RUGH, 1962) with associated behavioural deficits. However, there have been no studies of behavioural effects in children without gross deformities although experiments in rats suggest that low levels of X-irradiation in early or late gestation may markedly alter offspring behaviour in novel environments or maze-learning situations (LEVINSON, 1952; FURCHTGOTT *et al.*, 1958; FURCHTGOTT and ECHOLS, 1958; WERBOFF *et al.*, 1962).

Intrauterine infections may be behavioural teratogens, cytomegalovirus infection during gestation being one of the more important *known* causes of mental retardation in children (DUDGEON, 1973). Congenital rubella (MARSHALL, 1973) and the rarer disease of congenital toxoplasmosis (FLECK, 1973) also cause brain damage and mental subnormality.

Pesticides, herbicides, fungicides and industrial pollutants have also been indicted. In the early 1960's in Minamata Bay in Japan, the effluent containing methylmercury from a plastics factory was discharged into the sea. This accumulated in fish which, when consumed by the villagers living alongside the bay, led to an epidemic of degenerative neurological disease in adults, and of cerebral palsy in children whose mothers had consumed the contaminated fish during pregnancy. Six percent of births in the area were affected at the time and another similar, though less severe, episode subsequently occurred some hundreds of miles away at Niigata (MILLER, 1974). In animal studies, methylmercury exposure during pregnancy in the mouse has been reported to affect offspring open field behaviour (SPYKER *et al.*, 1972) and similar findings have been reported after treatment of pregnant rats with the herbicide 2-4-5 trichlorophenoxy-acetic acid (SJODEN and SODERBERG, 1972).

In the future, attention will undoubtedly be focussed on the behavioural effects of prenatal drug administration. In humans, premedication with sedatives or narcotic analgesics prior to delivery may depress motor activity, suckling, heart rate and respiration rate for up to a week after birth (BRAZELTON, 1970) and maternal consumption of psychotropic drugs (opiates, tranquillisers and alcohol) during pregnancy may disturb neonatal behaviour with particular effects persisting into infancy (DESMOND *et al.*, 1969).

There is considerable evidence from animal experiments to suggest that drug administration, particularly during the neonatal period, may give rise to permanent behavioural abnormalities in otherwise normal individuals. Two major groups of drugs have been studied so far, the cytotoxic drugs, certain of which have been discussed elsewhere (Chapter 4) and the psychotropic drugs. Tranquillisers such as reserpine, chlorpromazine and meprobamate administered to rats during pregnancy may affect offspring activity, impair maze-learning ability and the acquisition of conditioned avoidance responses (HOFFELD *et al.*, 1968; CLARK *et al.*, 1970; WERBOFF, 1962; WERBOFF and HAVLENA, 1962) and render the young more susceptible to stress (YOUNG, 1965). Occasionally, drugs with pharmacologically dissimilar effects on brain amine levels are found to have similar effects on the behaviour of offspring. Prenatal reserpine, which decreases the levels of monoamines in the central nervous system, has been shown to increase offspring activity and susceptibility to audiogenic seizures. However, the monoamine oxidase inhibitors, iproniazid and isocarboxazid, and 5-hydroxytryptophan, which increase brain amine levels, produce similar effects (WERBOFF *et al.*, 1961 a; WERBOFF *et al.*, 1961 b). Studies by TONGE (1973 b) have shown that while similar effects may be produced on *total* brain amines, the effects in discrete areas of the brain may be very different. Variable local levels of amines in the brain suggest that total values are the mean of a large number of different concentrations. Because of the misleading information which whole brain assays produce, it is important to study effects at specific brain loci in order to allow the proper interpretation and correlation with behavioural effects. The dangers of extrapolation from chemical studies on peripheral nerves have also been demonstrated (COYLE *et al.*, 1973).

Other drugs given to pregnant rats, such as salicylate (BUTCHER *et al.*, 1972), sodium bromide (HARNED *et al.*, 1940; HARNED *et al.*, 1944), and barbiturates (ARMITAGE, 1952) all impair the maze-learning ability of the offspring in the absence of any gross CNS deformities. Prenatal and preweaning exposure to morphine impairs shock-elicited escape behaviour in mice (ZIMMERBERG *et al.*, 1974) and even chronic exposure of rats to trifluoperazine during infancy may impair escape responses in the subsequent generation of undrugged offspring (GAURON and ROWLEY, 1973).

Hormone administration during gestation or the early postnatal period may also affect brain development and behaviour, not always adversely. Prenatal administration of growth hormone (BLOCK and ESSMAN, 1965; CLENDINNEN and EAYRS, 1961; SARA and LAZARUS, 1974) or thyroid hormone (DISPENSA and HORNBECK, 1941; SCHAPIRO, 1971) accelerates development of the CNS in rodents, a phenomenon which may be correlated with improved performance in learning tests. Alternatively, the apparent advancement of maturation of the CNS may be associated with a premature termination of cell proliferation with a reduction in ultimate cell number in the brain. Thus although innately organised behavioural patterns may emerge earlier than expected following treatment with thyroid hormones, the performance of such animals in tests of adaptive behaviour in later life may be permanently impaired (BALÁZS, 1972). Neonatal corticosteroids have also been shown to retard physical maturation (ORNOY and HOROWITZ, 1972) and functional development of the CNS (SCHAPIRO, 1971) The effects of prenatal exposure to gonadal hormones on sexual and related behaviours are reviewed elsewhere (JOFFE, 1969) and general aspects of hormonal treatment on brain development have been interestingly reviewed by BALÁZS (1972). In man it has been reported that prenatal exposure to androgenic substances is responsible for the better school performance and higher I.Q. of children from pregnancies where the mother received progestogens for threatened abortion (MONEY, 1971).

Behavioural Teratology Testing

It is not possible in this account to outline any comprehensive screening programme for developmental and behavioural abnormalities. We propose to discuss some of the practical difficulties and the many variables which may be encountered in behavioural teratology testing and to suggest methods of controlling certain of these variables. Wherever possible, references are given to papers and reviews where more detailed information may be obtained.

Premating and Prenatal Variables

Species

The choice of species will obviously influence the nature and sophistication of the behavioural tests which may be used and particular attention must be paid to the

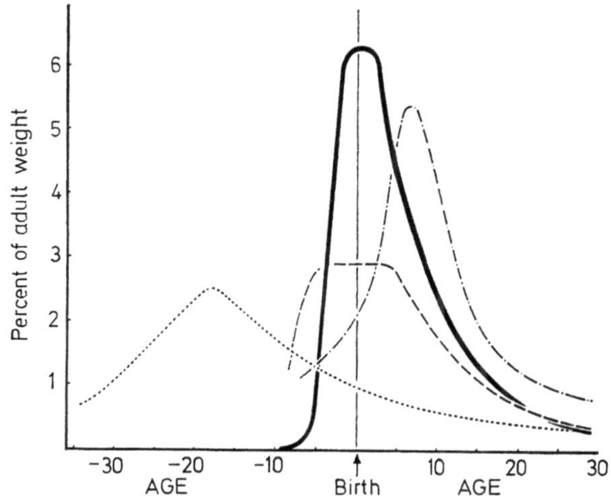

Fig. 1. Velocity of human brain growth (wet weight) compared with that in other species. Prenatal and postnatal are expressed as follows: human ——— in mounths, guinea pig ····· in days, pig — — — in weeks, rat —·—·— in days. Reproduced by kind permission of John Dobbing, taken from DOBBING, p. 567, 1974.

timing of the prenatal treatment in relation to the species used. The studies of DOBBING (1974) and his colleagues have shown that there is a "vulnerable period" in brain development at the time of the brain growth spurt, which varies from species to species depending largely on the state of maturity of the offspring at birth (see ALTMAN, 1970; DOBBING, 1974, and Fig. 1). Growth restriction or toxic insults during the vulnerable period may result in permanent deficits in brain structure and function. Observations also indicate that there are vulnerable periods for interference with the biochemical function of the brain during maturation of the biogenic amine transmitter systems (ENGEL *et al.*, 1974) and for interference with postnatal endocrine development (KŘEČEK, 1971). However, these vulnerable periods are not the only factor in species differences in behavioural teratology since animals such as rats and mice, with a similar chronology of brain development, may behave in a completely opposite manner after the same prenatal treatment (THOMPSON *et al.*, 1962; THOMPSON and OLIAN, 1961). The explanation for such differences, unless they are related to the particular strains chosen (see below), is not yet known.

As will be seen later, one of the most difficult problems in behavioural teratology is to separate the influences of prenatal factors from those of postnatal environmental factors. These latter include parental/offspring relationships, and one method of reducing them is to use birds. SPARBER has reported that the use of the common domestic chicken (Gallus domesticus) allows a separation of maternal and fetal effects both during development and after hatching. The chicken, he states (SPARBER, 1972) enters the world with a repertoire of several complex pieces of behaviour which can be used for estimation of behavioural deviation either directly or after moulding. The chicken may have a particular usefulness in attempts to correlate drug-induced behavioural changes with the biochemical changes induced in the brain at the same time (Sparber and Shideman, 1968). However, much useful information may also be gained from species such as the rat and mouse if suitable fostering techniques (see below) are used to separate prenatal from postnatal influences.

Strain

Strain differences in normal behaviour are evident in all species. Rats and mice, for example, may be selectively bred for particular characteristics such as low or high activity, low or high frequency of defecation, and good or poor performance on conditioned avoidance tasks (Broadhurst, 1960; Levine and Broadhurst, 1963). Using strains with contrasting behaviours, many workers have shown that the effects on offspring behaviour of a particular prenatal treatment vary with the "baseline" behaviour of each strain (Joffe, 1969 for review). The maternal and paternal genotypes are therefore important determinants of offspring behaviour in their interaction with prenatal treatments. The use of a variety of strains may also be useful in attempts to correlate behavioural and biochemical changes induced by treatment, and in the development of models for specific defects such as minimal brain dysfunction (Coyle et al., 1973; Kempf et al., 1974).

Experiences of Previous Generations

Postnatal development and behaviour is determined not only by the interaction of offspring genotype with the immediate prenatal and postnatal environment but may also be influenced by the experiences of previous generations, a phenomenon known as the nongenetic transmission of information (Denenberg and Rosenberg, 1967). Exposure of one generation to psychotropic drugs during infancy may not only adversely affect learning behaviour of the second undrugged generation but also of the third undrugged generation (Gauron and Rowley, 1971, 1973). Stress or handling may similarly affect the behaviour of the second and third generations (Denenberg and Whimbey, 1963; Wehmer et al., 1970). It is obviously necessary to standardise and to control rigorously the rearing conditions for the breeding stocks used in behavioural teratology testing.

Time of Treatment

In normal testing, administration of the compound under investigation is often restricted to the period of embryogenesis i. e. days 6—16 for mouse and rat, and days 6—18 for the rabbit. For behavioural teratology tests, these periods are inadequate. Substances may affect different aspects of brain development at all stages from original appearance of the neural crest to the final states of neural and glial cell proliferation, myelination and synapse formation. As shown in Fig. 1, the time of peak brain growth differs widely in different species and in the present state of knowledge treatment should continue in the mouse, rat or rabbit from day 6 of pregnancy through to weaning, though there may be advantages in separating prenatal and postnatal phases in different groups of animals.

Other Factors

Other factors such as selection of dose levels, ensuring adequate food intake and absence of severe maternal toxicity, avoidance of stress, drug interactions etc. must obviously be carefully controlled, as for normal teratogenicity tests (WILSON and WARKANY, 1965; ROBSON and SULLIVAN, 1968).

Postnatal Variables

Litter Size

The rate of growth and maturation of offspring will certainly vary with litter size, but it is not clear whether variations in litter size also affect behaviour. SEITZ (1954) and CARLSON (1961), working with rats, and PRIESTNALL (1973), using mice, all reported an increase in emotionality (defined as either frequent defecation or low activity) of offspring from large litters compared with offspring from small litters, but BROADHURST and LEVINE (1963 a) and LORE and AVIS (1970) found no differences in offspring from different sized litters of rats. If a full developmental and behavioural study is to be carried out it would seem advisable to cull all litters to similar size and equal sex ratio at birth or during the suckling period, particularly if the prenatal treatment causes substantial intrauterine or postnatal mortality. A difference in litter size of 2 or 3 pups only has not been found to be of any significance in the studies described above.

Type of Rearing Mother

It is important to ascertain whether the effects of any prenatal treatment are the result of interference with the offspring prenatally, postnatally, or both. Behavioural changes may be brought about not only by prenatal treatment affecting the developing organism during embryogenesis or fetal life but may also be induced postnatally, via some chronic effect of the treatment on the mother. For example, lactation, nesting behaviour or general standard of maternal care may be affected, or maternal recognition that a pup is in any way different or abnormal may alter her behaviour towards that pup (MEIER and SCHULTZMAN, 1968). Any alteration in maternal physiology or behaviour may in turn alter the development and behaviour of the offspring. To control for these possibilities, fostering and cross-fostering techniques should be employed. Litters may be reared in one of three ways: non-fostered, where the litter is reared by its own mother; cross-fostered, where the litter is reared by a mother from a different treatment group from that of its own mother; or fostered, where a litter is reared by a mother from the same treatment group as that of its own mother (Fig. 2). By comparing cross-fostered with fostered groups it can be determined whether the effects of the treatment were mediated prenatally, postnatally, or both, and comparison of non-fostered with fostered groups acts as a control for the fostering procedure, which itself may have induced behavioural changes. If there are

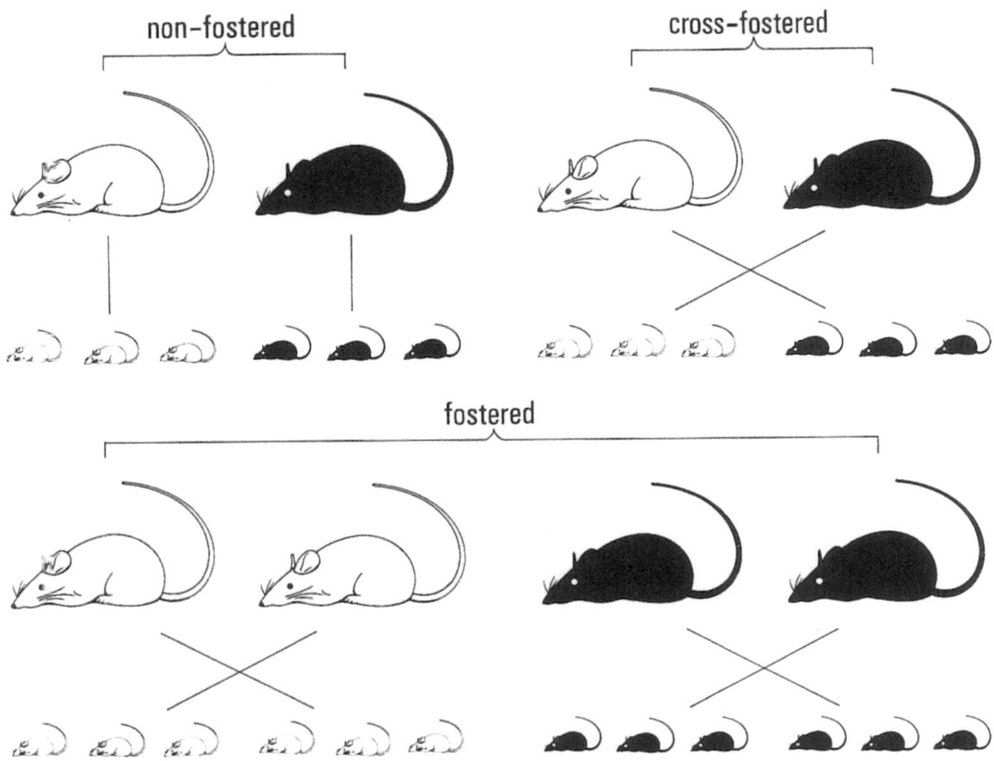

Fig. 2. Fostering and cross-fostering technique for separation of prenatal from postnatal effects. White mice — control group; black mice — treated group

several treatment groups, the fostering and cross-fostering technique becomes unmanageable and in these cases fostering of all the offspring onto mothers of a single type is preferable, either keeping litters of one type of pup together or mixing suitably identified pups so that each litter contains pups of all types, thus ensuring identical litter composition (JOFFE, 1969, for more detailed discussion).

Experiences of Offspring during Infancy

The experience of the offspring during infancy may markedly affect their later behaviour (NEWTON and LEVINE, 1968). For example, frequent handling of rats during infancy will alter their physiological responses to stress (LEVINE *et al.*, 1967) and their behaviour in tests for emotionality and learning (LEVINE and BROADHURST, 1963). Animals reared in enriched environments not only show behavioural changes but also have a heavier cerebral cortex, increased cholinesterase activity and altered levels of brain amines (ROSENZWEIG, 1971). To control for environmental experiences during infancy, the conditions under which the offspring are reared must be standardised within experiments with respect to such variables as temperature, humidity, noise level, lighting, cages, diet, handling and cage cleaning. Prenatal treatments may also interact with postnatal experiences to produce effects on offspring behaviour (YOUNG, 1964), and so variations in conditions of animal husbandry in different laboratories may be another confounding factor in the comparison of similar prenatal treatments by different workers.

Sex of Offspring

Sex differences in offspring behaviour are very common. In control animals, for example, males may exhibit high activity whilst females from the same litters are of low activity. The sex of the offspring also interacts with prenatal treatments to produce differential effects in males and females: prenatal X-irradiation has a more pronounced adverse effect on learning behaviour in female offspring than in males (WERBOFF *et al.*, 1962). Interactions between sex of offspring and postnatal rearing conditions are also found (ADER and CONKLIN, 1963; MEIER and SHULTZMAN, 1968). It is therefore important that results from the two sexes be separated in the analysis of results from behavioural teratology tests, otherwise effects may be masked.

Postnatal Assessment

There are a number of methods by which the effects of potential behavioural teratogens may be examined. These should not be thought of as competitive but as complementary and the choice depends largely on the expertise and experience of the experimenter. Roughly, they can be classified as follows:

1. The Anatomical method — this utilises measurement of brain weight, morphology, detailed microscopic and electron-microscopic studies.
2. The Behavioural method — an approach traditionally used by the psychologists and animal behaviourists. This has formed the basis for the development of "behavioural profiles" which have achieved such successful results in the field of psychopharmacology.
3. The Biochemical method — based on an increasing knowledge of the chemical basis of central neurotransmission and the modifications which can be induced by psychopharmacological agents.

Examples of the successful use of the anatomical approach are given in Chapter 11, and the others will be discussed below.

Behavioural Tests

Physical and functional development. There are innumerable tests for assessment of postnatal development and behaviour and the selection of tests to be used will depend on the information required. However, without adequate information on the physical and functional development of the offspring, the results of more complex behavioural tests may be misinterpreted. Many factors such as poor vision, olfaction or hearing, defective motor co-ordination, or overreaction to stress will adversely affect animal behaviour in particular types of learning task or exploratory situations. Thus some screening procedure to detect physical and functional deficits must first be used. Assessment of postnatal physical and functional development may include many variables, e. g. body weight, opening of ears and eyes, hair growth, appearance of reflexes, development of the senses of hearing, vision, smell, touch, temperature and pain, muscle tone and strength, motor co-ordination, endocrine status, sexual maturation, blood pressure, heart rate and respiration rate. The timing of normal development of some of these variables has been discussed by FOX (1965, 1966) for the mouse, by TILNEY and KUBIE (1931) for the rat, and both pre- and postnatal development of a variety of mammalian species by ALTMAN and DITTMER (1962). In behavioural teratology testing, using large numbers of offspring, it would be impossible to assess every developmental variable, however, IRWIN (1968) has devised a comprehensive, systematic assessment procedure which may be quickly learned, has good inter- and intra-observer consistency, and requires only 3 min to get 52 items of information on each animal. The system was originally devised for mice but may be easily adapted to other species, including man.

Choice of tests. There are many established tests devised by psychologists for the observation of animal behaviour. Some of these assess the animal's interaction with its environment, for example, locomotor activity, exploratory activity, emotional reactivity, grooming activity, learning and problem-solving, responses to stress and to drugs. Others look at interactions between animals as in play, aggression, sexual behaviour, maternal and paternal behaviour. Clearly, there is no single test which gives a comprehensive behavioural assessment suitable for behavioural teratology testing, and so a battery of tests is preferable and should be chosen having regard to the normal behaviour pattern of the species used. In primates, mother-infant interactions, play, establishment of social hierarchies and problem-solving abilities are predominant. In more solitary species, establishment of territories, involving activity, aggression, defecation and urination, is an important behaviour pattern and small animals will spend much of their waking hours in exploratory activity for food. (BARNETT, 1963, for an excellent introduction to rodent behaviour.)

When deciding the order in which tests are to be carried out it is important to bear in mind the stages of development of the offspring at the time of testing. For example, during the normal course of development of the neonatal rat, activity levels undergo considerable fluctuations (CAMPBELL and MABRY, 1973) and the development of learning and memory occurs postnatally in both the rat and the mouse (CAMPBELL and CAMPBELL, 1962; NAGY and SANDMAN, 1973). Adverse effects apparent in early life may later disappear (THOMPSON, 1957) and so will only be detected by incorporation of repeat testing into the experimental design. It is also important to ensure that all offspring within an experiment are exposed to the same tests in the same order since previous experience will modify their responses and changes in test order may modify the results obtained (LEVINE and BROADHURST, 1963). The animal's responses will also be conditioned by the time of day at which the test is carried out. Waking of animals during their normal sleep period is hardly likely to produce typical behaviour. Nocturnal animals should be tested at night or more conveniently reared under reversed lighting conditions and tested under red light during daytime.

It is desirable to assess animals by as wide a variety of tests as posible but with large numbers this is difficult. The most useful tests are those where several types of behaviour may be observed in a relatively short time, such as the open field test (see below) which contrasts with a time-consuming investigation such as the conditioned avoidance shuttlebox, in which the animals should not be observed whilst performing the test. Hence information on only one variable at a time is obtained. Since there is wide individual variation in animal behaviour, it is essential that large numbers of offspring are tested. Ideally, all individuals from each litter should be tested since, as with structural teratogens, only one or two individuals in a litter may be affected.

Types of test. Tests for activity include the open field (HALL, 1934, 1936), Y-maze (STEINBERG *et al.*, 1961), hole board (BOISSIER and SIMON, 1964) and tunnel board (SHILLITO, 1970), all of which normally require an observer present during the test. Automated methods are also available which permit observations to be made over long periods without the presence of an observer, such as "jiggle" cages, rotating drums and wheels (RILEY and SPINKS, 1958 a), and electronic activity meters which permit monitoring of a single individual within a group (SVENSON and THIEME, 1969). Some of these tests, e. g. the tunnel board, allow the observer to distinguish between simple locomotor activity and the more purposeful exploratory activity, giving useful information about the normality or abnormality of any changes in activity observed. Exploratory activity in novel environments may be influenced by many factors (BARNETT, 1958) but ultimately may be regarded as the net result of the opposing forces of curiosity and drive tending to promote activity, and fear tending to inhibit activity. The conditions under which the test takes place will therefore greatly influence the results and factors such as lighting, noise level and the observer used must be standardised. A number of other behaviour patterns, such as grooming, sniffing, rearing, jumping, freezing, repetitive activity, defecation and urination, may also be observed during activity tests. Most of these tests give some assessment of emotionality. The concept of emotionality is based on observations that in the open field, defecation increases and activity decreases in response to increased light and noise levels. Scoring of these two responses therefore gives a measure of the animal's "emotionality". However, the validity of this concept has recently been questioned in a review of the experimental evidence by ARCHER (1973). Furthermore, one must ensure that the pharmacological actions of drugs under test do not, for example, interfere with normal gut function and so give misleading results if defecation is one of the parameters measured.

Learning, which may be defined as a relatively permanent change in behaviour brought about by previous experience, can be assessed in many different ways. Use has been made of aversive reinforcement techniques, e. g. water-escape mazes, conditioned emotional responses (HUNT, 1961; RILEY and SPINKS, 1958 b), conditioned avoidance of electric shocks (WARNER, 1932; SIDMAN, 1953; RILEY and SPINKS, 1958 b), or positive reinforcement techniques where the animal is rewarded usually with food or water, e. g. T-maze, HEBB-WILLIAMS maze (RABINOVITCH and ROSVOLD, 1951) or lever-pressing tasks. Learning is however influenced by many other factors apart from the so-called "intelligence" of the animal. For example, emotionally reactive strains of rats learn less quickly than non-reactive strains, apparently because freezing and other emotional responses interfere with the response to be learned, particularly when aversive reinforcement is used (BROADHURST and LEVINE, 1963 b).

Similarly, in a positive reinforcement situation, an animal's performance will also depend on the physiological drive to seek the reward. Other influences on learning are discussed elsewhere (Hunt, 1961; Kimble, 1967).

Feeding behaviour, social and sexual behaviour (Barnett, 1963), maternal behaviour (Richards, 1967), aggressive behaviour (Levine *et al.*, 1965; Cook and Kelleher, 1963), experimental neuroses (Hunt, 1961), behavioural and endocrine responses to stressful situations (Brain, 1972) and to drugs (Steinberg, 1964) may all be useful in behavioural teratology testing. As yet, however, there has been little comparative evaluation of the usefulness of the various behavioural tests and there remains much dispute over the interpretation of results from individual tests.

Interpretation of results. As in other fields of toxicology the ability to interpret the results obtained in the foregoing tests depends largely on the skill and experience of the operators. Because of the complexities of the interactions between physical development, maternal influence, environmental factors and behaviour it is worthwhile attempting to define whether any effects observed are primary or secondary. Primary effects would be a result of direct interference with brain development. Secondary effects would be those resulting from effects of the substances tested on the mother and which can be controlled by the fostering procedures described above. Other secondary effects could be for example an interference with hormonal regulation in the offspring producing effects of the type described by Balázs (1972).

A further problem is in the statistical evaluation of the results of tests where effects may be confined to single litters or single pups in litters. Abbey and Howard (1973) have discussed some of the appropriate methods for analysis of such data.

Biochemical Assessment

Although we are still a long way from understanding the relationships between prenatally or neonatally induced modifications in brain anatomy and behaviour, there is an increasing amount of information on the relationships between the activity of certain neurotransmitters and behaviour (Kempf *et al.*, 1974). The development of psychoactive drugs during the past 20 years has emphasised the important role of catecholamines (noradrenaline and dopamine) and of 5-hydroxytryptamine in behaviour and mood. These transmitters play important roles in other aspects of brain function such as locomotor activity and exploratory behaviour (Essman, 1971) and hypothalamic functions such as control of sleep rhythms and gonadotrophin release. One method for examining animals for effects of behavioural teratogens would thus be to see whether any changes could be detected in the levels of activity of neurotransmitters. This may reveal effects which may not be observed during behavioural screening procedures.

In early studies the actual concentrations of the neurotransmitters in either whole brain or specific brain areas were studied. It has since become clear that the results of such studies can be very misleading, since there may be large increases in turnover of transmitters without any change in their concentration. It is impossible to interpret isolated observations of low or high levels of transmitters since these may be affected by changes in synthesis rate, storage capacity, rate of release, rate of metabolism and rate of excretion from the site, and it is necessary to study several of the variables mentioned above for each transmitter, in order to give some idea of the rate of turnover. This can be done by a variety of techniques. Levels of the transmitters and their metabolites may be measured; TONGE (1973 a, 1973 b) showed that the offspring of rats treated with methylamphetamine and chlorpromazine had permanent alterations in the levels of noradrenaline, dopamine and the metabolite normetanephrine, and of 5-hydroxytryptamine (5-HT) and its metabolite 5-hydroxyindoleacetic acid, (5-HIAA), in specific areas. CURZON and his coworkers have shown that in the study of 5-HT turnover it is important to measure as many precursors and metabolites as possible. For example, during stressful procedures in rats which produced no change in total plasma tryptophan or in brain 5-HT concentration, they were able to show marked changes in plasma free (ultra filterable) tryptophan, and in brain tryptophan and 5-HIAA levels. These results indicated that a marked increase in 5-HT turnover had in fact occurred (KNOTT *et al.*, 1973).

Another method of study is to block the metabolism of the transmitters and measure the rate of increase in transmitter concentration in the brain or rate of exit of preformed metabolite. BLISS *et al.* (1972) used this technique with a monoamine oxidase inhibitor to study the turnover of 5-HT in the mouse and rat brain during stress. They also investigated the possibility that changes may have occurred in the rate of transport of the acid metabolite 5-HIAA out of the brain by preinjections of probenecid which blocks the active transport of this compound from cerebro-spinal fluid via the choroid plexus. Similar techniques have been used to study the metabolism of noradrenaline and dopamine in the brain. KELLOGG and LUNDBORG (1973) analysed the rate of disappearance of noradrenaline and dopamine in the developing rat brain by inhibition of the rate limiting enzymes in the synthetic pathway. This technique may give information on changes in the release and metabolism of the transmitters and has been used by LUNDBORG and his coworkers to demonstrate that noradrenaline containing neurones become functional at an earlier age than the dopaminergic neurones in both rats and rabbits (ENGEL *et al.*, 1974).

Other techniques which have been used to study the activity or development of aminergic neurones include histofluorescence (LOIZOU, 1972), measurement of uptake of tritiated amines into specific sites (IVERSEN, 1967) and urinary excretion of catecholamines (BERNET and DENIMAL, 1970). The role of the cholinergic system has been less extensively studied but similar techniques have been used (BROWN and KING, 1971).

Conclusion

There is still no clear conception of what constitutes normal or abnormal behaviour in animals other than man. Thus attempts to extrapolate the results of behavioural teratology tests from animals to man will present just as many problems as do tests for structural teratogens. IRWIN believes that many of the basic units of behaviour as measured by his screening techniques (IRWIN, 1968) are common in different animal species, including man, and if this is so, then inter-species extrapolation might be appropriate. Arguments about the choice of species to be used will also be relevant; the closeness of primate behaviour to that of man versus the difficulties of carrying out reproductive tests in these animals, and the greater number of rodents which may be tested are factors which will need to be considered. However, from the evidence accumulated so far, it can be seen that carefully controlled behavioural teratology tests on any species may reveal the presence of severe behavioural disorders resulting from prenatal influences in otherwise normal individuals.

References

ABBEY, H., HOWARD, E.: Statistical procedure in developmental studies on species with multiple offspring. Dev. Psychobiol. **6,** 329 (1973).

ADER, R., CONKLIN, P. M.: Handling of pregnant rats: effects on emotionality of their offspring. Science **142,** 411 (1963).

ALTMAN, J.: Postnatal neurogenesis and the problem of neural plasticity. Developmental Neurobiology, p. 197, W. A. HIMWICH, Ed. Illinois: C. C. Thomas 1970.

ALTMAN, P., DITTMER, D. S.: Eds. Growth. Washington D.C.: Biological Handbooks, Federation of American Societies for Experimental Biology 1962.

ARCHER, J.: Tests for emotionality in rats and mice: a review. Anim. Behav. **21,** 205 (1973).

ARCHER, J. E., BLACKMAN, D. E.: Prenatal psychological stress and offspring behaviour in rats and mice. Dev. Psychobiol. **4,** 193 (1971).

ARMITAGE, S. G.: The effects of barbiturates on the behaviour of rat offspring as measured on learning and reasoning situations. J. comp. physiol. Psychol. **45,** 146 (1952).

BALÁZS, R.: Hormonal aspects of brain development, The Brain in Unclassified Mental Retardation. p. 61, J. B. CAVANAGH, Ed. Edinburgh and London: Churchill Livingstone 1972.

BARNETT, S. A.: Exploratory behaviour. Brit. J. Psychol. **49,** 289 (1958).

BARNETT, S. A.: A Study in Behaviour. London and Southampton: Methuen & Co. Ltd. 1963.

BERNET, F., DENIMAL, J.: Comparaison de deux lots de rats présentant une émotivité différente. C. R. Soc. Biol. (Paris) **164,** 2543 (1970).

BLISS, E. L., THATCHER, W., AILION, J.: Relationship of stress to brain serotonin and 5-hydroxyindoleacetic acid. J. psychiat. Res. **9,** 71 (1972).

BLOCK, J. B., ESSMAN, W. B.: Growth hormone administration during pregnancy: a behavioural difference in offspring of rats. Nature (Lond.) **205,** 1136 (1965).

BOISSIER, J. R., SIMON, P.: Dissociation de deux composantes dans le comportement d'investigation de la souris. Arch. int. Pharmacodyn. **147,** 372 (1964).

BRAIN, P. F.: Mammalian behaviour and the adrenal cortex — A review. Behav. Biol. **7,** 453 (1972).

BRAZELTON, T. B.: Effect of prenatal drugs on the behaviour of the neonate. Amer. J. Psychiat. **126,** 1261 (1970).

BROADHURST, P. L.: Experiments in psychogenetics: applications of biometrical genetics to the inheritance of behaviour. Experiments in Personality, vol. I, p. 1, H. J. EYSENCK, Ed. London: Routledge & Kegan Paul 1960.

BROADHURST, P. L., LEVINE, S.: Litter size, emotionality and avoidance learning. Psychol. Rep. **12,** 41 (1963 a).

BROADHURST, P. L., LEVINE, S.: Behavioural consistency in strains of rats selectively bred for emotional elimination. Brit. J. Psychol. **54,** 121 (1963 b).

BROWN, C. P., KING, M. G.: Developmental environment: variables important for later learning and changes in cholinergic activity. Dev. Psychobiol. **4,** 275 (1971).

BURCH, P. R. J.: Smoking and pregnancy. Nature (Lond.) **246,** 177 (1973).

BURKE, B. S., BEAL, V. A., KIRKWOOD, S. B., STUART, H. C.: Nutrition studies during pregnancy. Amer. J. Obstet. Gynec. **46,** 38 (1943).

BUTCHER, R. E., BRUNNER, R. L., ROTH, T., KIMMEL, C. A.: A learning impairment associated with maternal hypervitaminosis-A in rats. Life Sci. **2,** 141 (1970).

BUTCHER, R. E., VOORHEES, C. V., KIMMEL, C. A.: Learning impairment from maternal salicylate treatment in rats. Nature (Lond.) New Biol. **236,** 211 (1972).

BUTLER, N. R., GOLDSTEIN, H.: Smoking in pregnancy and subsequent child development. Brit. med. J. **4**, 573 (1973).

CAMPBELL, B. A., CAMPBELL, E. H.: Retention and extinction of learned fear in infant and adult rats. J. comp. physiol. Psychol. **55**, 1 (1962).

CAMPBELL, B. A., MABRY, P. D.: The role of catecholamines in behavioural arousal during ontogenesis. Psychopharmacologia (Berl.) **31**, 253 (1973).

CARLSON, P. V.: The development of emotional behaviour as a function of didactic mother-young relationships. Ph. D. Thesis. Purdue Univ. (1961).

CLARKE, C. V. H., GORMAN, D., VERNADAKIS, A.: Effects of prenatal administration of psychotropic drugs on behaviour of developing rats. Dev. Psychobiol. **3**, 225 (1970).

CLENDINNEN, B. G., EAYRS, J. T.: The anatomical and physiological effects of prenatally administered somatotrophin on cerebral development in rats. J. Endocr. **22**, 183 (1961).

COOK, L., KELLEHER, R. T.: Effects of drugs on behaviour. Ann. Rev. Pharmacol. **3**, 205 (1963).

COYLE, J. T., WENDER, P., LIPSKY, A.: Avoidance conditioning in different strains of rats: neurochemical correlates. Psychopharmacologia (Berl.) **31**, 25 (1973).

DENENBERG, V. H., ROSENBERG, K. M.: Nongenetic transmission of information. Nature (Lond.) **216**, 549 (1967).

DENENBERG, V. H., WHIMBEY, A. E.: Behaviour of adult rats is modified by the experiences their mothers had as infants. Science **142**, 1192 (1963).

DESMOND, M. M., RUDOLPH, A. J., HILL, R. M., CLAGHORN, J. L., DREESEN, P. R., BURGDOFF, I.: Behavioural alterations in infants born to mothers on psychoactive medication during pregnancy. Congenital Mental Retardation, p. 235, G. FARRELL, Ed. Austin and London: University of Texas Press 1969.

DISPENSA, J., HORNBECK, R. T.: Can intelligence be improved by prenatal endocrine therapy? J. Psychol. **12**, 209 (1941).

DOBBING, J.: Later development of the brain and its vulnerability. Scientific Foundations of Paediatrics, p. 565, J. A. DAVIS, J. DOBBING, Eds. London: William Heinemann Medical Books Ltd. 1974.

DOBBING, J., SMART, J. L.: Early undernutrition, brain development and behaviour. Ethology and Development, p. 16, S. A. BARNETT, Ed. London: William Heinemann Medical Books Ltd. 1973.

DUDGEON, J. A.: Chairman's summary. Intrauterine Infections, Ciba Foundation Symposium No. 10 (new series), p. 200, Amsterdam: Excerpta Medica 1973.

EBBS, J. H., BROWN, A., TISDALL, F. F., MOYLE, W. J., BELL, M.: The influence of improved prenatal nutrition upon the infant. Canad. med. Ass. J. **46**, 6 (1942).

ENGEL, J., AHLENIUS, S., BROWN, R., LUNDBORG, P.: Behavioural effects in offspring of nursing mothers given neuroleptic drugs. Experimental model systems in toxicology and their significance in man. Proc. Eur. Soc. Study of Drug Toxicity, vol. XV, p. 20, W. A. M. DUNCAN, Ed. Amsterdam: Excerpta Medica 1974.

ESSMAN, W. B.: Isolation-induced behavioural modification: some neurochemical correlates. Brain Development and Behaviour, p. 265, M. B. STERMAN, D. J. MCGINTY, A. M. ADINOLFI, Eds. New York and London: Academic Press 1971.

FERREIRA, A. J.: Emotional factors in prenatal environment. J. nerv. ment. Dis. **141**, 108 (1965).

FITZHUGH, O. G.: Reproduction tests. Modern Trends in Toxicology, p. 75, E. BOYLAND, R. GOULDING, Eds. London: Butterworths 1968.

FLECK, D. G.: The problem of congenital toxoplasmosis. Intrauterine Infections, Ciba Foundation Symposium No. 10 (new series), p. 45. Amsterdam, Excerpta Medica 1973.

FOX, M. W.: Reflex-ontogeny and behavioural development of the mouse. Anim. Behav. **13**, 234 (1965).

FOX, M. W.: Neuro-behavioural ontogeny: a synthesis of ethological and neurophysiological concepts. Brain Res. **2**, 3 (1966).

FURCHTGOTT, E., ECHOLS, M.: Activity and emotionality in pre- and neonatally X-irradiated rats. J. comp. physiol. Psychol. **51**, 541 (1958).

FURCHTGOTT, E., ECHOLS, M., OPENSHAW, J. W.: Maze learning in pre- and neonatally X-irradiated rats. J. comp. physiol. Psychol. **51**, 178 (1958).

Gauron, E. F., Rowley, V. N.: Cross-generational effects resulting from an early maternal chronic drug experience. Eur. J. Pharmacol. **15**, 171 (1971).
Gauron, E. F., Rowley, V. N.: Effects on offspring behaviour of parental early drug experience and cross-fostering. Psychopharmacologia (Berl.) **30**, 269 (1973).
Hale, F.: Pigs born without eyeballs. J. Hered. **24**, 105 (1933).
Hall, C. S.: Emotional behaviour in the rat. I. Defecation and urination as measures of individual differences in emotionality. J. comp. Psychol. **18**, 385 (1934).
Hall, C. S.: Emotional behaviour in the rat. III. The relationship between emotionality and ambulatory activity. J. comp. Psychol. **22**, 345 (1936).
Harned, B. K., Hamilton, H. C., Borrus, J. C.: The effect of bromide administration to pregnant rats on the learning ability of offspring. Amer. J. med. Sci. **200**, 846 (1940).
Harned, B. K., Hamilton, H. C., Cole, B. B.: The effect of administration of sodium bromide to pregnant rats on the learning ability of the offspring. II. Maze test. J. Pharmacol. exp. Ther. **82**, 215 (1944).
Harrel, R. F., Woodyard, E., Gates, A. E.: The effects of mothers diets on the intelligence of offspring: A study of the influence of vitamin supplementation of the diets of pregnant and lactating women on the intelligence of their children. New York: Teachers College, Columbia University 1955.
Hoffeld, D. R., McNew, J., Webster, R. L.: Effect of tranquillising drugs during pregnancy on activity of offspring. Nature (Lond.) **218**, 357 (1968).
Hunt, H. F.: Methods for studying the behavioural effects of drugs. Ann. Rev. Pharmacol. **1**, 125 (1961).
Irwin, S.: Comprehensive observation assessment: 1 a. Systematic quantitative procedure for assessing the behavioural and physiologic state of the mouse. Psychopharmacologia (Berl.) **13**, 222 (1968).
Iversen, L. L.: The Uptake and Storage of Noradrenaline in Sympathetic Nerves. Cambridge: Cambridge University Press 1967.
Joffe, J. M.: Prenatal Determinants of Behaviour. Vol. 7, International Series of Monographs in Experimental Psychology. Oxford: Pergamon Press 1969.
Kellogg, C., Lundborg, P.: Inhibition of catecholamine synthesis during ontogenic development. Brain Res. **61**, 321 (1973).
Kempf, E., Greilsamer, J., Mack, G., Mendel, P.: Correlation of behavioural differences in three strains of mice with differences in brain amines. Nature (Lond.) **247**, 483 (1974).
Kimble, G. A.: Foundations of Conditioning and Learning. Century Psychology Series. New York: Appleton-Century-Crofts 1967.
Knott, P. J., Joseph, M. H., Curzon, G.: Effects of food deprivation and immobilisation on tryptophan and other amino acids in rat brain. J. Neurochem. **20**, 249 (1973).
Křeček, J.: The theory of critical development periods and postnatal development of endocrine functions. The Biopsychology of Development, p. 233, E. Tobach, L. R. Aronson, E. Shaw, Eds. New York: Academic Press 1971.
Levine, S., Broadhurst, P. L.: Genetic and ontogenetic determinants of behaviour. II. Effects of infantile stimulation on adult emotionality and learning in selected strains of rats. J. comp. physiol. Psychol. **56**, 423 (1963).
Levine, S., Diakow, C. A., Barsel, G. E.: Interstrain fighting in male mice. Anim. Behav. **13**, 52 (1965).
Levine, S., Haltmeyer, G. C., Karas, G. G., Denenberg, V. H.: Physiological and behavioural effects of infantile stimulation. Physiol. Behav. **2**, 55 (1967).
Levinson, B.: Effects of fetal irradiation on learning. J. comp. physiol. Psychol. **45**, 140 (1952).
Loizou, L. A.: The postnatal ontogeny of monoamine-containing neurons in the central nervous system of the rat. Brain Res. **40**, 395 (1972).
Lore, R., Avis, H.: Effects of auditory stimulation and litter size upon subsequent emotional behaviour in the rat. Dev. Psychobiol. **2**, 212 (1970).
Marshall, W. C.: The clinical impact of intrauterine rubella. Intrauterine Infections, Ciba Foundation Symposium No. 10 (new series) p. 3. Amsterdam: Excerpta Medica 1973.
Meier, G. W., Schultzman, L. H.: Mother-infant interactions and experimental manipulations: confounding or misidentification? Dev. Psychobiol. **1**, 141 (1968).

MILLER, R. W.: How environmental effects in child health are recognised. Pediatrics **53**, 792 (1974).

MONEY, J.: Prenatal hormones and intelligence: a possible relationship. Impact Sci. Soc. **21**, 285 (1971).

NAGASAWA, H., YANAI, R., KIKUYAMA, S.: Irreversible inhibition of pituitary prolactin and growth hormone secretion and of mammary gland development in mice by monosodium glutamate administered neonatally. Acta endocr. (Kbh.) **75**, 249 (1974).

NAGY, Z. M., SANDEMAN, N. M.: Development of learning and memory of T-maze training in neonatal mice. J. comp. physiol. Psychol. **83**, 19 (1973).

NEWTON, G., LEVINE, S.: Eds. Early Experience and Behaviour. Illinois: Thomas Springfield 1968.

OLNEY, J. W.: Brain lesions, obesity, and other disturbances in mice treated with monosodium glutamate. Science **164**, 719 (1969).

OLNEY, J. W., SHARPE, L. G.: Brain lesions in an infant rhesus monkey treated with monosodium glutamate. Science **166**, 386 (1969).

ORNOY, A., HOROWITZ, A.: Postnatal effects of maternal hypercorticism on skeletal development in newborn rats. Teratology **6**, 153 (1972).

PAN AMERICAN HEALTH ORGANISATION: Nutrition, the nervous system and behaviour. Washington: Pan American Health Organisation (World Health Organisation), Scientific Publication No. 251, 1972.

POSWILLO, D. E., SOPHER, D., MITCHELL, S. J., COXON, D. T., CURTIS, R. F., PRICE, K. R.: Further investigation into the teratogenic potential of imperfect potatoes. Nature (Lond.) **244**, 367 (1973).

PRIESTNALL, R.: The effects of litter size and post-weaning isolation or grouping on adult emotionality in C3H mice. Dev. Psychobiol. **6**, 217 (1973).

RABINOVITCH, M. S., ROSVOLD, M. E.: A closed-field intelligence test for rats. Canadian J. Psychol. **5**, 122 (1951).

RICHARDS, I. D. G.: Congenital malformations and environmental influences in pregnancy. Brit. J. prev. soc. Med. **23**, 218 (1969).

RICHARDS, M. P. M.: Maternal behaviour in rodents and lagomorphs. Advances in Reproductive Physiology, vol. 2, p. 53, A. MCLAREN, Ed. London: Academic Press 1967.

RILEY, H., SPINKS, A.: Biological assessment of tranquillisers, Part I. J. Pharm. Pharmacol. **10**, 657 (1958 a).

RILEY, H., SPINKS, A.: Biological assessment of tranquillisers, Part II. J. Pharm. Pharmacol. **10**, 721 (1958 b).

ROBSON, J. M., SULLIVAN, F. M.: Teratology. Modern Trends in Toxicology, p. 86, E. BOYLAND, R. GOULDING, Eds. London: Butterworths 1968.

ROSENZWEIG, M. R.: Effects of environment on development of brain and behaviour. The Biopsychology of Development, p. 303, E. TOBACH, L. ARONSON, E. SHAW, Eds. New York: Academic Press 1971.

RUGH, R.: Low levels of X-irradiation and the early mammalian embryo. Amer. J. Roentgenol. **87**, 559 (1962).

SARA, V. R., LAZARUS, L.: Prenatal action of growth hormone on brain and behaviour. Nature (Lond.) **250**, 257 (1974).

SCHAPIRO, S.: Hormonal and environmental influences on rat brain development and behaviour. Brain Development and Behaviour, p. 307, M. B. STERMAN, D. J. MCGINTY, A. M. ADINOLFI, Eds. New York and London: Academic Press 1971.

SEITZ, P. F. D.: Effect of litter size during infancy upon adult behaviour in the rat. Amer. J. Psychiat. **110**, 916 (1954).

SHILLITO, E. E.: A method for investigating the effects of drugs on the exploratory behaviour in mice. Brit. J. Pharmacol. **40**, 113 (1970).

SIDMAN, M.: Avoidance conditioning with brief shock and no exteroceptive warning signal. Science **118**, 157 (1953).

SJODEN, P., SODERBERG, U.: Sex-dependent effects of prenatal 2-4-5 trichlorophenoxy-acetic acid on rats' open field behaviour. Physiol. Behav. **9**, 357 (1972).

SPARBER, S. B.: Effects of drugs on the biochemical and behavioural responses of developing organisms. Fed. Proc. **31**, 74 (1972).

Sparber, S. B., Shideman, F. E.: Prenatal administration of reserpine: effect upon hatching, behaviour, and brain stem catecholamines of the young chick. Dev. Psychobiol. **1**, 236 (1968).

Spyker, S. M., Sparber, S. B., Goldberg, A. M.: Subtle consequences of methylmercury exposure: Behavioural deviations in offspring of treated mothers. Science **177**, 621 (1972).

Steinberg, H.: Ed. Animal Behaviour and Drug Action. Ciba Foundation Symposium. London: J. & A. Churchill 1964.

Steinberg, H., Rushton, R., Tinson, C.: Modification of the effects of an amphetamine-barbiturate mixture by the past experience of rats. Nature (Lond.) **192**, 533 (1961).

Stott, D. H.: Physical and mental handicaps following a disturbed pregnancy. Lancet **I**, **1957**, 1006.

Svensson, T. H., Thieme, G.: An investigation of a new instrument to measure motor activity of small animals. Psychopharmacologia (Berl.) **14**, 157 (1969).

Thompson, W. R.: Influence of prenatal maternal anxiety on emotionality in young rats. Science **125**, 698 (1957).

Thompson, W. R., Olian, S.: Some effects on offspring behaviour of maternal adrenalin injection during pregnancy in three inbred mouse strains. Psychol. Rep. **8**, 87 (1961).

Thompson, W. R., Watson, J., Charlesworth, W. R.: The effects of prenatal maternal stress on offspring behaviour in rats. Psychol. Monogr. **76**, No. 38 (1962).

Tilney, F., Kubie, L. S.: Behaviour in its relation to development of brain. Bull. neurol. Inst. N.Y. **1**, 229 (1931).

Tonge, S. R.: Permanent alterations in catecholamine concentrations in discrete areas of brain in the offspring of rats treated with methylamphetamine and chlorpromazine. Brit. J. Pharmacol. **47**, 425 (1973 a).

Tonge, S. R.: Permanent alterations in 5-hydroxyindole concentrations in discrete areas of rat brain produced by the pre- and neonatal administration of methylamphetamine and chlorpromazine. J. Neurochem. **20**, 625 (1973 b).

Warner, L. H.: The association span of the white rat. J. genet. Psychol. **41**, 57 (1932).

Wehmer, F., Porter, R. H., Scales, B.: Premating and pregnancy stress in rats affects behaviour of grand pups. Nature (Lond.) **227**, 622 (1970).

Werboff, J.: Effects of prenatal administration of tranquillisers on maze learning ability. Amer. Psychologist **17**, 397 (1962).

Werboff, J., Gottlieb, J. S.: Drugs in pregnancy: Behavioural teratology. Obstet. Gynec. Surv. **18**, 420 (1963).

Werboff, J., Gottlieb, J. S., Dembicki, E. L., Havlena, J.: Postnatal effect of antidepressant drugs administered during gestation. Exp. Neurol. **3**, 542 (1961 a).

Werboff, J., Gottlieb, J. S., Havlena, J., Word, T. J.: Behavioural effects of prenatal drug administration in the white rat. Pediatrics **27**, 318 (1961).

Werboff, J., Havlena, J.: Postnatal behavioural effects of tranquillisers administered to the gravid rat. Exp. Neurol. **6**, 263 (1962).

Werboff, J., Havlena, J., Sikov, M. R.: Effects of prenatal X-irradiation on activity, emotionality, and maze learning ability in the rat. Radiat. Res. **16**, 441 (1962).

Wilson, J. G., Warkany, J.: Teratology Principles and Techniques. Chicago: University of Chicago Press 1965.

Young, R. D.: Effect of prenatal drugs and neonatal stimulation on later behaviour. J. comp. physiol. Psychol. **58**, 309 (1964).

Young, R. D.: Effects of differential early experiences and neonatal tranquillisation on later behaviour. Psychol. Rep. **17**, 675 (1965).

Zimmerberg, B., Charap, A. D., Glick, S. D.: Behavioural effects of *in utero* administration of morphine. Nature (Lond.) **247**, 376 (1974).

7. Teratological Investigations in Laboratory Primates: Why, When and How to Use Them

D. E. Poswillo and I. R. Phillips

With 3 Figures

Why Primates?

The value of using laboratory animals to predict the teratogenicity of drugs or chemicals in man is not yet certain. Nonetheless a great deal of time and money is devoted annually to exercises of this kind. For reasons of economy and availability laboratory rodents and lagomorphs are the most favoured species for this work, and the susceptibility of these lower mammals to the teratogenic effects of a large number of compounds in common use is undisputed. A dilemma arises when attempts are made to assess whether evidence of teratogenicity in rats, mice, hamsters and rabbits has any special relevance to similar situations in man. Many attempts have been made to resolve these problems of extrapolation (WHO, 1967); it has been argued, for example, that on the basis of phylogenetic similarity, simian primates should be employed for the screening of compounds that may be teratogenic in man. While such reasoning may appear logical, there is little reliable data, from scientific investigations, to confirm or deny this suggestion (Tuchmann-Duplessis, 1972).

While the characteristic inverted yolk sac placenta found in rodents and lagomorphs is accepted as being vastly different in function from the system of early placental nutrition in simian primates and man, it remains to be determined whether the greater permeability of the yolk sac placenta to chemical teratogens does not provide an added measure of sensitivity to tests designed to detect weak teratogenic action. On the other hand, however, there exists an obvious danger in using as a routine an oversensitive animal test system. Drugs and chemicals of great potential value to man may be placed on a restricted or prohibited list, or not developed because they fail to pass a standard test for teratogenicity. There also exists another hazard which reflects the opposite side of the coin; there is a danger that the species chosen, be it common or exotic, fails to respond to a drug that is later shown to be teratogenic in man. While it has often been said that the effects of thalidomide were not revealed in the laboratory animals in which it was tested, there is ample evidence to suggest that in tests on mice a high degree of toxicity had been revealed (Somers, 1963). If additional tests had been conducted at that stage, over realistic dose ranges, it is most probable that teratogenicity would have been foreseen.

It seems unlikely, therefore, that this second hazard, that of inadvertently overlooking an agent which is teratogenic in man, would occur when adequate routine tests had been carried out in lower laboratory mammals at dose ranges which are proportional to the embryonic (rather than maternal) LD50. The problem

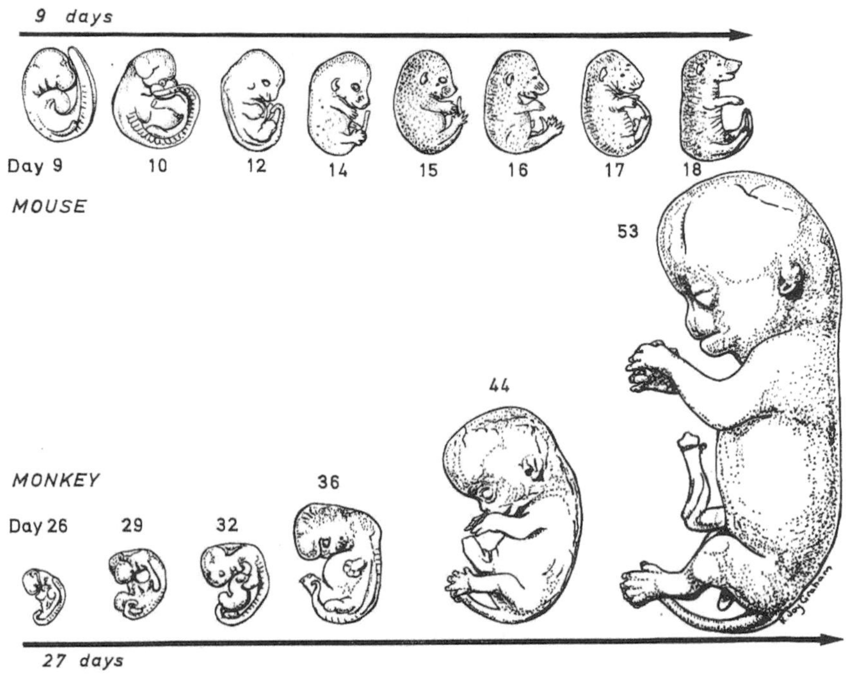

Fig. 1. The temporal scale of morphogenesis in the mouse compared with that in the M. irus monkey

of assessing the teratogenicity in man of new or suspected compounds appears, therefore, to be more one of interpretation of findings than of testing technique; of discerning from studies in laboratory rodents the relevance of a positive finding, of teratogenic activity. It revolves around the necessity to distinguish between the theoretical and the actual risk to the pregnant human being. In other words, does the agent shown to be of low teratogenicity in rat, mouse, hamster or rabbit induce dysmorphogenesis in the offspring of even the most genetically susceptible woman when taken over the teratogenosensitive period? The answer to this problem is not readily apparent from analysis of data from lower animal studies. This difficulty has led to the statement from the WHO (1967) that "there is urgent need for the provision of a suitable non-human model for research in teratology". General statements of this nature often provoke "logical" suggestions such as "because there is in man and monkey close correspondence between the metabolic patterns" (SMITH, 1968), therefore there is an obvious case for teratologic testing in non-human primates. While superficially logical, it is by no means certain that there are major or distinct differences at embryonic level between any of the species used for toxicological or teratological research. The anatomical differences in the early somite stages of rat, monkey and man are all comparatively small; it is only in the later stages of organogenesis that distinctive differences appear.

There is, however, one important aspect of simian primate morphogenesis which is seldom discussed, but of great significance to the problem of teratological testing. The temporal scale of morphogenesis in the monkey is distinctly similar to man and vastly different from that in lower mammals (Fig. 1). When the similarity of patterns of placental transfer, methods of maternal metabolism, and temporal scales of morphogenesis are considered together there emerges a significant case for serious consideration of the simian primate as a special model for malformation research. In this chapter it is intended to describe, on the basis of an 8 year experience with non-human primates, their advantages and disadvantages in this branch of medical research.

Which Primates should be Used?

A number of primate species have been investigated in recent years for suitability for teratological studies. Those which have commanded especial attention are M. mulatta, M. fascicularis, M. fuscata, M. radiata, M. arctoides, C. aethiops, P. cynocephalus, and C. jacchus. Limited studies have also been carried out on the prosimian Galago crassicaudatus. Wilson *et al.* have made a considerable contribution to the study and evaluation of teratogens in simians, and their reviews (1972, 1974) should be read by all contemplating studies of this nature.
All simian and prosimian species differ in certain small respects from each other and from man; notably there are differences in implantation, placentation, placental morphology, temporal scales of gestation and reproductive endocrinology. Nevertheless, as adequate baseline data are obtained for each of the species investigated, it is likely that they will come to be regarded as more closely comparable to man than any of the other species commonly used in teratological research. Although our present knowledge is far from complete on many points, it is likely that the eventual differences between man in general and monkeys in general will be no greater than the differences in susceptibility to birth defects or disease which are found in present human populations. It is unlikely that even if human testing for suspected teratogenicity became possible (and morally and ethically the possibility at present is remote) that all of the problems with the evaluation of teratogenic potential could be solved in reasonable time. Studies in the field of experimental teratology in humans, are even more unlikely. It remains essential therefore to explore the possibility of developing an economical and readily available suitable primate model for the study of teratogenesis.
Yet all simian species are threatened with rapidly diminishing populations in their natural environment even to the point of extinction in some areas. For many years the rhesus monkey has been the laboratory primate of choice; it is no longer readily available. The warnings of the conservationists are clear, and must be heeded. Primates are too costly, too precious, and too rare to be used for studies of large scale or a frivolous nature. The message for teratology is equally clear; primates should be chosen with great care and reserved for exceptional investigations only.
In choosing the most suitable primate model, attention should be paid to several important factors, some of which will become more obvious after reading the fol-

lowing sections on where and how to use them. Obviously the laboratory facilities available will influence the size and character of primate to be used; so also will the cost of the agent, be it drug or chemical, which is to be employed. When the compound is costly, the lower the body weight of the mature animal the smaller the amount of drug used to provide a suitable dose/body weight ratio, and the lower the overall cost. Furthermore, where twin studies or multiple progeny studies are desired, consideration will be given to the species known to produce multiple births. These are practical points, and although obvious, do to a large extent, determine the choice of species. There are, however, other more fundamental matters which should also be considered, the most important of which is metabolic similarity to man.

From a solely evolutionary point of view, no New World monkey is considered close to man, close to Old World monkeys, or necessarily even close to New World monkeys of other genera (WASHBURN and HARDING, 1970). The resemblances between New and Old World monkeys and man are due to the evolution, along parallel lines, of similar functional and anatomical features; because of this, the closeness of their metabolic relationship to man is capricious and varies from species to species, without following the pattern one might expect from their evolutionary hierarchy. DICZFALUSY (1972) who reviewed certain aspects of drug metabolism in laboratory animals and primates and compared them with man, remarked on these inconsistencies. On the other hand, studies of the basic correspondence of serum albumins (SARICH and WILSON, 1966) and the metabolism of quinic acid to hippuric acid supported the line of man followed by great apes, Old World monkey, New World monkeys, and prosimians in descending evolutionary order.

The metabolism of phenyl acetic acid in simian primates (JAMES *et al.*, 1972) suggests that the marmoset has an exceptional place in the scale, closer to the higher apes than M. fascicularis or M. mulatta. There is still some doubt about comparative plasma histaminase activity in various non-human primates; studies by PETERS and GORDON (1968) currently disputed, suggest that New World monkeys as a group are more similar to man than the great apes, Old World monkeys or prosimians. When the metabolism of steroids in pregnancy is studied, however, SHACKELTON and MITCHELL (1975) believe that primates other than the gorilla and chimpanzee differ so much from man that it is almost impossible to extrapolate from these animals to man with respect to steroid metabolism. The exception in their study was the marmoset which, while differing in steroid metabolism from man, was more closely comparable than the macaque or the baboon.

Until a great deal more is known of the general metabolic and toxicologic reactions of the various species of laboratory primates, the choice will remain somewhat arbitrary. For reasons of economy, size, availability and fecundity the common cotton-eared marmoset, which is readily adapted to small-animal facilities, has much to recommend it for general teratological investigations.

When should Primates be Used for Teratological Research?

Malformation research in the laboratory falls into two broad categories

a) Teratological screening,

b) Experimental teratology.

In both of these groups there arise situations where non-human primate models can be of great value to the scientist. The situations will be considered separately.

a) The screening of new or suspected compounds for teratogenic activity. Under most circumstances routine screening for teratogenicity can be conducted on at least two of the species rat, mouse, hamster or rabbit. When tests on two of these species give no cause for concern then it would not appear essential for further tests to be conducted in the primate. However, occasions will arise, when, after well designed and conducted tests on adequate numbers of rodents and rabbits (see Chapter 8) the results of trials in lower mammals are unsatisfactory or difficult to interpret. On such occasions there is a clear indication for a teratological study in another species, and especial consideration should be given to the selection of a laboratory primate. At this stage of the investigation sufficient data should be available from the pilot studies to enable an accurate estimate of the likely teratogenic dose range to be tested in the primate. WILSON (1971) has proposed an admirable and practical method for producing a reasonably comprehensive test of embryotoxicity in 30 pregnant monkeys based on the examination of one conceptus per treated female. Although there are those that argue that the number of tests used for statistical evaluation should be the total treated females rather than the total offspring, little would be lost and something gained by using a species of primate e. g. marmoset, in a Wilson-type test where the incidence of multiple births would more than double the number of offspring examined for abnormality (POSWILLO *et al.*, 1972). There is a longer span of morphogenetic activity in the primate than in the rat. Because of this it would appear reasonable to dose the monkey with the test material on alternate days rather than daily throughout the teratogenosensitive period. In this way the problems of excessive induction or inhibition of drug-metabolizing enzymes are probably avoided, yet realistic blood levels of the agent maintained. In addition, the stress associated with the dosing procedure is reduced to a minimum; this is of particular importance when primates of low body weight are employed. Resistance to stressful situations appears less in the marmoset, for example, than in the macaque, and less in the macaque than in the baboon.

Embryotoxicity in the primate may manifest itself in different ways. Known toxic teratogens such as thalidomide, which produces malformations in the primate closely comparable with those in man (Fig. 2), can effect intrauterine absorption or abortion in about one third of treated animals at dose levels which induce deformity in those embryos that survive to term. These phenomena are readily recognised during regular examination of the uterus by palpation. Following such events the affected animal can be released from the experiment. A proportion of embryos in the treated series will show abnormal development when examined at 100+ days of development; occasionally no gross anatomical changes are observed yet obvious growth retardation is present. At this lesser end of the scale, where gross changes are minimal, experiments can be designed to permit neonatal examination of the experimental animals, and continuing comparison with control subjects, until sexual maturity is reached (POSWILLO *et al.*, 1973). Delivery of primate fetuses by Caesarean section and hand-rearing to six months of age provides a reliable system for comparative studies on the effects of test compounds on growth, development, and maturation.

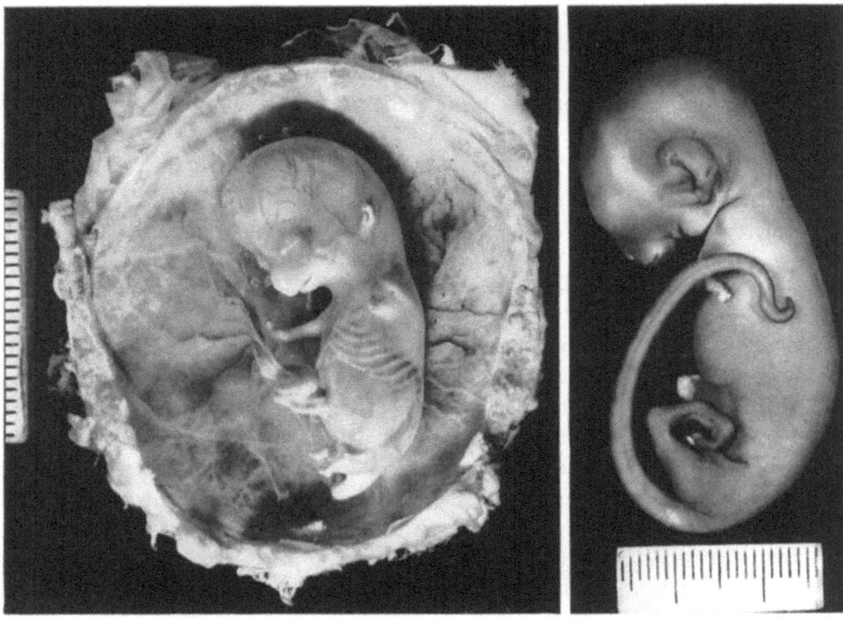

(a) (b)

Fig. 2. (a) M. irus fetus of 60 days showing otomandibular and appendicular defects induced by maternal thalidomide ingestion between days 20 and 30 of embryonic development. (b) Thalidomide-induced defects in marmoset fetus of 120 days

In the routine screening of compounds for teratogenicity the results from a standard series of tests may appear ambiguous or inconsistent; negative results in one species may conflict seriously with positive results in another species of lower mammal. Under such circumstances it would again seem desirable to extend the tests to laboratory primates, not so much in the expectation that a clear and unequivocal explanation of the differences in behaviour of the drug in the lower species can be obtained but in the hope that the effects of the compound on an embryo developing at much the same rate as man can be determined. There is considerable evidence that minor degrees of damage in the embryo can be repaired without permanent effects on normal morphogenesis; "catch-up" growth and differentiation can occur after repair provided that there exists sufficient time for such recovery. When the temporal span of morphodifferentiation is condensed into a short period two factors can upset the reliability of a drug-screening system. First, damage, inflicted by the teratogen may be sufficiently severe to be beyond the capacity of the mechanism to repair in the limited time available before morphodifferentiation is "switched-off". Examples of this phenomenon are seen in cases of induced focal haematoma in the mouse (Poswillo, 1975 b). When morphodifferentiation is spread out over many days, the capacity for repair without blemish i. e. normal development after teratogenic insult, becomes much greater.

Second, when morphodifferentiation takes place at speed, as it does in the rat and mouse, it is possible that a target-specific teratogen (and it is probable that such exist, POSWILLO, 1975 a) will miss the objective because of small errors in the time of arrival at the site of action. FRAZER (1968) believes that many of the common malformations are caused by threshold factors which are capable of disorganising morphogenetic movements. That being so, then the more rapidly the developing system moves towards complete differentiation the better the chance of escaping disorganisation by a time-specific teratogen. Where time/dose relationships are critical for the induction of deformity, slow rate morphogenesis which exposes the system to a longer period of risk may provide optimum conditions for the detection of weak teratogenicity.

Conversely, when morphogenesis is complete in a few days, agents which are metabolised only slowly by the mother may act on many different embryological systems before they are eliminated. In this way multiple malformations may be induced in the embryo with a rapid growth rate whereas a similar agent acting in the slow-growing primate may have little or no effect on morphogenesis.

While the parallels which exist between the metabolism and placentation of the monkey and man may vary, it seems likely that there exists close comparability between the gradients of embryonic development in most simian species and man, at least until the stage of closure of the palate about day 48 of development. Thus by comparison with rat, mouse and rabbit the similarities between man and monkey far outweigh the differences when their values as models for teratogenic testing are compared. There is a good case, based on present knowledge, for the investigation of special situations in teratological screening in selected laboratory primates, especially when the results from rodent and rabbit tests are inconclusive or restrictive. Good drugs and chemicals should not be discarded because of inconclusive tests in animals. But monkeys are scarce and expensive to maintain. It is not reasonable to expect that they could be used for routine drug screening or in sufficient quantities to detect, with assurance, marginal teratogenic risks. There is some hope that in future simple and inexpensive animal models may be developed to detect some of the lesser environmental agents incriminiated in polygenic multifactorial malformations (see Chapter 5). Nevertheless there will occasionally arise in the examination of new or suspected drugs, the need for a system of examination that has closer comparability to man than that provided by routine rodent tests. In these exceptional situations the laboratory primate will play a necessary and useful role. As the physiological and pharmacological features of small laboratory primates become better understood, there is the likelyhood that their role in deciding equivocal situations will become much more significant than it is today.

b) Experimental teratology. The laboratory primate has much to offer the experimental teratologist with interests in mechanism studies, the problems of abnormal growth and development induced by birth defects, and the intrauterine correction of dysmorphology (see Chapter 10). Although only a small proportion of the drugs in common use have been positively implicated as human teratogens, there still exists the probability that in a susceptible case, with a familial predisposition to deformity, the cumulative effects of weak teratogens may tip the scale of development beyond the threshold of normality. In such circumstances it may be impossible for man to establish the degree of teratogenic risk for thousands of agents which influence the course of embryonic development. On the brighter side, however, it is likely that many of these environmental teratogens of minor but cumulative effect will precipitate similar or identical pathogenetic mechanisms of malformation. While the number of actual mechanisms of dysmorphogenesis remains unknown, it is likely to be very small by comparison with the number of potential teratogenic agents. That being so it would appear profitable for preventive teratology to ascertain the actual mechanisms which operate in man as a first step towards the ultimate identification of the agents which may initiate them. When such things as molecular structure and biological activity of teratogens have been linked without doubt, the search for like compounds will become scientific and systematic. It seems obvious that the first step in this direction should be the identification of the pathogenetic mechanisms, primary, secondary, and so on, of the known human teratogens which act in a similar fashion in both animal and man. Three such teratogens, thalidomide, androgenic steroids, and ionizing radiations have been shown to act in a similar fashion in monkey and man (Wilson, 1974; Poswillo *et al.*, 1972).

It is surprising that more than ten years after the withdrawal of thalidomide from the market no definitive description of the pathogenetic mechanism of action of this drug has yet been reported. In like manner, while the anatomical defects induced by androgenic steroids in macaque monkeys have been reported in some detail (Wharton and Scott, 1964) no clear description of the pathogenetic mechanism has been reported in the literature. Recent studies on the effects of thalidomide on the developing otomandibular region and the limbs (Poswillo, 1973) have contributed to some understanding of the pathogenesis of these anomalies. By describing the pathogenesis, both the role and the limitations of reconstructive surgery for correction of thalidomide defects has become better understood. There exists a rich field for embryological investigation of the pathogenesis of many more induced malformations in the laboratory primate in order to further our knowledge of spontaneous dysmorphogenesis in man and its therapeutic management.

It is unlikely that studies in the laboratory primate will prove profitable if confined to the investigation of the spontaneous malformations observed in these species. These anomalies occur only rarely in primates in captivity, with a frequency less than that observed in man. An excellent review of both spontaneous and induced defects in non-human primates has been published by Wilson (1972). Dominant inheritance of defects in laboratory primates has not yet been described. There remains great scope for the investigation of stage-by-stage development of deformity in primate models and the effects of malformation on the growth and development of both fetus and neonate. The size, shape and anatomical similarity of the primate embryo commends it for studies of this kind. The developmental horizons in the macaque have been described in detail by Heuser and Streeter (1941), and in the baboon by Hendrickx *et al.* (1971); both show close correspondence to the stages of development in man.

In some primates multiple births are common; when malformation is induced the littermates show differences in dysmorphology comparable with those recorded in human twins. These models are invaluable, both for the study of pathogenesis and for growth and development investigations. In contrast to lower mammals, primate models of human malformations may be reared to maturity. Thus they are suitable for a wide range of studies related to postnatal growth retardation, behavioural deficits, and the rehabilitation of deformity. Primates have the exceptional and additional advantage over lower mammals in such studies of both anatomical and developmental features similar to man. Thus careful extrapolation of research findings becomes a possibility, and warrants the use of expensive and exotic species for laboratory studies designed to relieve the suffering of man.

Where and How should Primates be Used?

The basic principles of animal husbandry relating to the common species of laboratory animals also apply to primates. Simians however, present an additional problem due to the exacting nature of their environmental requirements and also because of their ability to transmit a wide variety of infectious agents to man and other species. The risk from zoonotic diseases has been well documented by PERKINS and O'DONOGHUE (1969) and COID (1972). It is a common misconception that the greatest obstacle to the establishment of a primate colony is the cost of the animals and their accommodation (COHEN, 1971). The purchase price of a monkey is higher than that for many common experimental animals, but in any colony the initial outlay is relatively unimportant compared to the expense of its upkeep i. e. feeding, lighting, cleaning materials, staff salaries, etc. It is of prime importance that the accommodation provided for the larger species of laboratory primate be specifically designed for that purpose and should not be a haphazard conversion of existing premises. The environment required for the New World species should be no less carefully controlled, but their smaller size means that they may be more readily accommodated in an existing laboratory facility. Up to 6 marmosets may be caged in the space occupied by one adult macaque (POSWILLO and RICHARDS, 1972), Fig. 3.
Of the several species available, it is important that the right animal is used in relation to a particular experiment. Macaques and baboons are large animals in the adult state and with few exceptions are difficult to handle without sedation. It has been claimed that M. fuscata and M. arctoides are more tractable than other macaque species. Cercopithecus aethiops, the grivet monkey, has been used by HENDRICKX (1975) but is reportedly a very excitable species. The Callithricidae are small and can be readily handled without sedation. Regardless of the species chosen it is the responsibility of all engaged in research on primates to maintain breeding colonies of the species used, thereby providing some of their own replacement animals and thus reducing further depletion of wild populations.
Teratological experiments demand a species with a high reproductive potential. In their wild state, most female primates undergo a seasonal cycle of sexual activity; regular sexual cycles are followed by periods during which sexual cycles do not occur, or occur infrequently. VALERIO *et al.* (1969) reported marked attenuation of seasonal breeding in M. mulatta following adaptation to a laboratory environment. HENDRICKX and KRAEMER (1971) observed births in Papio spp. in all months of the year with the majority of births occurring during the autumn and winter months. PHILLIPS (1975) noted no breeding season in a closed colony of Callithrix jacchus over a four year period.
The age of sexual maturity and the age at which the first pregnacy occurs are clearly important factors in the choice of an animal model for studies in reproductive biol-

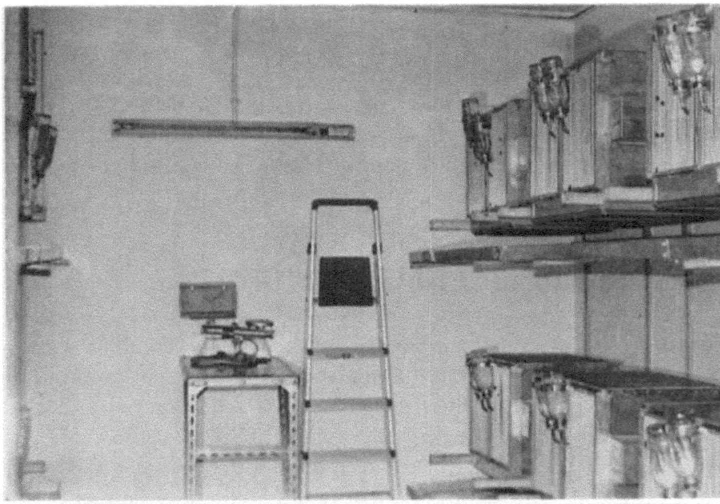

a

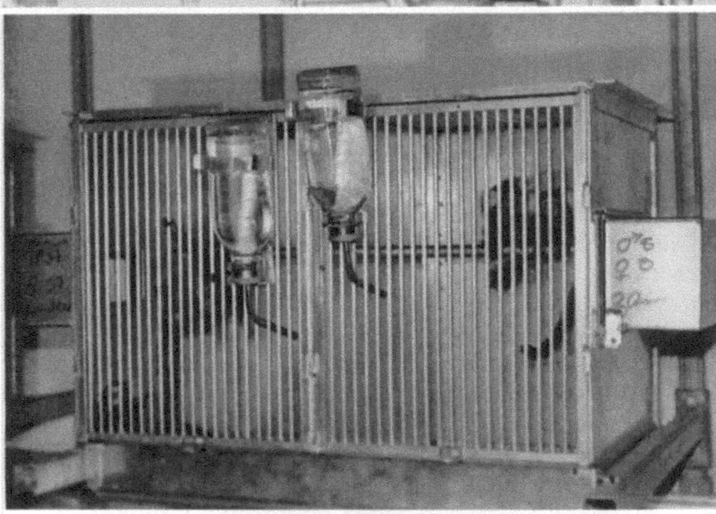

b

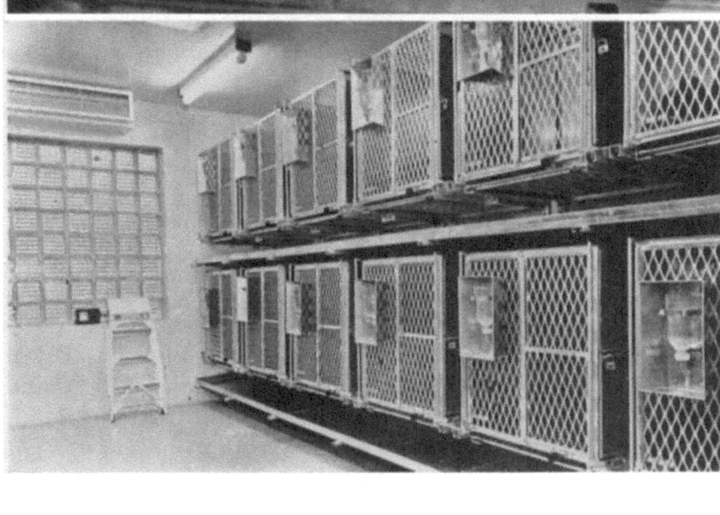

c

ogy. ASANOV (1972) stated that sexual maturity in Papio hamadryas was reached at a mean of 30.1 months. Sexual maturation was reached somewhat earlier in both the rhesus and grivet monkeys. The mean interval length between sexual maturity and the attainment of the first pregnancy was 15 months for rhesus monkeys and 10 months for baboons and grivets. NOMURA *et al.* (1972) gave the average time of the first pregnancy as 55 months for M. fuscata, 46 months for M. irus and 53 months for Papio anubis. The average time of first pregnancy in the RCS colony of Callithrix jacchus is 13$^{1}/_{2}$ months, although two individuals have conceived at 11 months and carried their pregnancies to term.

The mean gestation and ovarian cycle lengths for the four primate species most commonly employed in teratological investigations are given in Table 1.

Table 1

Species	Gestation	Ovarian Cycle	Reference
M. mulatta	165	28	VALERIO *et al.* (1969)
M. fascicularis	165	30.8	DUKELOW *et al.* (1971)
P. cynocephalus	175	33	HENDRICKX and KRAEMER (1971)
C. jacchus	148 ± 4.3	16.4 ± 1.7	HEARN and LUNN (1975)

Marmosets are to some degree a reproductive enigma in that they exhibit neither the conspicuous oestrus cycle of lower species, nor a detectable menstrual cycle characteristic of other primates (PRESLOCK *et al.*, 1973). The lack of overt signs of menstruation or ovulation is therefore a problem with these species when embryos of known gestational age are required. Macaques and baboons follow a menstrual cycle that closely resemble that of the human female and mating periods as short as two hours have enabled HENDRICKX *et al.* (1975) to reduce the variation in the assessment of embryonic age.

A review of the methods of determining ovulation time in macaques has been given by MAHONEY (1975). Ovarian activity can be monitored by determining changes in a) uterine and ovarian size and texture, b) physicochemical properties of cervical mucus, c) intensity of sex skin colouration, d) plasma concentrations of oestradiol, progesterone and luteinising hormone. Definitive evidence of ovulation may be obtained by laparotomy or laparoscopy, recovery of tubal ova, or pregnancy following a single mating.

A variety of methods exist for determining pregnancy in primates. Biological tests utilising the level of chorionic gonadotrophin in the urine can be carried out in most species although they tend to be inaccurate and are laborious to use on a colony

◀ Fig. 3. (a) Cage arrangement suitable for marmoset accommodation in a small laboratory. (b) Individual marmoset cage, as illustrated in Fig. 3 a, showing two conjugal pairs of animals with offspring in units separated by a median division, so that one cage accommodates up to eight animals. (c) Caging arrangements for M. irus monkeys; each cage holds one, or at the most, two animals

basis. Radioimmunoassay techniques have improved the speed and accuracy of hormone evaluation. Bimanual rectal palpation of the uterus and ovaries is commonly used to diagnose pregnancy in large primates and is probably the method of choice for general colony management.

Fertility and parity of a given species are important features in the management of primate colonies for teratological studies. Papio and Macaca spp. are generally monotocous but occasionally twinning occurs. Hendrickx *et al.* (1968) observed four sets of twins out of 730 deliveries in P. cynocephalus and Valerio *et al.* (1969) observed only three cases of twinning in over 900 births in M. mulatta. In the Royal College of Surgeons colony, one set of twins has occurred in 207 pregnancies in M. fascicularis. By contrast, twinning is the rule rather than the exception in marmosets. In the R.C.S. colony of C. jacchus there have been 148 pregnancies where the number of offspring was recorded resulting in 100 sets of twins, 31 triplets and 17 singletons.

Pregnancy may be interrupted by hysterotomy or flushing of tubal ova in Papio and Macaca spp. Hysterotomy may also be performed in the marmoset but flushing of tubal ova has not been recorded in this species. Up to 8 surgical procedures have been conducted in Papio spp. (Hendrickx and Kraemer, 1971) and up to six in C. jacchus (unpublished observations of the authors). The productivity of the R.C.S. colonies of M. fascicularis and C. jacchus is shown in Table 2.

Table 2

Species	Time Scale	Number of Females	Number of Abortions	Number of Hysterotomies	Number of Caesarian Sections	Number of Vaginal Births	Total Preg.
M. fascicularis	$10^1/_2$ yrs.	74	43	52	43	69	207
C. jacchus	$4^1/_2$ yrs.	41	30	85	3	82	200

Pickering (1968) and Wilson (1969) suggested that pre-term hysterotomy affected the subsequent fertility of primates. This does not appear to be true in the two species in the R.C.S. colony. Valerio *et al.* (1969) observed that in M. mulatta most females resume menstruation within the first 45 days after parturition. Hendrickx and Kraemer (1971) stated that the average recycling time in the baboon was 44 days, with a range of 21—67 days. They noted that surgical intervention involving removal of the embryo tended to shorten the recycling time. It is unusual to obtain more than one to two pregnancies per year in the larger primates. A post-partum oestrus occurs in marmosets (Phillips and Grist, 1975) and two to three litters per year may be obtained in these species.

It would be desirable to develop inbred strains of primates such as exist for other laboratory species, but the possibilities of realising this ideal are, at present, remote. It would be true to say that virtually no systematic screening of individuals can be carried out in most instances. Records of multiple generation births, that is, breeding of individuals born only to parents that have themselves been born in captivity, are

not encouraging. The International Zoo Yearbook (1973) recorded the following numbers of full generations born in captivity: C. jacchus, 2; M. fascicularis, 2; M. mulatta, at least 4; Papio cynocephalus, at least 4.
Further intensive study into long-term breeding programmes for primates are required before the research worker can be truly confident of the reproducibility of his results.

Conclusion

The human primate is the most studied animal from almost all biomedical aspects except teratology. This field remains an exception, and is likely to continue to do so. For at least a decade there has been an increasing interest in the selection and use of non-human primates for research into the problems of human reproduction. While many original questions have been answered, there remains no simple solution to the problem of the best animal model for predictive research in developmental pathology.
One can not say yet, with assurance, that simian primates are the best animal models for the study of these problems. Nevertheless much information has been obtained both on the role of primates in this field of research, and the selection of the most appropriate species. It is likely that there will always be subtle differences between optimum animal models and man; scientists who extrapolate from the animal to man will continue to do so with reservation and care.
The difficulties associated with the provision and maintenance of simian primates for laboratory purposes will always restrict their use in medical research. Nonetheless, when carefully selected and used for the investigation of specific problems in the field of teratology, non-human primates can make a unique contribution to our understanding of reproductive processes in man.

References

ASANOV, S. S.: In: The use of non-human primates in research on human reproduction, WHO Symposium, Sukhumi 1971, Eds. E. DICZFALUSY and C. C. STANDLEY, pp. 458—471, Stockholm: Karolinska Institute (1972).

COHEN, B.: The monkey colony at Downe. Ann. roy. Coll. Surg. Engl. 48, 46—53 (1971).

COID, C. R.: Infectious agents and the management of simians in a medical research institute in Medical Primatology, Proc. 3rd Conf. exp. Med. Surg. Primates, Lyon 1972, part III, pp. 39—44. Basel: Karger 1972.

DICZFALUSY, E.: In: The use of non-human primates in research on human reproduction, WHO Symposium, Sukhumi 1971, Eds. E. DICZFALUSY and C. C. STANDLEY, pp. 422—427. Stockholm: Karolinska Institute (1972).

DUKELOW, W. R., HARRISON, R. M., RAWSON, J. M. R., JOHNSON, M. P.: Natural and artificial control of ovulation in non-human primates in Medical Primatology. Proc. 3rd Conf. exp. Med. Surg. Primates, Lyon 1972, part I, pp. 232—236. Basel: Karger 1972.

FRASER, F. C.: Genetic factors in experimental teratology. Congenital Anom. 8, 78—79 (1968).

HEARN, J. P., LUNN, S. F.: The reproductive biology of the marmoset monkey in: Breeding simians for developmental biology Lab. Anim. Handbook 6 Eds. F. T. PERKINS and P. N. O'DONOGHUE, Laboratory Animals Ltd., London, pp. 191—202 (1975).

HENDRICKX, A. G.: Embryology of the Baboon. Chicago and London: University of Chicago Press (1971).

HENDRICKX, A. G., SAWYER, R. M., LASLEY, B., BARNES, R. D.: Comparsion of developmental stages in primates with a note on the detection of ovulation, Lab. Anim. Handbook 6. Eds. F. T. PREKINS and P. N. O'DONOGHUE, Laboratory Animals Ltd., London, pp. 305—315.

HEUSER, C. H., STREETER, G. L.: Development of the macaque embryo, Carnegie Inst. Wash. Pub. 525, Contrib. to Embryol., 29 (1941).

International Zoo Yearbook (1973) vol. **13** Ed. N. DUPLAIX-HALL, Zoological Society of London p. 406.

JAMES, M. O., SMITH, R. L., WILLIAMS, R. T., REIDENBERG, M.: The conjugation of phenylacetic acid in man, sub-human primates and some non-primate species. Proc. roy. Soc. Lond. B. **182**, 25—35 (1972).

MAHONEY, C. J.: Practical aspects of determining early pregnancy, stages of foetal development and imminent parturition in the monkey in Breeding simians for developmental biology, Lab. Anim. Handbook **6**, Eds. F. T. PERKINS and P. N. O'DONOGHUE, Laboratory Animals Ltd., London pp. 261—274 (1975).

NOMURA, T., OHSAWA, N., TAJIMA, Y., TANAKA, T., KOTERA, S., ANDO, A., NIGI, H.: In: The use of non-human primates in research on human reproduction, WHO Symposium, Sukhumi 1971, Eds. E. DICZFALUSY and C. C. STANDLEY, pp. 473—482. Stockholm: Karolinska Institute.

PERKINS, F. T., O'DONOGHUE, P. N.: Eds. Hazards of handling simians Lab. Anim. Handbook **4** Laboratory Animals Ltd., London (1969).

PETERS, J. H., GORDON, G. R.: Histaminase activities in the plasma of sub-human primates and man. Nature (Lond.) **217**, 274—275 (1968).

PHILLIPS, I. R.: Macaque and marmoset monkeys as animal models for the study of birth defects in Breeding simians for developmental biology, Lab. Anim. Handbook **6**, Eds. F. T. PERKINS and P. N. O'DONOGHUE, Laboratory Animals Ltd., London pp. 293—302 (1975).

PHILLIPS, I. R., GRIST, S. G.: The use of transabdominal palpation to determine the course of pregnancy in the marmoset (Callithrix jacchus) J. Reprod. Fert. **43**, 103—108 (1975).

PICKERING, D. E.: Reproduction characteristics in a colony of laboratory confined mulatta macaque monkeys. Folia primat. **8**, 169—179 (1968).

POSWILLO, D. E.: Otomandibular deformity: pathogenesis as a guide to treatment. J. Max. fac. Surg. **8**, 34—41 (1973).

POSWILLO, D. E.: The pathogenesis of the Treacher Collins Syndrome. Brit. J. Oral Surg. **13**, 1 (1975).

POSWILLO, D. E.: Haemorrhage in development of the face, in Morphogenesis and Malformation of the brain and face. Ed. J. LANGMAN. Williams and Wilkins, Baltimore, National Foundation Birth Defects Series (1975 b).

POSWILLO, D. E., HAMILTON, W. J., SOPHER, D.: The marmoset as an animal model for teratological research. Nature (Lond.) **239**, 460—462 (1972).

POSWILLO, D. E., RICHARDS, T.: Maintaining an environment for marmosets in the laboratory. Eng. Med. 1972 I, 86—88.

POSWILLO, D. E., SOPHER, D., MITCHELL, S., COXON, D. F., CURTIS, R. F., PRICE, K. R.: Investigations into the teratogenic potential of imperfect potatoes. Teratology **8**, 339 (1973).

PRESLOCK, J. P., HAMPTON, S. H., HAMPTON, J. K.: Cyclic variations of serum progestins and immunoreactive estrogens in marmosets. Endocrinology **92**, 4, 1096—1101 (1973).

SARICH, V. M., WILSON, A. C.: Quantitative immunochemistry and the evolution of primate albumin; microcomplement fixation. Science **154**, 1563—1566 (1966).

SHACKLETON, C. H. L., MITCHELL, F. L.: The comparison of perinatal steroid endocrinology in Simians, with a view to finding a suitable animal model to study human problems. Lab. Anim. Handbook **6** Eds. F. T. PERKINS and P. N. O'DONOGHUE, Laboratory Animals Ltd., London, pp. 159—181 (1975).

SMITH, C. C.: In: VOGTBORG, H. ed. Use of non-human primates in drug evaluation pp. 469—478. Austin and London: Univ. of Texas Press 1968.

SOMERS, G. F.: The fetal toxicity of thalidomide. Proc. Europ. Soc. Study Drug Toxicity **1**, 49—58 (1963).

TUCHMANN-DUPLESSIS, H.: Teratogenic drug screening: Present procedures and requirements. Teratology **5**, 271—284 (1972).

VALERIO, D. A., MILLER, R. L., INNES, J. R. M., COURTNEY, K. D., PALOTTA, A. J., GUTTMACHER, R. M.: Macaca mulatta — management of a laboratory breeding colony. New York and London: Academic Press 1969.

WASHBURN, S. L., HARDING, R. S. O.: The selection of non-human primates in biological research in: Feeding and nutrition of non-human primates, Ed. R. S. HARRIS, pp. 1—13. New York and London: Academic Press 1970.

WHARTON, R., SCOTT, R. B.: Experimental production of genital lesions with norethindrone. Amer. J. Obst. Gynec. **89**, 701—715 (1964).

WHO Wld. Hlth Org. Techn. Rep. Ser. 364 (1967).

WILSON, J. G.: Teratological and reproductive studies in non-human primates. Proc. Int. Workshop Teratol. **2**, 16—33 (1969).

WILSON, J. G.: In: The use of non-human primates in research on human reproduction, WHO Symposium, Sukhumi 1971, Eds. E. DICZFALUSY and C. C. STANDLEY, pp. 261—292. Stockholm: Karolinska Institute 1972.

WILSON, J. G.: Teratologic causation in man and its evaluation in non-human primates in: Birth Defects, Eds. A. G. MOTULSKY and W. LENZ, Excerpta Medica, Amsterdam, pp. 191—203 (1974).

8. Screening Medicines for Teratogenicity: Problems of Interpretation

F. M. ATKINSON

With 6 Figures

It is some 12 years since screening for teratogenicity became an important part of the toxicity tests on new substances, especially medicines. Yet tests in use until now are not generally regarded as satisfactory, and the degree of protection they afford to mankind is unknown.

This situation results from the way that the tests came to be designed. By use of known teratogens it was possible to identify certain now familiar factors that influence the production of teratogenic effects in laboratory animals. This led to recommendations on experiment design, such as the number and nature of species to be tested, the duration and timing of dosage, and the route of administration. Various reviews of recommended procedures have been published (CAHEN, 1964; TUCHMANN-DUPLESSIS, 1965, 1972; W.H.O., 1967; WILSON, 1974). BRENT (1972) has reviewed critically the current empirical teratogenicity screening methods, and concluded that they do not reliably fulfil their purpose, the prediction of the human response. Tests must remain unsatisfactory until there is a greater knowledge of how teratogens exert their action, and until by the application of this knowledge it becomes much more certain that unknown teratogens will be detected by newly designed tests.

Not only are protocols for teratogenicity screening empirical, but they are also more difficult to implement in practice than is usually realised; and the more detailed the recommendations, the more difficult they are to perform. PALMER (1974 a) has reported some of the practical problems that are encountered in the screening of new compounds for teratogenicity.

Attempts are made from time to time to improve existing screening schemes. During 1974, for example, the British Committee on Safety of Medicines proposed a screening protocol for teratogenicity and other reproduction tests. Little in the new scheme can be regarded as an advance scientifically: the suggested tests are as empirical as those from which they were derived.

Apart from changes to the design of screening schemes, it is now thought that drug metabolism studies should be performed on pregnant experimental animals and fetuses. This seems likely to yield, in the long term, fundamental knowledge that will help to improve testing methods. Unfortunately, such metabolism studies are not likely to enhance the value of tests on new medicines in the short term, because comparative metabolism studies in pregnant human volunteers are not to be contemplated: however, comparative studies are necessary to establish the relevance of tests in animals.

Until now, attempts to improve teratogenicity testing methods have tended to neglect the problem of interpreting each screening test — yet before deciding that a new medicine is unlikely to present teratogenic hazards for mankind, a decision must be made about its teratogenic potential for the laboratory test species. It is therefore necessary to define what observations should be made as measures of the state of the progeny, and what statistical methods are appropriate for their analysis, lest there be dispute about the interpretation of the results.

Measurements

The gestation may be assessed by observations on the mother, by counting fetuses and resorptions, and by determining the degree of normality of the fetuses (WILSON, 1973). Variation in rates of growth and development, and the existence of spontaneous minor and major abnormalities, require that many observations be made as indices of the state of the fetuses. Furthermore it is important to decide what observations are to be made before inspection of experimental material, in case an injudicious choice of measurements should bias the conclusions.

It has hitherto been the practice to confine attention largely to the macroscopic appearance of the fetuses — external appearance, soft tissues and skeletons. Were a toxicity test to be conducted on mature animals with the macroscopic appearance of those animals and of their organs as the sole criteria of normality, the test would be rightly regarded as inadequate; additional observations are regarded as essential, for example various measurements of the cellular and chemical constituents of the blood, and microscopic examination of the tissues. Why are similar routine measurements and examination not recommended for diagnosis of the condition of a fetus?

The need to consider what measurements are appropriate for the proper recording and interpretation of teratogenicity tests is thus our first outstanding problem. A scientist charged with responsibility for screening new products cannot await a rational solution to this problem. Instead he must select his list of observations empirically, as likely as not following current fashion.

Statistical Analysis

Careful statistical analysis of results is particularly important in toxicity tests, including tests for teratogenicity. This arises from the fact that products submitted to toxicity testing become acceptable when no effect is detected. Biologists with a disinclination for mathematics are apt to claim that important effects are obvious without statistical analysis. Even if this were always so, it is an unsuitable approach for toxicity tests, in which the detection of small effects is important and in which lack of effect is a desirable result.

The statistical analysis of teratogenicity tests is beset with difficulties. For instance, it may be thought that the greater the number of observations made on each experimental animal the more reliable and clear are the conclusions that can be drawn. However, this creates problems with the statistical analysis. If significance tests between groups are performed for each observation separately, as is customary, and if the conventional 5 per cent level of probability is taken as indicating statistical significance, it follows that about 5 per cent of the analyses should reveal a statistical significance that is wholly spurious — thus the more observations the greater the chance of anomalies. It is not possible to predict precisely how many anomalous significant results to expect, because 5 per cent would be anticipated only when the observations made on a fetus are uncorrelated; but many measurements are correlated in practice.

This confusing situation arises from failure to deal adequately with a multivariate problem. When more than one measurement is made on each experimental subject, some form of multivariate analysis seems more appropriate than individual analyses on the observations. Multivariate techniques avoid the confusion that arises from separate analysis of observations and from their correlation. The average biologist finds multivariate methods difficult to understand. They are indeed complex; even a short text (MARRIOTT, 1974) "... intended for anyone who has to interpret collections of multivariate data" is not easy for the average biologist to follow. Probably because of their complexity, multivariate techniques have been infrequently applied to teratological and other toxicological investigations.

There is a second reason to use multivariate analytical methods instead of simpler statistical analyses, namely that differences between groups may be apparent when the results are considered as a whole, even though the results taken singly give no indication of them. A simple artificial example[1] is illustrated by the two groups of mice in Fig. 1. The astute biologist recognises that, although there is substantial size variation within each of the groups, differences in shape between the groups may be present — see the means illustrated in Fig. 2. If, in an attempt to compare the groups, the lengths of the anterior ends of the mice are analysed, there is no significant difference (group 1 mean length = 16.02, standard deviation = 2.52; group 2 mean length = 14.12, S. D. = 2.53; Student's t = 1.958, 22 degrees of freedom, $P > 0.05$); comparison of widths likewise reveals no significant difference (means are 14.45 and 15.88, with S. D. = 2.65 and 2.42 respectively; t = 1.474, $P > 0.1$). Yet if the two measurements are considered simultaneously, as when (Fig. 3) length is plotted against width, a clear distinction between the groups can be seen.

In Fig. 3, each individual is represented by a point in 2-dimensional space, because two measurements were made, and each group of subjects is represented as an elliptical swarm of points. By analogy, a new axis can be added for each extra measurement made, the axes being mutually perpendicular. So with multiple measurements, each subject is a point and each group an ellipsoid in multidimensional space (assuming Normal distribution). This abstraction cannot be visualized as can the 2-dimensional example in Fig. 3; but multivariate analytical techniques can be used to distinguish differences between groups despite the multiplicity of the variables.

---

[1] A similar simple example is treated mathematically by LI (1964).

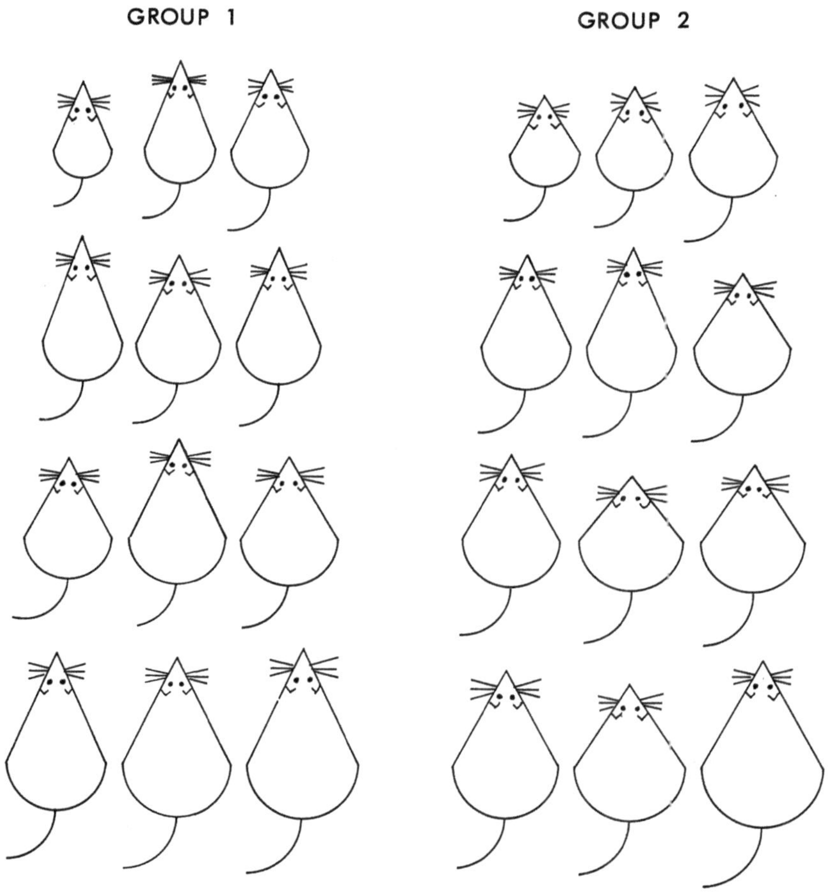

Fig. 1. Differences between groups are not always detectable when simple individual measurements are examined. The group mean lengths (of the anterior pointed ends) of these illustrative mice do not differ significantly; neither do group mean widths. (The data are artificial)

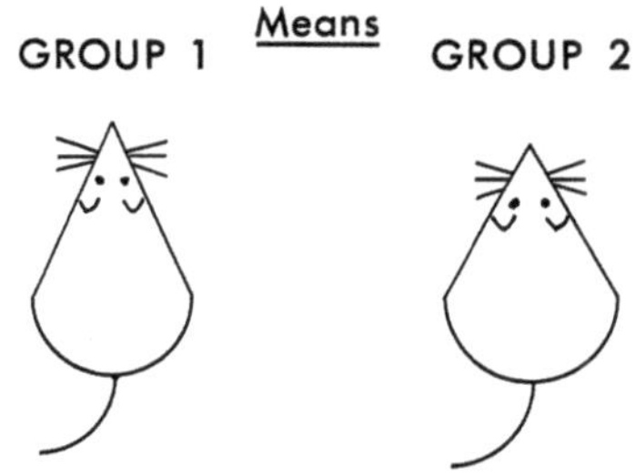

Fig. 2. Mice drawn to illustrate the mean lengths and widths from Fig. 1

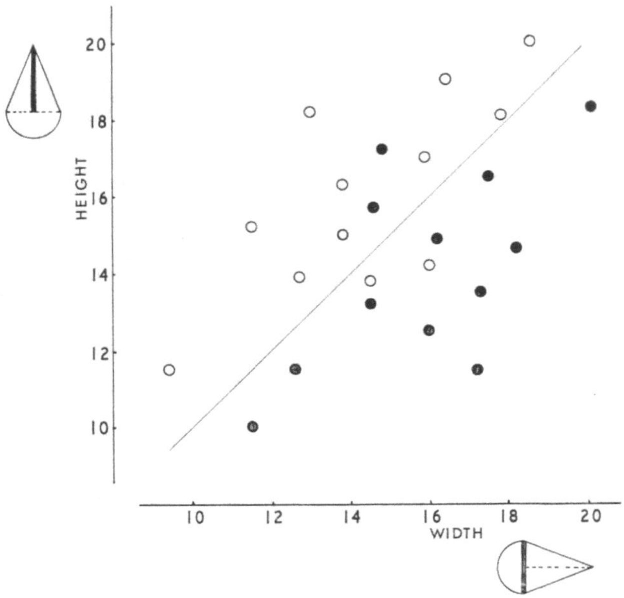

Fig. 3. Lengths of the mice in Fig. 1 plotted against their widths. The diagonal separates Group 1 (open circles) from Group 2 (closed circles)

The academic research worker often avoids the complexity of multivariate problems, by investigating treatment effects on single variables; but teratological screening, seeking as it does a negative result, must measure several variables if it is to be reliable.

Experimental Units

Another source of difficulty for those performing most types of teratogenicity test springs from failure to recognise the nature of the experimental unit, as pointed out by Weil (1970). The experimental unit is that which can be assigned to a treatment, independent of the assignment of all other experimental units. In the usual teratogenicity test, an individual fetus cannot be treated differently from its litter mates, and so it cannot be an experimental unit, whereas the pregnant animal (or its whole litter) can be independently assigned to treatment and therefore is an experimental unit. This might be considered a trivial matter; yet if it is ignored differences between group means tend to seem more significant than they really are. Thus, in a screening test, not only would there be a greater probability of judging a small chance effect to be statistically significant, but also each successful test would seem to be based on a large number of animals, and so to have an unwarranted predictive value.

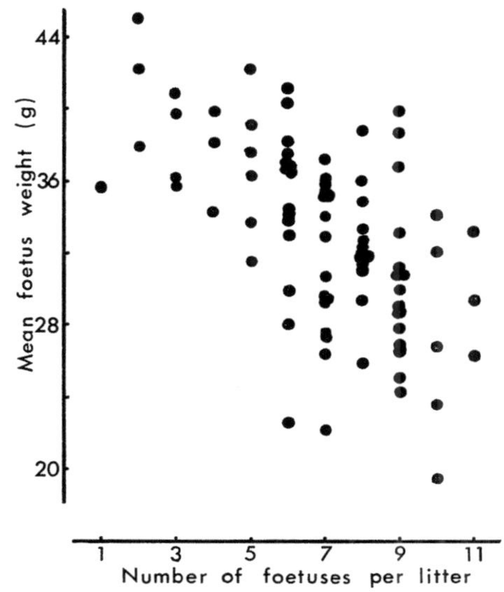

Fig. 4. Mean weight of fetuses from primigravid Dutch rabbits plotted against the number of fetuses in the litter

Many scientific reports on teratogenicity tests do not specify completely the method adopted for statistical analysis, although it may be deduced that some workers have analysed their results incorrectly. It is not possible to demonstrate from published work the practical consequences of incorrect analysis, because sufficiently detailed results are not available. As an alternative, therefore, the author has simulated for this purpose some simple teratogenicity test results on a computer.

Computer Simulation

To provide a basis for the simulation, body weights of 585 fetuses from 84 litters born to untreated primigravid Dutch rabbits were examined. The mean number of fetuses per litter was 6.96 (standard deviation = 2.12), and there were significant correlations between the number of fetuses in a litter and the mean fetal weight (Fig. 4), and between the number in a litter and the standard deviation of fetal weight within the litter.

By use of these relationships and the pseudorandom number generator of an ICL 1900 computer, it was possible to create realistic Normally distributed data representing body weights of litters of rabbits. In all, data for 100 mock experiments were generated, with 4 groups of 10 litters in each experiment. Analyses of variance of the data were then performed on the computer. Each experiment of 40 litters was analysed in two ways, the first with the fetuses and the second (by the method of HEALY, 1972) with litters as experimental units. A variance ratio (F) value for

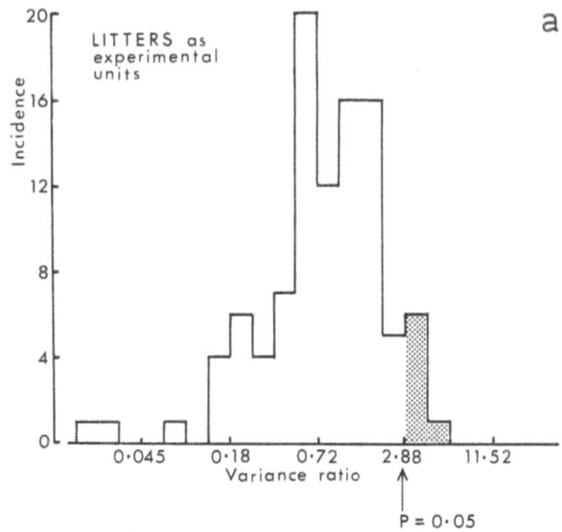

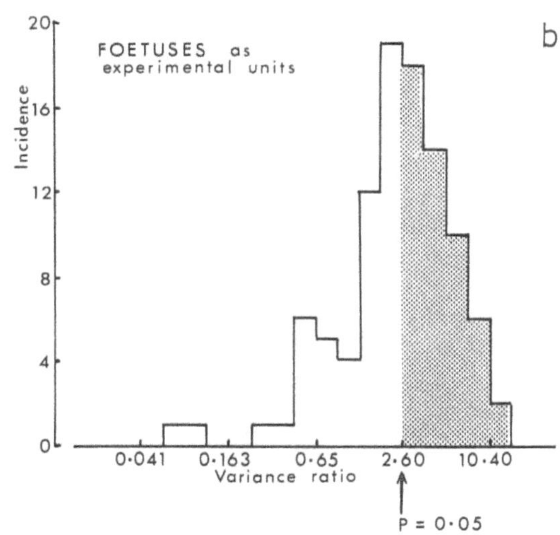

Fig. 5 a and b. Frequency distribution of variance ratios (plotted on a logarithmic scale) for between group differences in 100 simulated teratogenicity screening tests on fetal body weights. Each test had 4 groups of 10 litters, and each was analysed with litters and with fetuses as experimental units. The shaded areas to the right represent the chance occurrence of "significant" results

the difference between groups was calculated in each case, and Fig. 5 shows the distribution of the ratios so obtained.

Because the litters had been randomly allocated to groups, it was expected that in about 5 of the 100 experiments the differences between groups would be significant at the conventional 5 per cent probability level. With litters as observations, 7 such significant experiments were in fact observed; this is reasonably close to the 5 expected. However, with fetuses as experimental units no less than 50 of the 100 experiments showed significant differences between groups, dramatically more than the expected number. It seems therefore that the use of individual fetuses as though they are experimental units is liable to produce erroneous conclusions, contrary to the opinion expressed by WILSON (1973).

Not all biologists readily accept that the individual fetus is not an experimental unit. KALTER (1974) has argued that because the fetus itself may play a substantial part in the outcome of an experiment, it must be sometimes appropriate to regard it as an independent unit. This view is disputed by STAPLES and HASEMAN (1974), who assert that as long as the pregnant female plays any role whatever in the outcome she alone must be regarded as the experimental unit. They point out that the incidence of a change within the litter is an appropriate measure of effect — this ensures that information provided by individual fetuses is not lost. BECKER (1974) allows that a small incidence of an abnormality in several litters is probably more important than a large incidence in one litter; this would seem to favour the use of the litter as an experimental unit. But he then proposes that results should be inspected before deciding on an appropriate statistical treatment. WEIL (1974) and PALMER (1974 b) agree with STAPLES and HASEMAN. No doubt the correspondence on this subject will continue.

This controversy reflects the frequent misunderstanding between statisticians and biologists. In teratogenicity testing there is an obvious need (obvious to the biologist at least) for the information gained from individual foetuses to be utilised in drawing conclusions from the experiment. What biologists have failed to appreciate is that this is comparable with any other multivariate situation. A pregnant uterus may be thought of as containing an array of observations; each fetus is an "observation", a result of treatment, and the whole array of such observations is an experimental unit.

Unfortunately, the arrays of results arising in the various uteri do not all contain the same number of observations, which makes analysis difficult or impossible with presently available techniques. The ideal situation for analysis would arise if all pregnant uteri in teratogenicity screening tests could be made to contain the same number of fetuses, distributed comparably within the uteri. As this is not practicable, perhaps statisticians can devise a multivariate technique suitable for screening tests as they are in fact performed.

Distribution

Another source of complexity in the statistical analysis of teratogenicity screening tests is the distribution of the results. Analyses of variance, and significance tests related thereto, depend for their validity on Normal distribution of errors, and on equality of the error variances of the treatment groups; at least some reasonable approximation to these conditions is advisable. The observations from conventional toxicity tests on mature animals usually meet these requirements, but many of the observations from teratogenicity tests do not.

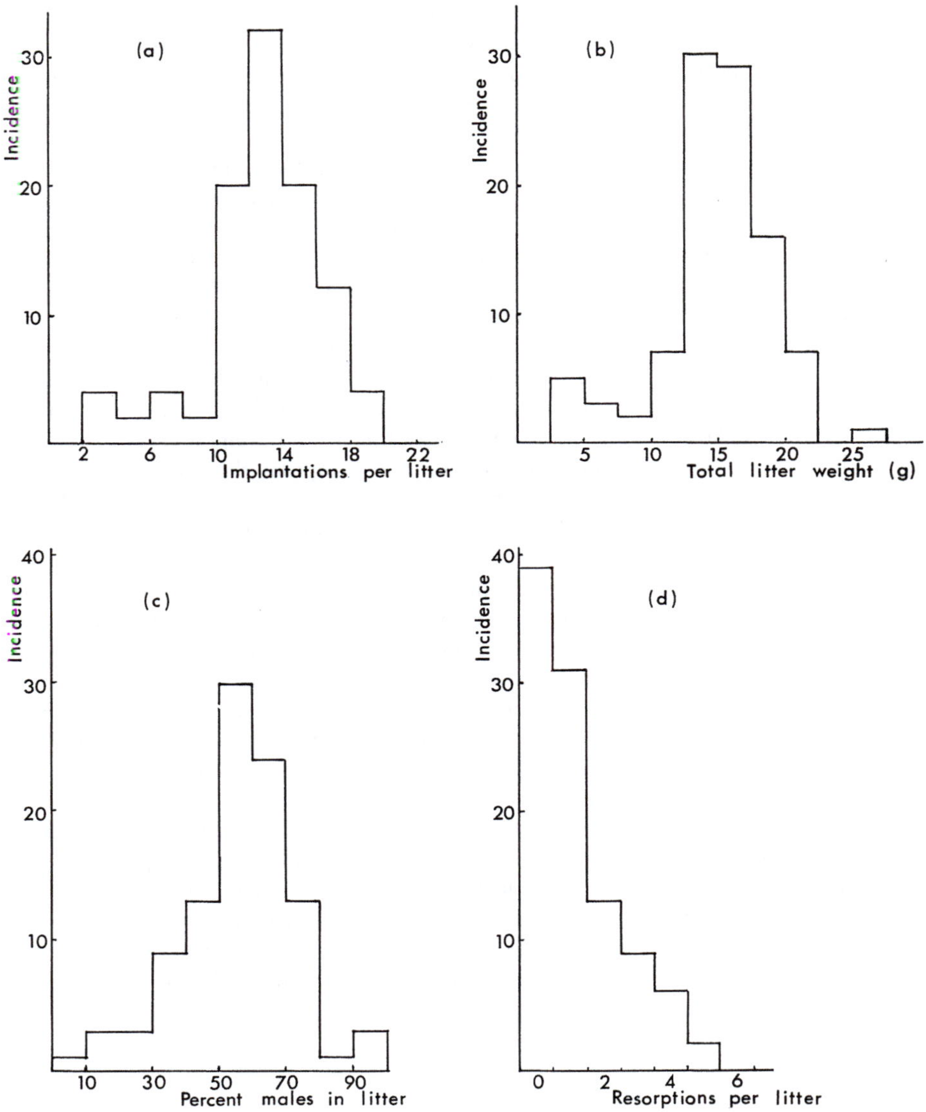

Fig. 6 a—d. Frequency distributions of four observations made on each of 100 litters of primigravid Charles River CD1 mice. The litters were delivered by Caesarian section on the 19th day of gestation. The observations on each litter were (a) the number of implantations, (b) the total body weight of the fetuses, (c) the sex ratio, (d) the number of resorptions. Not all distributions are Normal

Figure 6 illustrates the distributions of four observations made on each of 100 litters of untreated mice. An obvious departure from Normality is seen in the distribution of the number of resorptions per litter (Fig. 6 d); in fact resorptions follow a Poisson distribution. The standard texts on statistics (for example SNEDECOR and COCHRAN, 1967; SOKAL and ROHLF, 1969) recommend that such measurements should be transformed, after which analysis of variance becomes possible. The square root transformation is recommended for results following the Poisson distribution, and the addition of 0.5 to each result before taking the root is advised when there are zero observations. Mathematically expressed, the square root transformation is as follows:

$$y' = \sqrt{(y+0.5)}$$

where y is the original observation on the litter and y′ is the transformed observation to be analysed.

Proportions, which have been suggested above as suitable for measurements on the litter as a whole, follow the binomial distribution. When the proportion of responders is substantial, as when (Fig. 6 c) the sex ratio is measured for each litter, and also if the number of foetuses in a litter were to be large (say 30 or more), then proportions are sufficiently like the Normal in their distribution to present no problem. However, numbers per litter are small for conventional laboratory test species and usually there is a small expected frequency of response, as with abnormalities; marked departures from the normal distribution are then to be expected. For binomial distributions of this kind, the arcsine (angular) transformation is recommended:

$$p' = \text{arcsine}\ (\sqrt{p})$$

where p is the observed proportion and p′ is the transformed observation.

Some variates that can be measured in a teratogenicity test are continuous, such as the body weight of the litter. The distribution of litter weights (Fig. 6 b) tends to be Normal, and the number of implantations per litter, though discontinuous, is distributed nearly enough to Normal (Fig. 6 a) for satisfactory analysis of variance without transformation.

PALMER (1974 b) avoids difficulty with non-Normal distributions by use of nonparametric methods of analysis.

Conclusion

Toxicological screening methods should be improved whenever possible, as a matter of principle, and the need for improvement is nowhere greater than in teratogenicity tests. However, new methods should be soundly based on new knowledge, or unapplied existing knowledge, from all relevant disciplines. The time for empiricism has passed; "change" and "elaboration" are not synonymous with "improvement".

The resources available for testing new substances are limited, and the best possible use should be made of them. It is thus to be hoped that a cautious approach will be made by all those responsible for new teratological screening methods.

The author suggests that improved efficiency may result from research to determine what are the most appropriate observations to be made on pregnant experimental animals and their offspring, and to discover the best statistical methods for the complex results obtained.

References

Becker, B. A.: The statistics of teratology. Teratology **9**, 261—262 (1974).

Brent, R. L.: Drug testing for teratogenicity: its implications, limitations and application to man. pp. 31—43 in Klingberg, M. A., Abramovici, A. and Chemke, J. (Eds.): Drugs and Fetal Development. New York: Plenum Press 1972.

Cahen, R L.: Evaluation of the teratogenicity of drugs. Clin. Pharmacol. Ther. **5**, 480—514 (1964).

Healy, M. J. R.: Animal litters as experimental units. Appl. Statist. **21**, 155—159 (1972).

Kalter, H.: Choice of the number of sampling units in teratology. Teratology **9**, 257—258 (1974).

Li, C. C.: Introduction to Experimental Statistics. Ch. 30: Multiple measurements (pp. 403 to 415). New York: McGraw-Hill 1964.

Marriott, F. H. C.: The Interpretation of Multiple Observations. New York: Academic Press 1974.

Palmer, A. K.: Problems associated with the screening of drugs for possible teratogenic activity. Ch. 2 (pp. 16—33) in Woollam, D. H. M. and Morris, G. M. (Eds.): Experimental Embryology and Teratology **1**. London: Elek Science (1974 a).

Palmer, A. K.: Statistical analysis and choice of sample units. Teratology **10**, 301—302 (1974 b).

Snedecor, G. W., Cochran, W. G.: Statistical Methods. 6th Ed., pp. 324—329. Ames, Iowa: Iowa State University Press 1967.

Sokal, R. R., Rohlf, F. J.: Biometry. Ch. 13: Assumptions of the analysis of variance (pp. 367—402). San Francisco: Freeman 1969.

Staples, R. E., Haseman, J. K.: Selection of appropriate experimental units in teratology. Teratology **9**, 259—260 (1974).

Tuchmann-Duplessis, H.: Design and interpretation of teratogenic tests. pp. 56—87 in Robson, J. M., Sullivan, F. M. and Smith, R. L. (Eds.): A Symposium on Embryopathic Activity of Drugs. London: Churchill 1965.

Tuchmann-Duplessis, H.: Teratogenic drug screening. Present procedures and requirements. Teratology **5**, 271—285 (1972).

Weil, C. S.: Selection of the valid number of sampling units and a consideration of their combination in toxicological studies involving reproduction, teratogenesis or carcinogenesis. Fd. Cosmet. Toxicol. **8**, 177—182 (1970).

Weil, C. S.: Choice of the number of sampling units in teratology. Teratology **10**, 301 (1974).

W.H.O.: Principles for the testing of drugs for teratogenicity. Wld. Hlth Org. techn. Rep. Ser., **364** (1967).

Wilson, J. G.: Environment and Birth Defects. Ch. 9: Collection and interpretation of results (pp. 173—193). New York: Academic Press 1973.

Wilson, J. G.: Factors determining the teratogenicity of drugs. pp. 205—217 in Elliott, H. W., Okun, R. and George, R. (Eds.): Ann. Rev. Pharmacol. **14**. Palo Alto, Calif.: Annual Reviews Inc (1974).

Influencing the Fetal Milieu

The placenta and fetal membranes are of primary importance in controlling the fetal environment. Changes in the type of implantation, alterations in placental growth and migration, and changes in the volume of amniotic fluid are important potential causes of malformation. Very little is known about the secretion, absorbtion and circulation of the amniotic fluid, nor about the reparative capacity of the fetal membranes. As more and more investigations are carried out *in vivo* on the fetus and its milieu there is a need for more information about the reaction to injury. Attempts to extend the scope of fetal surgery in animals and man will depend on the availability of this information.

9. Placental Causes of Maldevelopment

K. Benirschke

With 8 Figures

The placenta is a vital organ during development. Changes affecting placental tissues are often reflected in fetal growth disturbances, thus the malnutrition of the fetus whose placenta is infarcted may be readily understood. However, it might not be thought proper to label placental infarcts as an example of "placental disease", for their cause is decidual (maternal) vascular disease, the placenta being only secondarily involved. Similarly, the changes found in the placenta as a result of infection (e. g., syphilis, toxoplasmosis, or viral infections), while at times devastating to both the organ and the fetus, cannot be properly construed as a "placental cause of maldevelopment". Indeed, is there any evidence that such causes exist? Malimplantation of the ovum, leading to velamentous insertion, or to placenta accreta may not be simple "placental" diseases; such changes may have their origin in uterine inflammation or uterine anomalies. There are in fact very few diseases of the placenta that can be considered to be "primary" to this organ and to relate to possible maldevelopment. A specific and rare example would be placental sulfatase deficiency, probably one of the causes of familial postmaturity (France *et al.*, 1973). As a further example it has recently been suggested that the absence of amniotic fluid is the cause of Potter's facies and pulmonary hypoplasia, for when a normal monoamnionic twin supplies this liquid, the fetus with renal agenesis lacks these secondary features of the syndrome (Kohler, 1972).
It must be concluded from reviewing the extensive literature on placental pathology that few entirely placental causes of abnormal development can be singled out. This is not to deny that a host of placental pathological lesions exist which are correlated with abnormal fetal development or growth. It is the purpose of this chapter to review these disturbances and bring into focus the few animal models that have been employed in attempts to understand better maternal/placental/fetal interdependence, with special emphasis on teratological sequelae. A fuller discussion of the subject can be found in three texts (Boyd and Hamilton, 1970; Philippe, 1974; Benirschke and Driscoll, 1967).

Examination

Accurate observation by an experienced individual, keeping detailed records, is imperative for a better understanding of the relationships between placental change and fetal abnormality. The placenta must be inspected carefully and an attempt must be made to visualize how the organ may have lain in the uterus. Cord length and the number of cord vessels should be noted and sections taken if ambiguities exist. The cord and membranes should be trimmed off the placenta proper, loosely adherent clots removed and the weight of the organ recorded. The fetal surface is then examined: is it shiny, granular, opaque, green from meconium or brown from hemosiderin? The maternal surface is inspected to confirm that no fragment remains *in utero.* Is there calcification (maturity), are there hematomas, fresh or old (green; depression)? The organ is then sliced. Does it have normal red color (determined by *fetal* hemoglobin content), are there infarcts and how many, are there septal cysts (maturity), or tumors? When lesions or abnormal fetal findings require it, sections should be cut for histologic interpretation. They have been easier to prepare in my hands when the tissue is fixed in Bouin's solution, as it then becomes harder for secondary trimming than when it is fixed in formalin. These sections should include both surfaces, cord and a piece of rolled membrane.

Much more is known of the lesions in human placentas than in those from laboratory or other animals. In non-human species the placenta is often eaten and so little knowledge of its development is to hand that many investigators have neglected this organ. It is likely that an orderly investigation will be fruitful.

Amniotic Cavity

One of the most striking direct causes of fetal maldevelopment is the formation of amniotic bands. In Fig. 1 the only remnant of amnion was a band-like extension from the cord which had encircled the calf of the infant, nearly causing its amputation and resulting in amputation of several digits. A variety of amputations, syndactyly, and intrauterine death from encircling of the cord by such bands have all been documented (KRAG, 1974). There is some doubt whether a causal relationship to other malformations, e. g. facial clefts, exists, but bands have often been seen attached to the exencephalic remnants of brain in cranioschisis. Such bands are relatively uncommon, perhaps occurring once in 5000 deliveries, and they are not always constrictive or destructive. Their pathogenesis is uncertain. ORNOY *et al.* (1974) find a history of prenatal bleeding is often associated with their presence, but in other cases this is lacking. The amniotic sac does not become fully distended and passively applied to the chorion until the end of the first trimester. If rupture occurs before this the formation of bands is a possible sequel. The fetus then develops within the chorionic sac, whose surface is thickened and opacified, as shown in Fig. 1. The amount of fluid may be reduced, and as in this case, clubfoot and other positional anomalies may be secondary features.

The amnion may rupture long before birth, the chorion may stop growing after rupture and the fetus may escape and develop extrachorionically. This is a very unusual occurrence but one which gives clues as to the developmental need for amniotic fluid. In Figs. 2 and 3, such a case in shown. The 950 g fetus had developed essentially within the endometrial cavity, outside the membranes. There was no fluid and the hole in the amnion had a maximum diameter of 4 cm, through

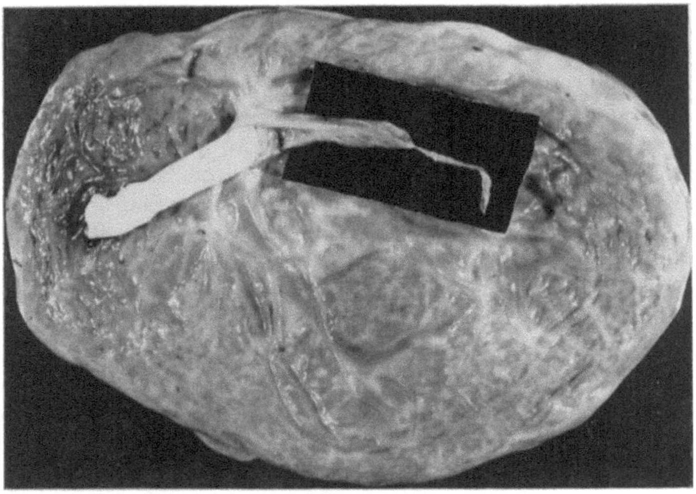

Fig. 1. Term placenta of baby with amputation of terminal phalanx of rt. index finger, several toes, severe constriction of right mid calf, and clubfoot. Patient was heroin addict; no diseases known during pregnancy; 60 ml of dark yellow amniotic fluid only. Note only remains of folded amnion, terminating in thin band, on black paper. Chorionic membrane is thick and opaque

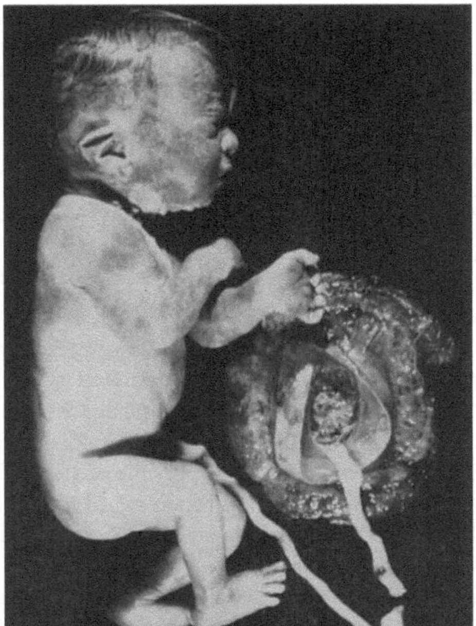

Fig. 2. Infant and placenta showing extramembranous development. The 950 g infant died immediately after birth from pulmonary hypoplasia and has low set, malformed ears. The placental membranes are held open by cardboard and can be seen better in Fig. 3

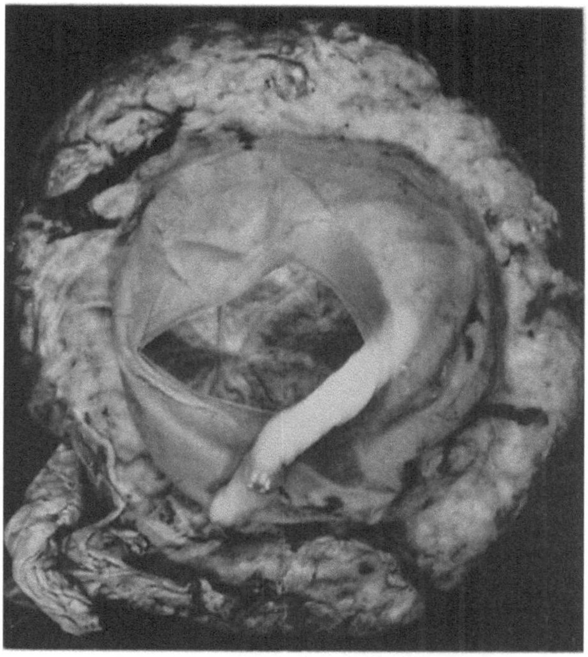

Fig. 3. Placenta of previous infant. Note the circumvallate nature of membrane attachment and peripheral old hemorrhages. The membranes have a 4 cm opening, much smaller than the large fetus who developed outside the membranes. Unlike other cases (DELLENBACH *et al.*, 1967), no amnion nodosum had developed here

which the umbilical cord passed. The placenta was circumvallate, and periodic prenatal bleeding had been recorded. The premature infant had positional deformities of the feet and a facies that reminded one of the "Potter" facies associated with renal agenesis. At autopsy a normal urinary tract was present; the lung, however, was hypoplastic.

Other evidence suggests that for the normal development of lungs and facies an adequate amount of amniotic fluid must be present. Thus, in monozygotic twins, symmelia (sirenomelia, sympodia) develops most commonly in only one (DAVIES *et al.*, 1971) and occasionally the fetuses develop in a single amnion as discordant monoamnionic twins. In such a twin, KOHLER (1972) has found that the typical features associated with renal agenesis ("Potter's syndrome") were lacking. Despite an absent urinary tract, the sympus had normal facies and lung, presumably because amniotic fluid was supplied by the normal twin.

Amniotic fluid may be lost by premature continuous leakage of fluid from ruptured membranes and fetal sequelae vary; they may be serious. In such a case oligohydramnios finds its pathologic expression in the placenta in the form of amnion nodosum, a characteristic lesion secondary to absent fluid (BAIN *et al.*, 1964). These small nodules of debris at sites of degenerate amniotic epithelium are diagnostic. Their pathogenesis is related to defective nutrition of the avascular amnion once

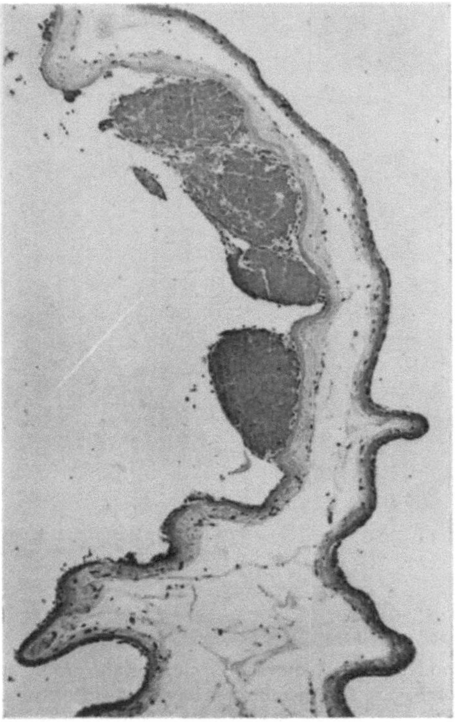

Fig. 4. Diamnionic "dividing membranes" of monochorionic placenta. The right amnion is normal and the fetus was living. The left fetus was dead, amnion is undergoing necrosis and gray debris is attached in balls, ultimately becoming amnion nodosum. (H&E × 60). (From BENIRSCHKE and DRISCOLL, 1967, with permission of publisher)

the liquor is gone. It can readily be observed on the "dividing membranes" of diamnionic monochorionic twins, when one has died (Fig. 4).

When amniotic fluid is removed experimentally in rats, characteristic anomalies develop. In early gestation it results in cleft palate, later the fetus is compacted, has clubfeet and other peripheral anomalies whose genesis must be attributed to the absent fluid (POSWILLO, 1966). It is interesting to note that these fetuses also have short cords. Nothing is known about factors that determine the very variable length of cords, whose extremes are often associated with fetal death or complications at delivery. Perhaps one factor regulating the length is fetal mobility and, indirectly, the amount of fluid.

Umbilical Cord

The variations in length just referred to are not known to correlate with fetal maldevelopment; however, excessive length is responsible for the higher incidence of knots, which may cause fetal death. Excessively short cords are encountered in fetuses with omphalocele. A possibly causal relationship in this latter event is difficult to assess (KHUDR and BENIRSCHKE, 1972). Fetal death is also occasionally related to ectopia of various tissues (e. g., stomach, pancreas) in the umbilical remnant of the omphalomesenteric duct. Such tissue may ulcerate and lead to fetal exsanguination (BLANC and ALLAN, 1961). Another uncommon pathologic feature of umbilical cords is vascular calcification with thrombosis and fetal death. Its pathogenesis is not understood.

Much the most common anomaly of the cord is the single umbilical artery (SUA) whose relationship to fetal maldevelopment is no longer in dispute. The anomaly is now so well known that a note of the number of umbilical vessels is made at birth in many hospitals. Pediatricians are also attuned to perform a specially detailed examination of the newborn in such cases. SUA occurs with a frequency of about 1% in newborns and is more common in whites and in twins than in negroes or singletons. About 25% of the infants have low birth weight. The literature on this subject has become voluminous since its rediscovery in 1955. Most pertinent aspects are considered in a recent follow-up study of survivors of this anomaly by FROEHLICH and FUJIKURA (1973). In their large population (344 infants) there was a 14% perinatal mortality, 53% of which infants had associated malformations. Of the 0.7% survivors, anomalies were identified in 4%. No specific anomaly was more common. When 266 survivors were matched with acceptable controls and followed to age 4 years, no significant differences in development were seen, with one exception: inguinal hernias occurred significantly more often in the SUA survivors. It thus appears that most malformed infants with SUA die neonatally and that those found normal on careful physical examination may be expected to develop normally.

SUA is an interesting anomaly from an embryologist's point of view. MONIE (1970) has suggested that the anomaly may represent the persistence of the originally single artery in the 3—4 mm embryo which in failing to foreshorten, does not allow for the development of the second vessel. Experimental support for this thesis comes from experiments with rats given retinoic acid (MONIE and KHEMMANI, 1973). Alternatively, it has been suggested that the anomaly may arise from atrophy of one vessel. Evidence for this hypothesis has come from human case material and the study of armadillos in which cord vessels vary greatly (BENIRSCHKE *et al.*, 1964). Remnants of a second vessel (muscle or diminutive vessel with lumen) are often found on sections of anomalous cords. One must be careful, however, to exclude remnants of the generally non-muscular vitelline vessels. Moreover, the anomaly has been found in several cases of thalidomide embryopathy and is here construed as atrophy. The suggestion that fetal prognosis may differ in cases of aplasia as opposed to those of atrophy has not been supported (ALTSHULER, G. A., personal communication). The anomaly is also more commonly associated with altered placental forms, particularly velamentous insertion of the cord and it is almost invariably found in the cord of acardiac twins. It has a very high incidence in the cord of autosomal trisomics and other chromosomal errors (PHILIPPE, 1974) and is the rule in the sympus malformation. Whether it represents a vitelline or allantoic vessel in this situation is yet to be decided (MONIE, 1970). In a recent study of three severely malformed infants CHAURASIA (1974) finds the distal aorta replaced by the single umbilical artery and suggests a causal relationship of the vessel anomaly to the visceral maldevelopment. This disagrees with Monie's theory based on dissection specimens and emphasizes the need for detailed dissection of the anomalous vessels.

Apart from the rats and armadillos mentioned, SUA has been found in normal and thalidomide treated baboons (Hendrickx and Katzberg, 1967). When one umbilical artery is experimentally ligated in the fetal lamb severe growth retardation affects those surviving; when the procedure is undertaken late in pregnancy the fetus dies (Hobel *et al.*, 1970). These experiments support the notion that the low birth weight of infants with SUA may be the result of the vascular anomaly.

Insertion of the Umbilical Cord

The umbilical cord has a central or near central insertion in nearly 80% of deliveries. In 10% it is at the margin and in 1% of singleton placentas its insertion is on the membranes, "velamentous" by common terminology (Krone *et al.*, 1965). Velamentous insertion of the cord is more common in specimens from early pregnancy (15%) and is highly correlated with fetal anomalies (Monie, 1965). From his relatively small collection of material, this author found 25% of conceptuses with velamentous cords, 11% of those with marginal cords, and 7% with central or paracentral insertion of the cord to be malformed. The material studied by Krone concerns delivered infants and, on much larger numbers, it was shown that malformations of all types occur much more frequently in association with velamentous and marginal cord insertions than in babies with centrally inserted cords. He suggests that the pathogenetic mechanism for the development of eccentric insertion is to be sought in early interference with the expansion of the placenta. A number of findings support this contention of "trophotropism", *i. e.*, the migration of the placenta to sites of best nourishment. Thus, in low-lying placentas, including placenta previa, marginal and velamentous insertion is much more common than in fundal positions. In twins and notably in higher multiple births, the anomaly is common. Krone found a slightly higher maternal age and an increased frequency of prior curettage in women with this anomaly. We found that in three of seven placentas in whose membranes an intrauterine plastic contraceptive device was found, velamentous insertion of the cord was present.

These hypotheses assume that in man embryonic implantation always takes place in such a manner that the embryo is closest to the endometrium. If it were on the opposite pole or hemisphere of the implanting blastocyst, velamentous insertion could also be expected, as McLennan (1968) argues. In fact, the precise mechanism is not understood, but the concept of trophotropism is preferred in view of the observations made to date. Recent support for this explanation has come from ultrasonography. Contrary to past notions of a statically implanted placenta, King (1973) finds from serial ultrasonographs that placentas may migrate during pregnancy. This finding also explains the areas of marginal atrophy, succenturiate lobes, etc. which are commonplace. Thus, velamentous and marginal cords presumably denote a significant interference with early placental expansion. Since this period of early development coincides with the teratogen-sensitive period, a true cause and effect may be seen between these placental anomalies and fetal maldevelopment.

SUA is also more common with velamentous cords, as is atrophy of one artery. Thrombosis often occurs in the unprotected membranous vessels and the threat to the infant's life from disruption of the vasa previa in this condition is well known, particularly in twin deliveries. The thrombosis of velamentous vessels, as well as that occurring in the vessels of the most unusual furcate cord insertion, may be so extensive that consumption of coagulation factors leads to a transitory neonatal purpuric state. Finally, in monozygotic twins discordant for some congenital anomaly, it has been suggested that this abnormal cord insertion may be a placental indication of the disturbance that led to abnormal fetal development (BENIRSCHKE and HOEFNAGEL, 1970). It is proposed that for anomalies with a multifactorial basis and threshold effect, *e. g.*, cleft lip and palate, the anomalous placental development reflects the early growth disturbance which placed the affected individual beyond the threshold. The normal infant, having a normal placenta and being a monozygotic twin, serves as a valid control.

Circumvallation

The typical circumvallate insertion of membranes is seen in Fig. 3. Peripheral to the membranes is a ring of old blood, which also contains degenerate decidua and frequent villi; the membranes are often folded over. Partial circumvallation may also occur. About 2% of deliveries are associated with this anomaly which has been recognized as early as the 16th week of pregnancy. Its pathogenesis has been widely discussed and the divergent views are considered in detail elsewhere (BENIRSCHKE and DRISCOLL, 1967). The most likely mechanisms are recurrent episodes of vaginal bleeding and reduced amniotic fluid pressure; evidence for both conditions exists in many instances. Thus bleeding during pregnancy is often recorded and BAIN *et al.* (1964) find a history of hydrorrhea in many of their cases. The case shown in Fig. 2 further supports the contention. Prematurity and positional fetal anomalies are related to these events, and occasionally growth retardation is observed.

The relative frequency of circumvallates in rhesus monkey placentas (15%) has been noted recently (MYERS, 1972) and because of its common occurrence in single-disced organs the old theory of excessively deep implantation has been revived. Normally, the superficially implanting rhesus blastocyst develops 2 discs. Single discs occur in 20% of normal pregnancies, but in the majority these organs are normal (CHEZ *et al.*, 1972).

There is frequent confusion between the true circumvallate placentation and circummarginate placentas, a related form of "extrachorial" placenta. Here the placental tissue extends beyond the disc margin, but there is no plica. It is another expression of marginal placental growth and is frequently encountered in twins. Differences between amniotic sac pressures and placental growth are presumably responsible for this development.

Circumvallate placentas have been noted to recur and a genetic hypothesis has been advanced recently by DEACON and his colleagues (1974). They report a pedigree with three sisters who died in the neonatal period from respiratory distress and with many minor anomalies, including CNS disease. Hydramnios was present with all three and in the last case, in which the placenta was examined, a typical circumvallate was found.

Tumors

Only one tumor of the placenta has a direct relationship to fetal development, the chorangioma. This tumor is common and has significant implications for the fetus. An unusually large chorangioma is shown in Fig. 5; it weighed 400 g, and was found in the placenta of a premature stillbirth. Larger tumors have been recorded (542 g and 600 g) and they are often multiple. When careful examinations are made perhaps 1% of placentas possess small angiomas; larger ones are present in 0.1% or at an even lower frequency.

Chorangiomas are hamartomas, masses of excessively proliferated fetal villous vessels. Their lobular surfaces are covered with trophoblast, and fetal blood circulates through their capillary or sinusoidal vessels. Extramedullary hematopoietic foci are common, as are areas of infarction or thrombosis.

The effects upon fetal development are related principally to an increased cardiac load. Many cases with fetal cardiac hypertrophy and heart failure have been reported, and the frequent hydramnios associated with large tumors may be a direct sequel of heart failure, although other explanations have been given. In carefully studied cases the fetus has often been found to possess other angiomas; on occasion it has had cardiac anomalies. We observed a set of fraternal twins one of which subsequently became severely retarded. Multiple chorangiomata were found in the placenta and the child also had a *de novo* chromosomal translocation. In other cases normal karyotypes were found. Sandstedt (personal communication, 1974) who has studied a large number of placentas from babies with growth retardation, reports that this change may be associated with chorangioma.

There is little doubt that the tumor may have considerable effects on fetal development, particularly when it is large. Less well understood is "chorioangiosis", a term coined by v. Meyenburg (1922). Its pathogenesis is unknown but fetal death in midpregnancy is almost a rule. The entire villous capillary bed appears enormously overgrown, not merely congested as in diabetes. Fetal anomalies do not occur, but few cases have been studied in detail.

Infections

Numerous infections affect placental structures and most maternal organisms have gained access to the fetus at one time or another. Bacteria and fungi usually pursue an ascending path, through vagina, endocervix and membranes into the amniotic fluid and thence the fetus. Only listeria and, rarely, tubercle bacilli may reach the fetus through the villous tissue from endometrium or maternal hematogenous dis-

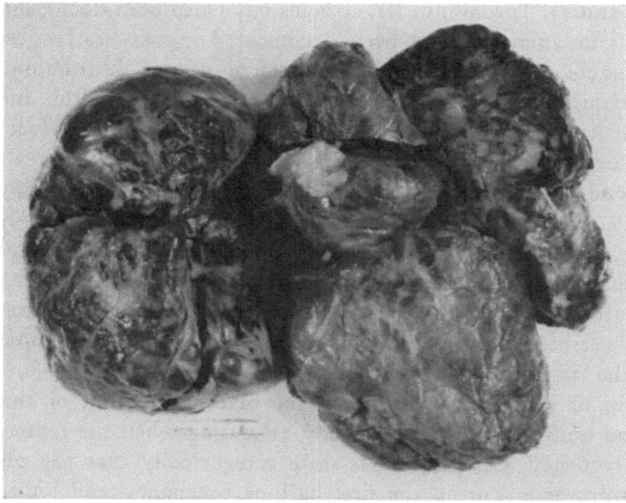

Fig. 5. Excessively large chorangioma of the placenta. This tumor weighed 400 g, had dark areas of plethoric capillary beds and light areas consisting of proliferated endothelium. The premature fetus was stillborn

semination. This is the route usually taken by viruses, spirochetes and trypanosomes. Infections often have serious fetal consequences. They may cause both generalized disease and focal infections, a few must be considered to cause fetal maldevelopment syndromes. Of these, best known is rubella embryopathy. Toxoplasma-induced hydrocephaly, cytomegalovirus-produced cerebral destruction and congenital syphilis with their various sequelae are other examples. In general these infections leave traces in the placenta that are pathognomonic; these lesions are not usually considered to be causal although circumstantial evidence warrants cautious interpretation. For some organisms the placenta serves as an effective barrier, for others this is not so. Thus, while several cases of extensive placental infection with the Californian fungus *Coccidioides immitis* have been described, the fetus has never been involved. Likewise, rubella and toxoplasma infection of the placenta may occur in the absence of fetal infection. The reasons for these discrepancies are not fully understood.

A direct relationship between placental lesions and destructive events in embryonic rubella has been suggested by Töndury (1962). This author observed villous endothelial necrosis and thrombus formation and suggested that microemboli originating in the placenta may be responsible for some of the fetal lesions in this disease. Others consider direct viral action on cells or chromosomes more likely. Another potential placental influence upon fetal development has been suggested in association with the lesions of cytomegalovirus, an agent which causes frequent and typical placental disease. Villi show an infiltration by lymphocytes, plasma cells, areas of hemorrhage and thrombosis, or complete necrosis. In later stages the affected villi undergo hyalinization, show pigment deposits and are effectively destroyed as exchange membranes (Figs. 6 and 7). Thrombi in larger veins have also been documented. Placental cytomegalovirus inflammation has been documented in very early gestation and it is not unreasonable to assume that such scattered villous destruction may be one cause of the frequent fetal growth retardation associated with this infection (ALTSHULER and MCADAMS, 1971). Other villous virus infections may act in a similar manner. In future the significance of a histologically similar lesion whose etiology is not understood, referred to as "villitis of unknown etiology" may be assessed (ALTSHULER, 1973). It is a relatively common entity and definitely related to recurrent stillbirths and/or growth retardation. It has recurred in several families we have studied and in those reported by DOLLMANN and SCHMITZ-MOORMANN (1972). Although an infectious etiology is supported by the histologic features, no responsible agent has yet been identified. Immunologic phenomena of unknown nature are considered by the last authors as possible causative factors.

The relationship of syphilitic infection of the placenta to that of the fetus is not fully understood and deserves further study at a time when the maternal disease is increasing in frequency. Obstetric texts state categorically that the placenta is impermeable to spirochetes during the first half of pregnancy and only the thinning membrane in later gestation allows the organism to pass. The facts are otherwise and have recently been reviewed (BENIRSCHKE, 1974). Placental/fetal spirochetes have been identified in abortion specimens, indeed syphilis has been held to be one cause of abortion. The search is difficult, however, and complicated by preparations that are difficult to stain. The spirochete invokes a severe plasmacellular reaction, and since the fetus reacts immunologically in this way only after the first trimester, the disease "congenital syphilis" as we know it histologically, will be recognized only in the later fetus. This is not to say that the spirochete has not "seeded" the placenta and fetus long before; all the available evidence suggests that this is so.

Growth Retardation

Repeated reference has been made to placental lesions that might have a restraining effect upon fetal growth, and tumors, infections and malposition have been described as such influences. By far the most common placental lesions found in association with small-for-dates infants are infarcts. Placental infarcts result from occlusion of decidual (maternal) vessels and most commonly occur as part of the pre-eclampsia complex. In pre-eclampsia the decidual arterioles are thickened, show fibrin imbibition, have endothelial swellings and a characteristic "atherosis" of the intima. Thrombosis is a frequent sequel which, if the vessel is a significant one, may lead to placental infarction. It is important to realize that numerous vessels in the placental bed are involved, thus reducing the overall blood delivery to the intervillous space. These lesions antedate the clinical recognition of "toxemia" as a disease entity. Thus, NADJI and SOMMERS (1973) recognized such lesions in 14% of the curetted specimens from legal abortions in women who were not (as yet) clinically affected by this disease. Indeed, when no infarcts are found in the placenta, diagnostic features of the disease are not found by placental examination alone; retroplacental curettings are needed, for they contain the decidual vessels. Secondary placental and fetal

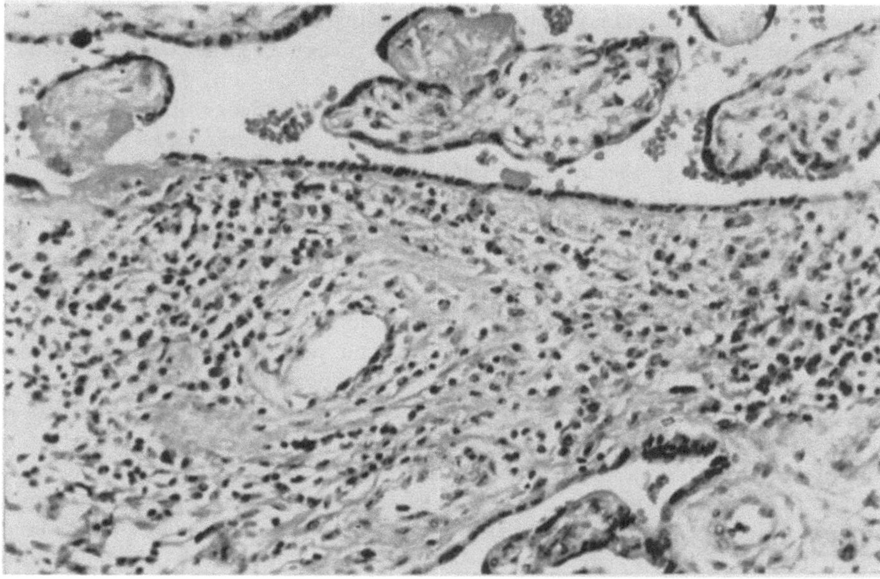

Fig. 6. Typical plasmacellular villitis of documented cytomegalovirus infection with growth retarded premature infant exhibiting purpura, hepatitis, seizures. Other areas were hyalinized (Fig. 7) and large venous thrombi were observed in major chorionic vessels. (H&E × 250)

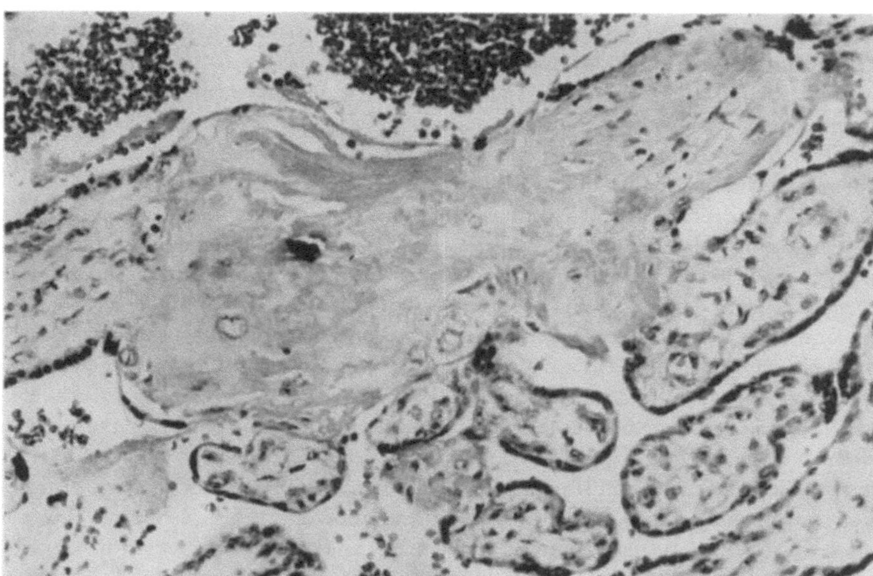

Fig. 7. Another area of same placenta as Fig. 6. Many larger villi were hyalinized with residual pigment testifying to former hemorrhage. These areas may contribute to growth retardation. (H&E × 250)

changes, such as increased syncytial buds, small placental size and evidence of growth restraint (from postnatal growth curves) have been documented (CIBILS, 1974).
How the vascular lesion develops is not certain but knowledge of its pathogenesis will be of potential benefit in view of the high frequency of this disease. The changes are clearly confined to the implantation site, they are exaggerated in molar and twin implantations, and are probably one consequence of trophoblastic immigration into the vascular lumena. Such trophoblastic cells, now shown to be derived from fetal tissues by fluorescent identification of the Y chromosome in male conceptuses, infiltrate into the intima. It is suggested that local antigen-antibody reactions may be important mediators of the disease state (KITZMILLER and BENIRSCHKE, 1973). The vascular damage can at times be shown to extend deep into the myometrium on occasions when such tissues become available at autopsy of eclamptic women.
WIGGLESWORTH (1964) has ligated one of the four uterine arteries in rat pregnancies and reproduced the embryonic growth retardation that is the overall sequel of reduced placental perfusion. In sheep, by restricting uterine perfusion by microembolization with spheres, CREASY *et al.* (1972) have achieved similar results, and other vascular restrictions in the rhesus monkey have attained similar results (MYERS *et al.*, 1971). Little doubt exists that a prolonged reduction of decidual vascular perfusion has invidious consequences for the growth of the conceptus.

Twinning

In twin pregnancies an unusual opportunity exists to make correlations between placental disease and fetal development. Not only is perinatal mortality related to placental form in twins (more so than to obstetric management) but, in addition, in monozygotic twins the hereditary aspects of possible malformations can be assessed. It is thus of interest, for instance, that symmelia is most frequently discordant, as are many other anomalies in twins (FOGEL *et al.*, 1965).
The most remarkable placental influence upon fetal development is found in the twin transfusion syndrome. This syndrome is confined to monochorionic, and hence monozygotic twins. It develops as a consequence of the haphazard vascularization of the placenta in early placentation. These twins share one or more cotyledons and while one twin furnishes the arterial supply to a cotyledon, the other receives the venous effluent. If only a single such arterio-venous connection exists, then the recipient will become plethoric, edematous, hypertrophied, while the donor is anemic, growth retarded and hemoconcentrated. Remarkable size differences have been recorded and NAEYE (1965) has given a precise definition of the various organ abnormalities that ensue. The differential development commences in the first trimester and at midpregnancy may lead to severe hydramnios of the recipient's sac. He may die, in which event a fetus papyraceous forms and the remaining twin develops normally for the remainder of gestation. Expression of the syndrome is extremely variable. This is presumably due to the fact that in many such placentas several cotyledons are shared, with shunts occurring in different directions. Direct artery-to-artery anastomoses also exist and these may equalize pressures. Although hyper-

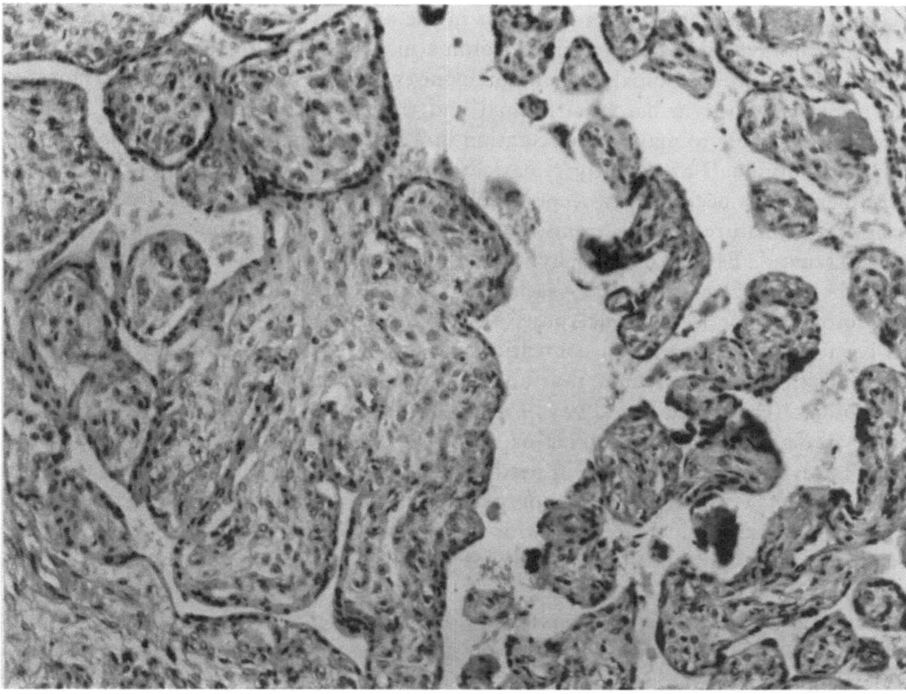

Fig. 8. Placenta of monozygotic twins with transfusion syndrome, at 34 weeks gestation. At left are villi of a cotyledon from the plethoric recipient, at right villi of the anemic donor. Note the marked difference in appearance of "maturity" of villi. (H&E × 160)

tension has been considered to have existed in the hypervolemic twin because of the blood vessel changes, measurements of pressures have not been recorded. Grossly uneven placental development occurs in such twins. In Fig. 8 the junction between two cotyledons (not shared) clearly demonstrates two entirely different villous structures. Those of the plethoric recipient are large and immature in appearance; those of the growth retarded anemic donor are small and have a very mature structure. It is of interest to see, in these monozygotic twins, how the vagaries of placental vascular development influence fetal growth profoundly and how, in turn, the fetal condition affects villous structure. The long-term effects of the runting caused by the transfusion syndrome are incompletely documented. BABSON and PHILLIPS (1973) find that in follow-up examination the deprived infant lags behind consistently.

Shared blood vessels may have other developmental sequelae. Several instances of disseminated intravascular coagulation have been described in surviving twins whose partner died *in utero* (DIMMICK *et al.*, 1971). It is suggested that thromboplastin-rich material from the circulatory bed of the dead fetus gained access to the survivor to initiate disseminated coagulation. There is no *a priori* reason why placental or cord vessel thrombi should not embolize in singletons and cause infarcts, although proof of such events is difficult to furnish. We have recently seen a fatal neonatal myocardial infarct caused by an embolus in the anterior coronary artery and believe its origin to have been a traumatic hematoma in the cord, with thrombosis.

A unique congenital anomaly of one of monozygotic twins is the acardiac monster. Invariably the co-twin has been normal and through two direct placental vascular anastomoses is able to maintain circulation in a reversed fashion through the monster. Affected individuals are usually remarkably malformed, with remnants of the heart and other organs occasionally recognizable, but severely disorganized. Because of the monozygotic nature of such twins, the formal genesis of the abnormality has been often discussed. Essentially two hypotheses have been held tenable: a) the anomaly ensues because of the placental vascular system (SEVERN and HOLYOKE, 1973), b) a chromosomal error is the basic cause (SCOTT and FERGUSON-SMITH, 1973). Evidence has been marshalled for both contentions. Thus it is only in ruminants with similar placental vasculature to man that anomalies of this kind have been observed and chromosomal errors are not always found. On the other hand, fibroblast cultures of some acardiacs have been trisomic or mosaic for different karyotypes. The problem is not resolved at present but is in need of further investigation. The fact that monozygotic twins with different karyotypes exist (the so-called heterokaryotic monozygotic twins) and that fraternal twins with blood vessel anastomoses rarely become blood chimeras underlines the need for detailed placental studies (BENIRSCHKE, 1971).

If what has been said so far about placental influences upon development of twins is true, it is possible that an examination of the placenta in twins may be useful in explaining other developmental errors that are perhaps less spectacular. It is true that velamentous cords and SUA are more common in twins, as are congenital anomalies. In addition there are frequent discordant monozygotic twin anomalies for which an explanation is yet to be found. Multifactorial causation is assumed for a majority of these. If placental anomalies coincide with such developmental disturbances in the fetus, it is not unreasonable to seek a common etiologic explanation. At this stage, and in the absence of appropriate animal models, it is important to collect appropriate data from detailed and informed placental studies. The hope is that eventually more will be known of how the placenta shapes the development of the embryo.

References

ALTSHULER, G.: Placental villitis of unknown etiology: Harbinger of serious disease? A four months' experience of nine cases. J. Reprod. Med. **11**, 215 (1973).

ALTSHULER, G., MCADAMS, A. J.: Cytomegalic inclusion disease of a nineteen week fetus. Amer. J. Obstet. Gynec. **111**, 295 (1971).

BABSON, S. G., PHILLIPS, D. S.: Growth and development of twins dissimilar in size at birth. New Engl. J. Med. **289**, 937 (1973).

BAIN, A. D., SMITH, I. I., GAULD, I. K.: Newborn after prolonged leakage of liquor amnii. Brit. Med. J. **1964 II**, 593.

BENIRSCHKE, K.: Chimerism, mosaicism and hybrids. In Human Genetics, Proc. Fourth Intern. Congr. Human Genetics. Amsterdam, Excerpta Medica. 212 (1971).

BENIRSCHKE, K.: Syphilis — The placenta and the fetus. Amer. J. Dis. Child. **128**, 142 (1974).

BENIRSCHKE, K., DRISCOLL, S. G.: The pathology of the human placenta. Berlin-Heidelberg-New York: Springer 1967.

BENIRSCHKE, K., HOEFNAGEL, D.: Structural development of the placenta in relation to fetal growth. Fetal Growth and Development, p. 1, H. A. WAISMAN and G. KERR, Eds. New York: McGraw-Hill 1970.

BENIRSCHKE, K., SULLIVAN, M. M., MARIN-PADILLA, M.: Size and number of umbilical vessels. A study of multiple pregnancy in man and the armadillo. Obstet. and Gynec. **24**, 819 (1964).

BLANC, W. A., ALLAN, G. A.: Intrafunicular ulceration of persistent omphalomesenteric duct with intraamniotic hemorrhage and fetal death. Amer. J. Obstet. Gynec. **82**, 1392 (1961).

BOYD, J. D., HAMILTON, W. J.: The Human Placenta. Cambridge: Heffer 1970.

CHAURASIA, B. D.: Single umbilical artery with caudal defects in human fetuses. Teratology **9**, 287 (1974).

CHEZ, R. A., SCHLESSELMAN, J. J., SALAZAR, H., FOX, R.: Single placentas in the rhesus monkey. J. med. Primat. **1**, 230 (1972).

CIBILS, L. A.: The placenta and newborn infant in hypertensive conditions. Amer. J. Obstet. Gynec. **118**, 256 (1974).

CREASY, R. K., BARRETT, C. T., SWIET, M. de, KAHANPÄÄ, K. V., RUDOLPH, A. M.: Experimental intrauterine growth retardation in the sheep. Amer. J. Obstet. Gyn. **112**, 566 (1972).

DAVIES, J., CHAZEN, E., NANCE, W. E.: Symmelia in one of monozygotic twins. Teratology **4**, 367 (1971).

DEACON, J. S. R., GILBERT, E. F., VISESKUL, C., HERMANN, J., OPITZ, J. M.: Polyhydramnios and neonatal hemorrhage in three sisters. A circumvallate placenta syndrome? In Malformation Syndromes, vol. 10, p. 41, D. BERGSMA, Ed. New York: Intercontinental Medical Book Corp. 1974.

DELLENBACH, P., SZWARCBERG, R., PHILIPPE, E., GILLET, J. Y.: Grossesse extramembraneuse avec amnion nodosum. Considérations cliniques et anatomiques. Rev. franç. Gynéc. **62**, 157 (1967).

DIMMICK, J. E., HARDWICK, D. F., HO-YUEN, B.: A case of renal necrosis and fibrosis in the immediate newborn period. Association with the twin-to-twin transfusion syndrome. Amer. J. Dis. Child. **122**, 345 (1971).

DOLLMANN, A., SCHMITZ-MOORMANN, P.: Rekurriende Plazentainsuffizienz durch villöse Plazentitis mit extremer fetaler Hypotrophie. (Geburtsgewicht 1030 g und 1000 g am Termin.) Geburtsh. u. Frauenheilk. **32**, 795 (1972).

FOGEL, B. J., NITOWSKY, H. M., GRUENWALD, P.: Discordant abnormalities in monozygotic twins. J. Pediat. **66**, 64 (1965).

FRANCE, J. T., SEDDON, R. J., LIGGINS, G. C.: A study of a pregnancy with low estrogen production due to placental sulfatase deficiency. J. clin. Endocr. **36**, 1 (1973).

FROEHLICH, L. A., FUJIKURA, T.: Follow-up of infants with single umbilical artery. Pediatrics **52**, 6 (1973).

HENDRICKX, A. G., KATZBERG, A. A.: A single umbilical artery in the baboon. Folia Primat. **5**, 295 (1967).

HOBEL, C. J., EMMANOUILIDES, G. C., TOWNSEND, D. E., YASHIRO, K.: Ligation of one umbilical artery in the fetal lamb. Experimental production of fetal malnutrition. Obstet. and Gynec. **36**, 582 (1970).

KHUDR, G., BENIRSCHKE, K.: Discordant monozygous twins associated with amnion rupture. A case report. Obstet. and Gynec. **39**, 713 (1972).

KING, D. L.: Placental migration demonstrated by ultrasonography. A hypothesis of dynamic placentation. Radiology **109**, 167 (1973).

KITZMILLER, J. L., BENIRSCHKE, K.: Immunofluorescent study of placental bed vessels in preeclampsia of pregnancy. Amer. J. Obstet. Gynec. **115**, 248 (1973).

KOHLER, H. G.: An unusual case of sirenomelia. Teratology **6**, 295 (1972).

KRAG, D.: Amnionic rupture and birth defects of the extremities. Hum. Pathol. **5**, 69 (1974).

KRONE, H. A., JOPP, H., SCHELLER, W.: Die Bedeutung anamnestischer Befunde für die verschiedenen Formen des Nabelschnuransatzes. Z. Geburtsh. Gynäk. **163**, 205 (1965).

McLennan, J. E.: Implications of the eccentricity of the human umbilical cord. Amer. J. Obstet. Gynec. **101**, 1124 (1968).
Meyenburg, H. v.: Über Hamangiomatosis diffusa placentae. Beitr. path. Anat. **70**, 510 (1922).
Monie, I. W.: Velamentous insertion of the cord in early pregnancy. Amer. J. Obstet. Gynec. **93**, 276 (1965).
Monie, I. W.: Genesis of single umbilical artery. Amer. J. Obstet. Gynec. **108**, 400 (1970).
Monie, I. W., Khemmani, M.: Absent and abnormal umbilical arteries. Teratology **7**, 135 (1973).
Myer, W. de, Baird, I.: Mortality and skeletal malformations from amniocentesis and oligohydramnios in rats: cleft palate, clubfoot, microstomia, and adactyly. Teratology **2**, 33 (1969).
Myers, R. E.: The gross pathology of the rhesus monkey placenta. J. Reprod. Med. **9**, 171 (1972).
Myers, R. E., Hill, D. E., Holt, A. B., Scott, R. E., Mellits, E. D., Cheek, D. B.: Fetal. growth retardation produced by experimental placental insufficiency in the rhesus monkey. I. Body weight, organ size. Biol. Neonat. **18**, 379 (1971).
Nadji, P., Sommers, S. C.: Lesions of toxemia in first trimester pregnancies. Amer. J. clin. Path. **59**, 344 (1973)
Naye, R. L.: Organ abnormalities in a human parabiotic syndrome. Amer. J. Path. **46**, 829 (1965).
Ornoy, A., Sekeles, E., Sadowsky, E.: Amniogenic bands as a cause of syndactyly in a young human fetus. Teratology **9**, 129 (1974).
Philippe, E.: Histopathologie placentaire. Paris: Masson 1974.
Poswillo, D.: Fetal posture and causal mechanisms of deformity of palate, jaws and limbs. J. dent. Res. **45**, 584 (1966).
Scott, J. M., Ferguson-Smith, M. A.: Heterokaryotypic monozygotic twins and the acardiac monster. J. Obstet. Gynaec. Brit. Cwlth **80**, 52 (1973).
Severn, C. B., Holyoke, E. A.: Human acardiac anomalies. Amer. J. Obstet. Gynec. **116**, 358 (1973).
Töndury, G.: Embryopathien. Berlin: Springer Verlag 1963.
Wigglesworth, J. S.: Experimental growth retardation in the foetal rat. J. Path. Bact. **88**, 1 (1964).

10. Future Prospects for Fetal Surgery

D. Sopher

With 11 Figures

Intrauterine surgery with fetal survival dates from the beginning of this century. Fetuses of the guinea pig (Mayer, 1918) and of the rabbit (Wolff, 1919) survived for several days after being transferred from the uterus to the maternal peritoneal cavity. Surgery on the fetus itself was first performed in 1925; through a small uterine incision, limb amputation was successfully accomplished in the guinea pig (Bors, 1925) and normal delivery of viable offspring followed ablation of an eye, leg or tail in the rat (Nicholas, 1925). Since these early beginnings a wide variety of surgical techniques have been used on several species of animals with varying degrees of success. Procedures such as spinal cord section (Hooker and Nicholas, 1930) adrenalectomy (Tobin, 1939), gonadectomy (Moore and Bodian, 1940; Jost, 1946) and decapitation (Foote and Foote, 1949; Domm and Leroy, 1951) have been carried out on mammals such as rat, rabbit, guinea pig, opossum and hamster.

Earlier studies employed immediate or relatively short-term fetal observations on small mammals. With the increase in complexity of attempted surgical procedures came the need for larger species such as dog, pig, goat, sheep and monkey. The longer gestational period in such species made long-term and serial studies possible and increasing emphasis was placed on achieving prolonged intrauterine survival. The work of Barcroft and Barron (1937, 1939, 1942) on the physiology and behaviour of the ovine fetus saw the beginning of experiments designed for fetal survival. In their operations the fetus was approached *via* a window-like opening in the wall of the gravid uterus and fetal membranes. Techniques using amniotic or uterine purse-string sutures (Hall and Schneiderhan, 1945; Barron, 1945) and tamponade of the uterine incision with the fetal body (Barnard, 1957) were developed to prevent excessive loss of amniotic fluid. Marsupialization of the fetus to the uterine wall with a running suture around the field of surgery (Jackson and Egdahl, 1960) allowed exploration of the fetal peritoneal and thoracic cavities with minimal leakage of amniotic fluid. All these techniques have been used to provide easy access to the fetus without removing it from the uterus; in addition, partial or total exteriorization of the fetus from the uterine cavity has also been successfully employed (Kraner, 1965).

Fetal surgery, initially developed for the study of intrauterine development, has become an important tool in other fields such as immunology and pathology. In studies of the ontogeny of the immune response in the fetus the use of prolonged and complex procedures *in utero*, without termination of pregnancy and with postnatal survival, has been particularly valuable. Skin grafting, thymectomy and splenectomy have been carried out in the sheep and in the monkey (SILVERSTEIN *et al.*, 1964; PARSHALL and SILVERSTEIN, 1969). In these experiments some fetuses were subjected to as many as four consecutive procedures. The results of these studies lend further support to an already appreciable body of evidence (STERZL and SILVERSTEIN, 1967) suggesting that the mammalian fetus is capable of active immunologic responses *in utero*. The fetus has also been used as a model for the study of clinically important congenital abnormalities, in particular those of the gastrointestinal tract. Ligation of the fetal mesenteric vessels in the dog (LOUW and BARNARD, 1965) produced anomalies identical to intestinal atresia. Biliary atresia (HOLDER and ASHCRAFT, 1966; MORGAN *et al.*, 1966) diaphragmatic hernia (DE LORIMIER *et al.*, 1967), and coarctation of the aorta (JACKSON *et al.*, 1963) have also been studied.

Human Fetal Surgery

In the 1960's clinical interest in fetal surgery was stimulated by the lack of adequate therapy for fetuses suffering from erythroblastosis. The first reported attempt at human fetal surgery was made on such a fetus (FREDA and ADAMSONS, 1964). Through a small incision in the uterus a leg was delivered and an exchange transfusion performed via the femoral artery. The fetus was aborted on the second post-operative day. Two years later two successful cases of human fetal surgery were reported (ASENSIO *et al.*, 1966; SEELEN *et al.*, 1966). Viable babies were delivered following transfusion through the saphenous vein in the first case and through a placental vein in the second.

Since these events there have been several references in the literature to the possibility of the *in utero* correction of congenital anomalies (KRANER, 1965; ADAMSONS, 1966; ROSENKRANTZ, 1969; VALENTI, 1972). Although most abnormalities can be dealt with in the postnatal period certain anomalies would best be treated before birth, particularly those which cause severe secondary changes. Examples of such anomalies are obstructive hydrocephalus, diaphragmatic hernia (leading to hypoplasia of the lungs), urinary tract anomalies, severe spina bifida (leading to development of paraplegia and incontinence) and severe cases of cleft lip and palate. The last example illustrates particularly well how an anomaly seen at birth can represent only one stage in the abnormal growth pattern initiated *in utero*. It has been suggested (BURSTON, 1964) that most of the deformity associated with cleft lip and palate occurs during the late stages of gestation when rapid unrestrained growth of the facial tissues and abnormal tongue behaviour, result in widening of the cleft. In young fetuses facial distortion, apart from the cleft dehiscence, is minimal with few of the characteristic stigmata seen at birth. Even in premature births facial distortion is much reduced.

Apart from its role in the prevention or alleviation of secondary deformities which derive from the original defect, surgical correction *in utero* would also offer the chance of post-operative recovery under optimum conditions, particularly in those cases where surgery in the neonate carries a high morbidity. The congenitally deformed infant may be unable to make all the necessary adaptations demanded by the transition from fetal to extrauterine existence, and may also sustain physical

and biochemical injuries at delivery. Death of those fetuses with cardiovascular anomalies which survive into late gestation rarely occurs until new conditions are imposed by the circulatory changes associated with extrauterine life. Intrauterine surgery would give such fetuses the added advantage of post-operative recovery in a near-ideal environment and post-operative complications associated with inadequacies in respiration, nutrition or thermoregulation would be virtually eliminated.
Recent advances in the field of prenatal diagnosis (HARRIS, 1971) have made the concept of intrauterine diagnosis and treatment of congenital anomalies increasingly plausible. Cytological and biochemical analysis of amniotic fluid can reveal certain conditions which are due to chromosome anomalies (e. g. Down's syndrome) and to specific inborn errors of metabolism (e. g. galactosemia). Some conditions which are not diagnosable by amniocentesis but which are associated with grossly abnormal morphology can be recognised with the use of techniques such as 2-dimensional ultrasound photography and fetoscopy (VALENTI, 1972; SCRIMGEOUR, 1973). Diagnostic ultrasound has been used in the recognition of neural tube effects and renal lesions (CAMPBELL, 1973; GARRETT *et al.*, 1970). The fetoscope, an instrument which is inserted into the amniotic sac via a small incision in the uterus, allows direct visualisation of the fetus. To date, there has been at least one reported case of its use in the human followed by live birth (LAURENCE *et al.*, 1974). In this case fetoscopy was performed at 18 weeks gestation in an attempt to establish the presence or absence of the digital anomalies associated with Hirschsprung's disease. The mother had previously given birth to two infants bearing the stigmata of the syndrome. Fetoscopy revealed that both hands and one foot were normal. Delivery of a normal infant took place at the 35th week.

Fetal Wound Healing

One important prerequisite for the successful application of fetal surgery to the treatment of congenital defects is an understanding of the response of fetal tissues to injury. As yet there is little information on wound healing mechanisms in the mammalian fetus. The results of fetal wound healing studies that have been carried out so far present a confusing picture. The differences in the size, nature and location of the wounds studied, together with the interspecies variation that must exist, may have been important factors in the production of a wide spectrum of fetal responses.
In the work reported by HESS (1954) the vertebral columns of guinea pig fetuses from 37—48 days of gestational age were severed with scissors. Extensive granulation tissue formation was observed and complete epithelialisation of the wounds occurred in 4—6 days. It was concluded that, considering the severe nature of the induced wounds, the healing time was rapid, although the process of healing was essentially the same as in postnatal animals. The wounds of younger fetuses did not heal more rapidly than those of older ones.
Studies on the effects of skin burns in fetal and neonatal rats (DIXON, 1960) showed a clear gradation of response from a fetal to an adult pattern. The essential difference between fetal and adult reactions to injury was manifested in the phase of

acute inflammation. In the younger fetuses ($16^1/_2$—$17^1/_2$ days old) rapid "filling-in" of the wounds with fast proliferating local mesenchymal cells was accompanied by absence of vascular dilatation and of exudation of fluid from the blood vessels. After the 18th day of gestation the blood vessels were observed to play an active role, and repair by mesenchymal cells of the fetal type was diminished. With increasing gestational age there was also a gradual decrease in the rate of muscular and epithelial regeneration.

In contrast to the results of the studies so far described is the apparent lack of intra-uterine healing in the rabbit fetus (SOMASUNDARAM and PRATHAP, 1970). Circular excisional wounds were made in the skin of fetuses ranging from 14—25 days gestational age. The fetal response was compared to that of the newborn rabbit and several major differences were observed. The fetal wounds displayed none of the phenomena associated with the healing open wound in the postnatal period viz. scab-formation, contraction, epithelialisation and granular tissue formation. In addition, the inflammatory response was insignificant. It was suggested that contact with amniotic fluid may be one of the main factors responsible for the lack of healing. The results of later studies (SOMASUNDARAM and PRATHAP, 1972), appeared to support this suggestion. Covering of the open wounds with silastic grafts resulted in rapid healing by mesenchymal proliferation and epithelialisation accompanied by wound contraction.

The study of fetal fractures in the rabbit (MUSA RIS and WRAY, 1972) has been compared with fracture healing in the newborn. Section of the femur was carried out in fetuses 23—27 days old and in neonatal animals. After 24 hrs there was less tissue disruption and a weaker inflammatory reaction at the fracture site in the fetus. Callus formation began after 2 days in the fetus and after 6 days in the neonate. Differentiation into cartilage occurred more rapidly in the fetal callus. The authors speculated on the relationship between diminished inflammatory reaction and the more rapid fracture healing of the fetus.

Comparative Fetal Wound Healing Studies

Experiments designed to compare the fetal response to similar forms of injury in two species have only recently been carried out (SOPHER, 1972, 1975). Both species studied, the rat and the cynomolgus monkey, make good animal models for investigations into intrauterine healing. In the rat, surgery is well tolerated by both the mother and the fetus, and this species is particularly suitable for short-term studies. Use of the relatively larger monkey fetus allows the study of the healing process over longer post-wounding intervals.

In the comparative study mentioned above the response to simple surgical incisions and excisions, and to conventional suture materials was examined. As all intra-uterine surgical procedures would involve the incision of fetal membranes and of fetal skin particular attention was paid to the response of these tissues to injury. In both species access to the fetus was obtained via window-like openings in the uterus. In the case of the rat, expulsion of the fetus was prevented by the placing of a purse-string suture around the uterine incision, and in the monkey a modification of the marsupializing incision was used (Fig. 1).

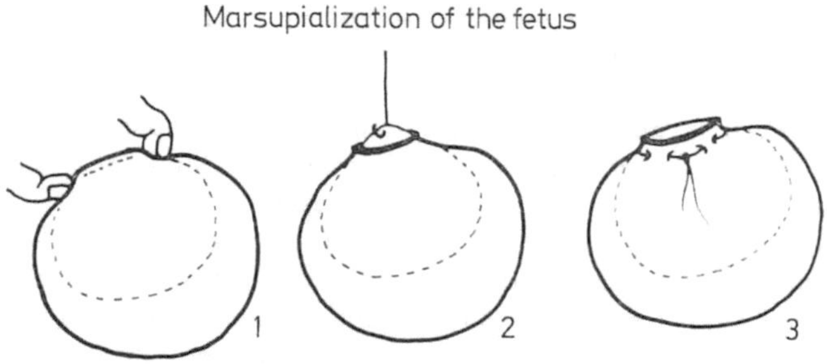

Fig. 1. 1. Manipulation and positioning of the fetus before incision of the uterus. 2. Tamponade of the uterine wound with the fetal body. 3. Purse-string suture marsupializing the fetus to the uterine wall

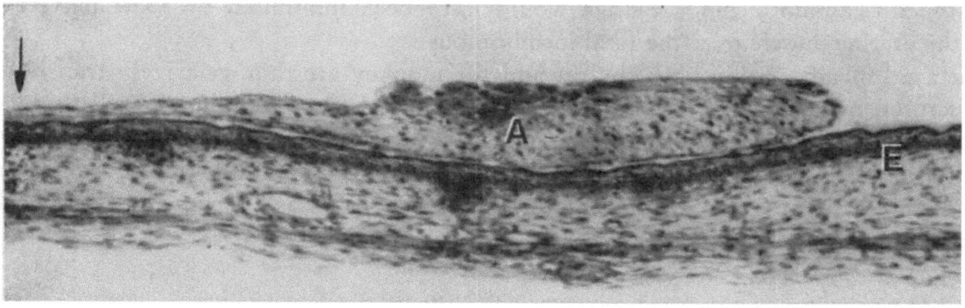

Fig. 2. Margin of a puncture wound in the amnion of the rat 48 hrs after wounding. The amnion (A) lies closely apposed to the fetal epidermis (E). The edge of the lesion is considerably thickened compared with the unwounded amnion (arrow). H and E., × 100

Healing in Fetal Membranes

Puncture of rat fetal membranes on the 16th day of gestation resulted in an immediate gaping of the wounds, with the formation of oval-shaped holes. By the end of the first post-operative day the thickened edges of the lesions could be clearly distinguished as opaque rims standing out against the surrounding translucent non-traumatised tissue. This thickening of the wound margins was particularly marked in the amnion. In section this area of the amnion consisted of accumulated fibroblast-like cells with fibrillar elements in an eosinophilic ground substance (Fig. 2). During the post-wounding interval (5 days) until the end of gestation, increasing cellularity in the wound area was accompanied by a gradual reduction in the size of the lesions in the amnion; by the end of the fifth post-operative day there was usually a marked difference between the sizes of the puncture wounds in the two membranes (amnion and yolk-sac). This process of wound contraction observed in the amnion would seem to support the suggestion (CHURCH and WARREN, 1968) that multiplying fibroblasts in the edge of a circular wound in a membranous tissue could be responsible for a contracting mechanism, orientated in a ring in the plane of the membrane. In this study complete closure of the puncture wounds in the rat fetal membranes was not observed. However, loss of amniotic fluid was minimized by a valve-like sealing action of the contracting uterine muscle moving over the underlying membranes, and by clot formation over the lesions. The clot formation was probably the result of coagulation of embryonic fluids and plasma proteins released from the damaged uterine and vitteline vessels.

In the monkey, puncture of the amnio-chorion, five to seven weeks before term, resulted in the formation of ovoid holes with rounded-off edges. These holes appeared to bear a close resemblance to the chorio-amnion fenestrations described in some clinical reports of premature rupture of membranes (BURNETT, 1957; REISFIELD, 1958). The peripheral zone of the puncture wound in the amnion contained hypertrophic fibroblasts and accumulated ground substance but there were no signs of the intense proliferative activity that was observed in the wounded area of the rat amnion. The edges of the lesions in the chorion were smoothed off by proliferation of trophoblast cells which tended to roll over the exposed stromal tissue. As in the rat, amniotic fluid leakage would have been minimised by some movement of the uterine muscle over the fetal membranous sac.

The fetal membranes in both the rat and the monkey are thin, relatively translucent structures, normally existing under tension. One would expect that in full-thickness wounds of these tissues the tension acting on the wound edges would prevent closure of the lesions. However, the cellular events following wounding can be interpreted as definite attempts at closure, and in the case of the case of the rat amnion the response was particularly effective.

Healing of Excised Wounds in Fetal Skin

The response to injury was rapid in a small excised wound made in the skin of the rat fetus on the 18th day of gestation. Within 24 hrs "filling-in" of the wound base had been achieved by the accumulation of mesenchymal cells and mononuclear cells, and the surface of the wound had been epithelialised by cells which had migrated from the cut edges of the epidermis (Fig. 3).

In contrast to this, the healing of a similar wound in monkey fetal skin (Fig. 4) was remarkably slow. Eight days after wounding, at about day 125 of gestation, the wound floor had still not been epithelialised. Although epidermal proliferation at the wound edges was particularly marked there were no signs of migratory activity from these points. However, some covering of the exposed wound base was provided by spindle-shaped epithelial-type cells which appeared to be derived from the damaged epidermal appendages in the dermis. There was no "filling-in" of the wound with granulation tissue. Epidermal migration in a skin wound of the fetal monkey was clearly evident in a 27 days old excision site (Fig. 5). The tissue filling the partially epithelialised wound base was dense and cellular, rich in ground substance and with some fibrous material. The connective tissue of the wound was comparable to that found in similar wounds in mature tissue after some resolution of the granulation tissue has taken place.

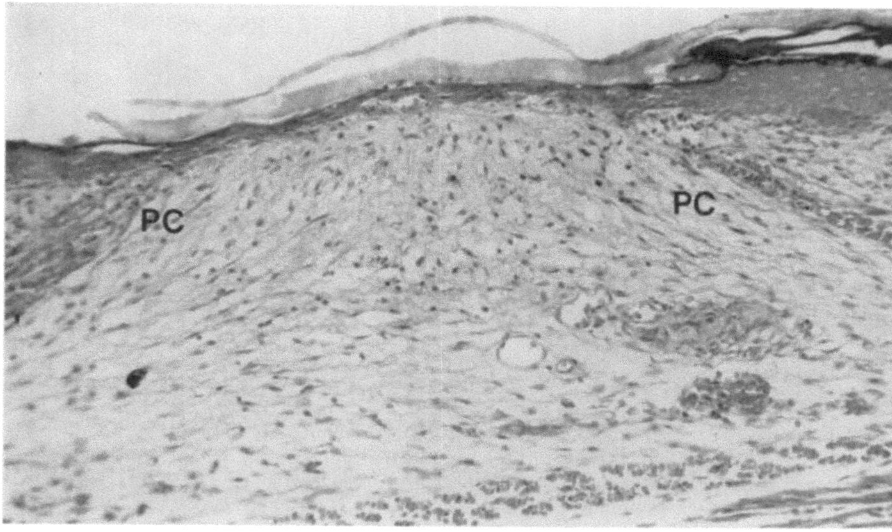

Fig. 3. Excisional wound in the skin of a 19 days old rat fetus 24 hrs after wounding. The dimension of the wound is indicated by the cut ends of the panniculus carnosus (PC). "Filling-in" of the wound with proliferating mesenchymal cells has taken place and the wound base has been epithelialised, with overlying fibrin and coagulated extraembryonic fluids. H and E., × 115

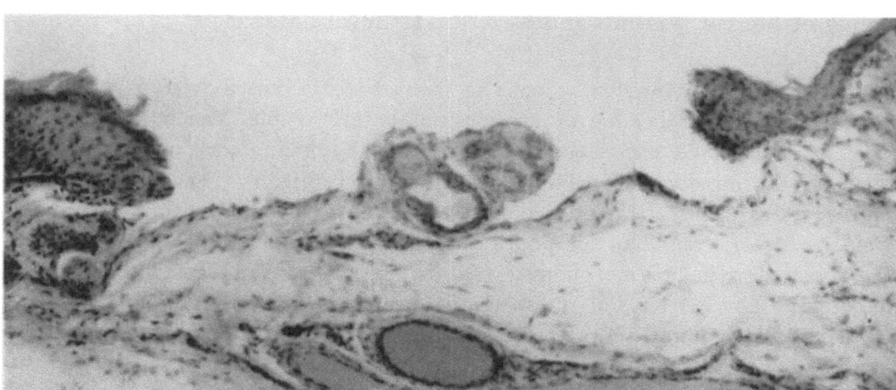

Fig. 4. Full thickness skin excisional wound after eight days of intrauterine healing in the monkey fetus. The epidermal cells are piled up at the wound margin and have not yet migrated across the wound base. The connective tissue is oedematous and there is no accumulation of granulation tissue. H and E., × 100

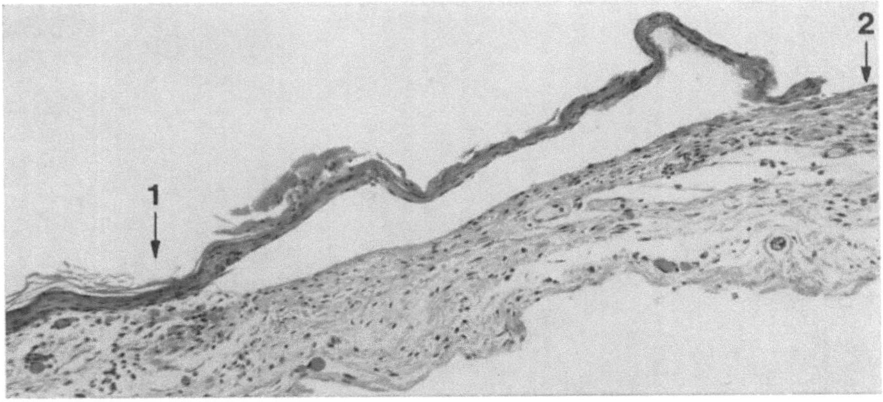

Fig. 5. Excisional site in fetal monkey skin after 27 days of intrauterine healing. The arrows 1 and 2 point to the approximate position of the original edge of the wound and to the mid-point of the wound floor respectively. The length of regenerated epidermis has become detached from the base of the wound. H and E., × 115

The gross appearance of the excisional wounds was similar in both rat and monkey. The wounded area was pale rather than inflamed, and the wound base was smooth and glistening. The lack of formation of a scab was conspicuous although the rat wounds developed fibrin clots in the early stages of healing. Accurate measurements of the dimensional changes were not made but, as far as it could be ascertained, the excisional wounds showed little or no contraction.

Healing of Incised Wounds and Reaction to Suture Materials

Sutured full-thickness incision wounds in monkey fetal skin showed rapid healing. Even after five days the line of incision was barely visible. The most remarkable histological feature of such wounds was a minimal inflammatory response, both at the site of the incision and around the suture tract (Fig. 6). The diminished perisutural reaction seen in fetal skin contrasted sharply with that seen in neonatal skin. Within 24 hrs of wounding, the perisutural space in neonatal (Fig. 7) skin was densely populated with polymorphonuclear cells. No similar infiltrate was seen in the skin of a 130 day old fetus at the same post-wounding interval (Fig. 8).
The perisutural reaction in rat fetal skin showed the additional feature of rapid encapsulation of the suture material. Three days after a length of silk suture had been embedded in the skin of an 18 days old rat fetus, the silk fibres had been almost completely encapsulated by epithelium which had grown down from the epidermis (Fig. 9).
The open incised skin wound in the monkey fetus showed delayed healing. The cut edges of a full-thickness incised wound in the skin of a 120 day old fetus did not

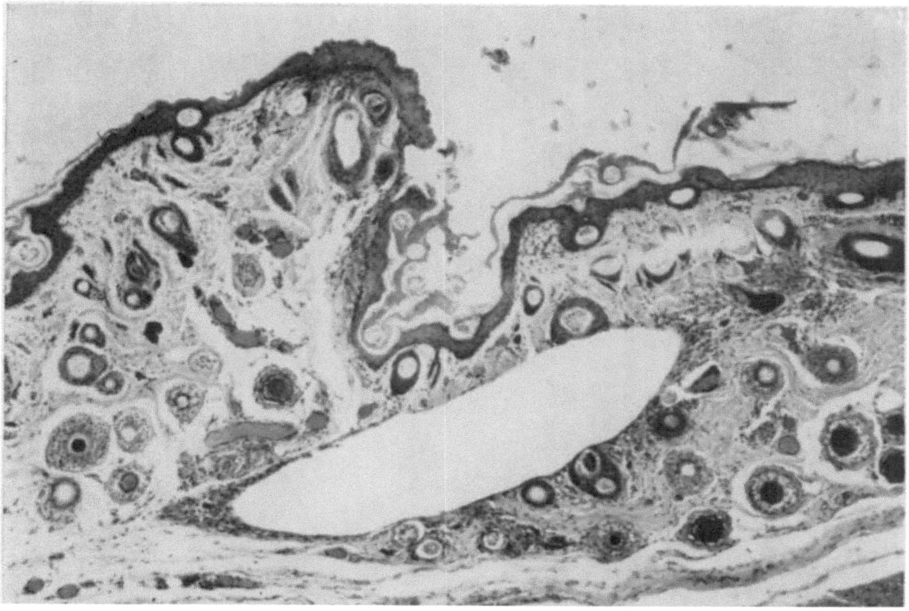

Fig. 6. Skin of the monkey fetus showing a sutured incision eight days after wounding. Epithelial cells have grown out from the transected hair follicles and have partially lined the suture space (the suture material — chromicised gut — has fallen out). The inflammatory response is negligible. H and E., × 75

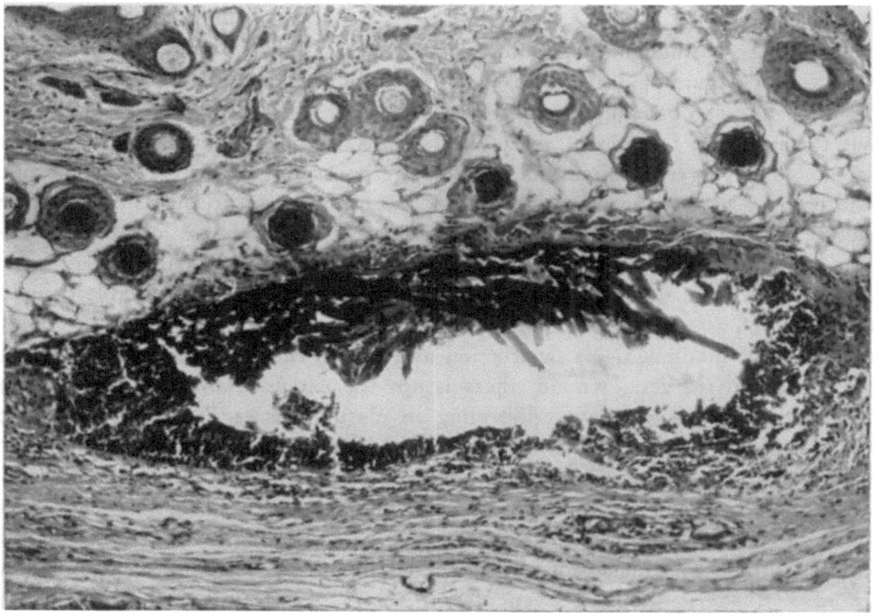

Fig. 7. Suture (silk) tract in the skin of neonatal monkey 24 hrs after wounding following delivery. There is a heavy infiltration of inflammatory cells around the suture space (compare with Fig. 8). H and E., × 100

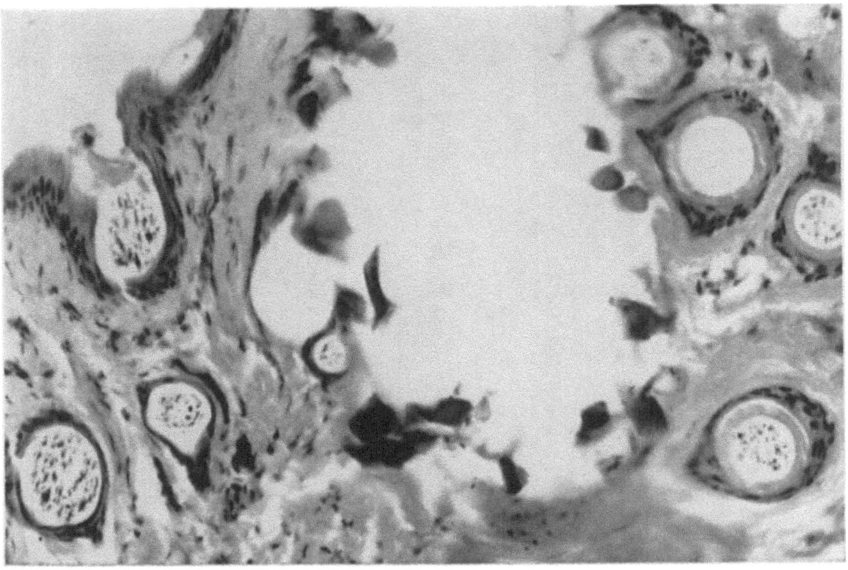

Fig. 8. Suture tract in the skin of the monkey fetus less than 24 hrs after wounding in utero. Most of the suture material has been lost during processing but a few fibres of silk remain. Note the lack of inflammatory cell infiltration around the tract. H and E., × 215

remain apposed although tissue adhesive had been applied to the wound (Fig. 10). After a post-wounding interval of five days the epidermis had grown down the sides of the incision but the wound base was still exposed.

Thus the principle features of the fetal response to injury, common to both the rat and the monkey, were minimal inflammatory response absence of infection and failure to develop a scab in open wounds. The last feature is not surprising as one important function of a scab in a skin wound is the prevention of continued loss of body fluids when the epidermal barrier has been broken. The fluid environment of the mammalian fetus precludes the need for scab-formation; there is no loss of viable tissue due to dehydration as in air-exposed skin wounds.

In the face of minimal tissue destruction and the absence of infection it is not surprising that, in the fetal wound, there is not the extensive inflammatory infiltrate normally associated with wound healing in mature tissues. It has been suggested (SCHWARTZ and OSBURN, 1974) that the limited inflammatory response of the monkey fetus is primarily due to the low level of circulating white blood cells. However, the fluid, sterile environment of the fetus may be the most important factor involved. The changes seen in a fetal wound exposed to air (SOPHER — unpublished) seem to support this suggestion. The exposed floor of an excisional wound in the skin of a full-term monkey, even after 22 days of intrauterine healing, becomes heavily infiltrated with leucocytes within 24 hrs of birth (Fig. 11).

The differences observed between the healing of skin excisional wounds in the rat and in the monkey could be a reflection of the difference in degree of maturation

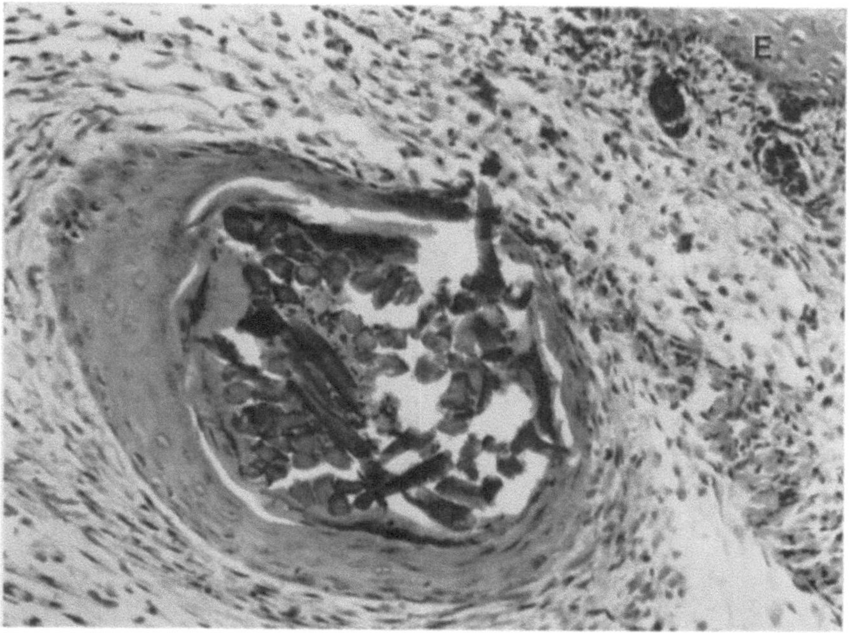

Fig. 9. Skin of a 21 days old rat fetus 3 days after embedding of silk suture material. The latter has been almost completely encapsulated with epithelium which has grown down from the epidermis (E). H and E., × 250

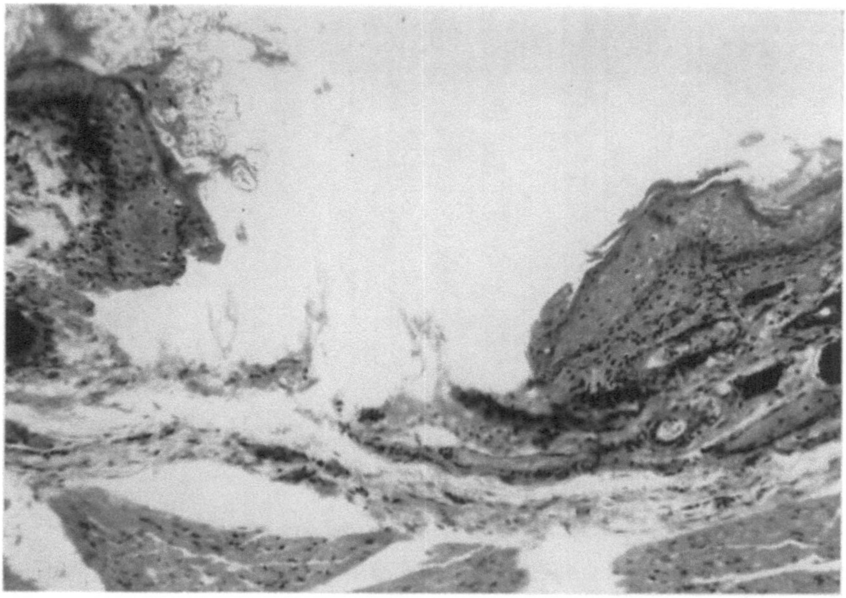

Fig. 10. Open full-thickness skin incision five days after wounding. There is some epidermal proliferation at the wound margins which are inverted. In the top left hand corner the epidermis is still covered with tissue adhesive (painted on at the time of wounding). The wound base remains denuded and is covered with loosely held collagenous strands. H and E., × 115

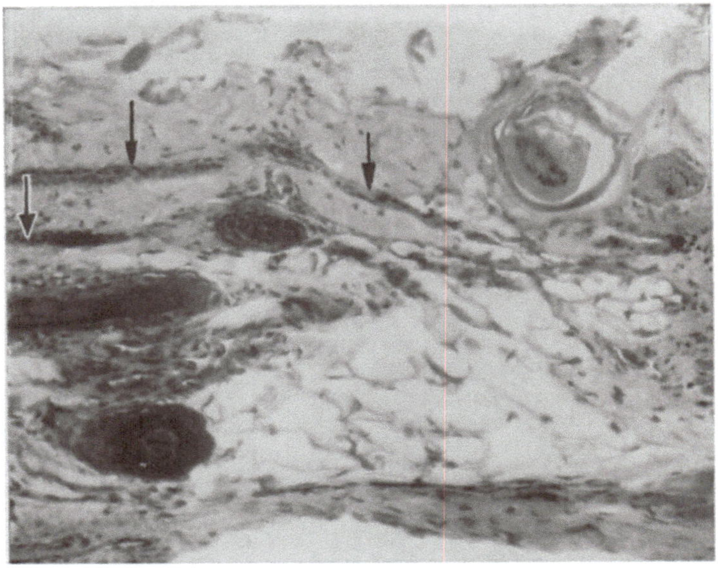

(a)

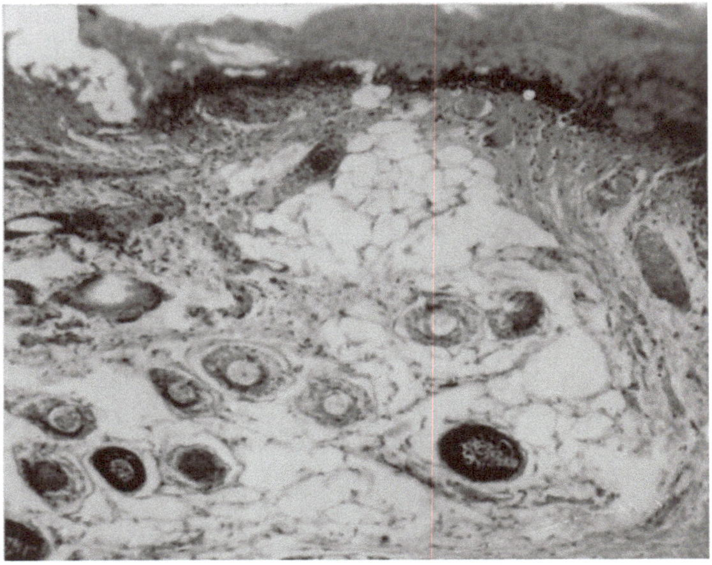

(b)

Fig. 11. (a) Biopsy of part of the floor of an excisional skin wound in a newly delivered monkey 22 days after wounding. Tongues of epithelium (arrows) are growing out from the wound edge (to the left). There are no signs of inflammatory cell infiltration. H and E., × 150. (b) Section of the same excisional wound as in (a) but 24 hrs after delivery. There is a heavy infiltration of leucocytes and the beginning of scab formation on the exposed surface of the wound. H and E., × 130

at birth. The fetal primate is relatively more mature at birth than is the fetal rat. It is not surprising that the process of rapid "filling-in" of skin wounds by proliferating mesenchymal cells, as observed in the rat, does not occur in similar wounds of the fetal monkey. Such wounds showed a distinct delay in the onset of fibroblastic activity and there was not the massive accumulation of tissue normally associated with granulating wounds in mature tissue. The delay in migration of epidermis from the wound edges and the lack of contraction observed may be related to the delayed fibroplasia. However, the outcome of slow intrauterine healing of excisional skin wounds need not be unfavourable. If healing by secondary intention in monkey fetal skin is indeed characterised by diminished neogenesis of connective tissue the amount of remodelling required in the cicatrization process should also be diminished. It is tempting to speculate that a major benefit of intrauterine healing in the primate would be minimal scarring.

The results of this study illustrate clearly the differences that can exist between two species in fetal response to wounding, and hence the value of comparative studies. If these differences are correlated primarily with the level of maturity of the fetal tissues at the time of wounding extrapolation to man may be possible, after further investigations using animals with a comparable length of gestation. Further studies of the reaction to suture materials and of the process of cicatrization would have particular relevance for human fetal surgery.

Conclusion

The human fetus can no longer be considered inviolate; the increasing sophistication of intrauterine diagnostic techniques has permitted safe and effective sampling of its immediate environs. It is likely that a new horizon in clinical surgery will be the development of diagnostic and reconstructive procedures for the intrauterine correction of birth defects. Advancement in these new areas will be all the more valuable when technical procedures are based on accurate information concerning the response of the fetus and its membranes to premeditated injury.

In the field of teratology the fetus has already proved to be a valuable model for the study of certain congenital anomalies. Similarities between simian and human gestation make the fetal monkey a particularly good model for further investigation of the asynchronous patterns of growth of the deformed fetus, and the response of its tissues to the process of intrauterine repair.

Interesting as the prospects may be for intrauterine correction of gross malformation, it remains to be shown that no long-term growth retardation is suffered by the patient as a result of these new techniques. Until such assurances can be given, based necessarily on additional experiments in the near-human primate, the prospects for fetal surgery in man cannot adequately be determined.

Acknowledgment: Figures 1, 4, 6, and 10 were reproduced from "Breeding Simians for Developmental Biology" (SOPHER, 1975) by courtesy of the editor of Laboratory Animal Handbooks.

References

Adamsons, K., Jr.: Fetal surgery. New Engl. J. Med. **275,** 204 (1966).

Asensio, S. H., Figueroa-Longo, J. G., Pelegrina, I. A.: Intrauterine exchange transfusion. Amer. J. Obstet. Gynec. **95,** 1129 (1966).

Barcroft, J., Barron, D. H.: Movements in midfetal life in the sheep embryo. J. Physiol. **91,** 329 (1937).

Barcroft, J., Barron, D. H.: The development of behaviour in the fetal sheep. J. comp. Neurol. **70,** 477 (1939).

Barcroft, J., Barron, D. H.: Observations on the functional development of the fetal brain. J. comp. Neurol. **77,** 431 (1942).

Barnard, C. N.: A method of operating on fetal dogs in utero. Surgery **41,** 805 (1957).

Barron, D. H.: The role of the sensory fibers in the differentiation of the spinal cord in sheep. J. exp. Zool. **100,** 431 (1945).

Bors, E.: Die Methodik der intrauterinen Operation am überlebenden Säugetierfoetus. Arch. Entwickl.-Mech. Org. **105,** 655 (1925).

Burnett, C. W. F.: Fenestrations of the fetal membranes. J. Obstet. Gynaec. Brit. Emp. **66,** 79 (1957).

Burston, W. R.: In symposium "Malformation of the face". Brit. dent. J. **116,** 285 (1964).

Campbell, S.: The antenatal detection of fetal abnormality by ultrasonic diagnosis. In "Birth Defects". Proceedings of the Fourth International Conference. A. G. Motulsky and W. Lenz, Eds. Amsterdam: Excerpta Medica 1973.

Church, J. C. T., Warren, D. J.: Wound healing in the web membrane of the fruit bat. Brit. J. Surg. **55,** 26 (1968).

De Lorimier, A. A., Tierney, D. F., Parker, H. R.: Hypoplastic lungs in fetal lambs with surgically produced congenital diaphragmatic hernia. Surgery **62,** 12 (1967).

Dixon, J. B.: Inflammation in the fetal and neonatal rat: The local reactions to skin burns. J. Path. Bact. **80,** 73 (1960).

Domm, L. V., Leroy, P.: A method for fetal hypophysectomy by decapitation in the rat. Anat. Rec. **109,** 395 (1951).

Foote, C. L., Foote, F. M.: Changes in the thyroid gland of hamster embryos hypophysectomized by decapitation. Anat. Rec. **105,** 79 (1949).

Freda, V. J., Adamsons, K., Jr.: Exchange transfusion in utero. Amer. J. Obstet. Gynec. **89,** 817 (1964).

Garrett, W. J., Grunwald, G., Robinson, D. E.: Prenatal diagnosis of fetal polycystic kidney by ultrasound. Aust. N. Z. J. Obstet. Gynaec. **10,** 7 (1970).

Hall, E. K., Schneiderhan, M. A.: Spinal ganglion hypoplasia after limb amputation in the fetal rat. J. comp. Neurol. **82,** 19 (1945).

Harris, A. (Ed.): Early diagnosis of human genetic defects: Scientific and ethical considerations. Washington, D.C., U.S. Govt. Printing Office 1971.

Hess, A.: Reactions of mammalian fetal tissues to injury. II. Skin. Anat. Rec. **119,** 435 (1954).

Holder, T., Ashcraft, K.: Production of experimental biliary atresia by ligation of the common bile duct in the fetus. Surg. Forum **17,** 356 (1966).

Hooker, D., Nicholas, J. S.: Spinal cord section in rat fetuses. J. comp. Neurol. **50,** 413 (1930).

Jackson, B. T., Egdahl, R. H.: The performance of complex fetal operations in utero without amniotic fluid loss or other disturbances of fetal-maternal relationships. Surgery **48,** 564 (1960).

Jackson, B. T., Piasecki, G. J., Egdahl, R. H.: Experimental production of coarctation of the aorta in utero with prolonged postnatal survival. Surg. Forum **14,** 290 (1963).

Jost, A.: Sur la differenciation sexuelle de l'embryon de lapin. I. Remarques au sujet de certaines operations chirurgicales sur l'embryon. C. R. Soc. Biol. **140,** 461 (1946).

Kraner, K. L.: Intrauterine fetal surgery. Advanc. vet. Sci. **10,** 1 (1965).

Louw, J. H., Barnard, C. N.: Congenital intestinal atresia. Observations on its origin. Lancet **1955 II,** 1065.

MAYER, A.: Über die Möglichkeit operativer Eingriffe beim lebenden Säugetierfötus. ZBL. Gynäk. **42**, 773 (1918).

MOORE, C. R., BODIAN, D.: Opossum pouch young as experimental material. Anat. Rec. **76**, 319 (1940).

MORGAN, W. W., ROSENKRANTZ, J. G., HILL, R. B., Jr.: Hepatic arterial interruption in the fetus — an attempt at simulating biliary atresia. J. Pediat. Surg. **1**, 342 (1966).

MUSA RIS, P., WRAY, J. B.: A histological study of fracture healing within the uterus of the rabbit. Clin. Orthop. **87**, 318 (1972).

NICHOLAS, J. S.: Notes on the application of experimental methods upon mammalian embryos. Anat. Rec. **31**, 385 (1925).

PARSHALL, C. J., Jr., SILVERSTEIN, A. M.: Surgical approaches to the study of fetal immunology in primate animals. Ann. N.Y. Acad. Sci. **162**, 254 (1969).

REISFIELD, D. R.: Congenital defect in the fetal membranes: A condition simulating spontaneous rupture. Bull. Sloane Hosp. Wom. N.Y. **4**, 16 (1958).

ROSENKRANTZ, J. G.: Foetal Surgery: In Recent advances in paediatric surgery, Chapter 2, p. 9, A. W. WILKINSON, Ed. London: J. A. Churchill Ltd. 1969.

SCHWARTZ, L. W., OSBURN, B. I.: An ontogenic study of the acute inflammatory reaction in the fetal rhesus monkey. I. Cellular response to bacterial and nonbacterial irritants. Lab. Invest. **31**, 441 (1974).

SCRIMGEOUR, J. B.: Fetoscopy. In "Birth defects". Proceedings of the Fourth International Conference. A. G. MOTULSKY and W. LENZ, Eds. Amsterdam: Excerpta Medica 1973.

SEELEN, J., VAN KESSEL, H., ESKES, T., BEEN, J., EVERS, J., VAN GENT, I., PEETERS, L., VAN DER VELDEN, W., ZONDERLAND, F.: A new method of exchange transfusion in utero. Amer. J. Obstet. Gynec. **95**, 872 (1966).

SILVERSTEIN, A. M., PRENDERGAST, R. A., KRANER, K. L.: Fetal response to antigenic stimulus. IV. Rejection of skin homgrafts by the fetal lamb. J. exp. Med. **119**, 955 (1964).

SOMASUNDARAM, K., PRATHAP, K.: Intra-uterine healing of skin wounds in rabbit fetuses. J. Path. **100**, 81 (1970).

SOMASUNDARAM, K., PRATHAP, K.: The effect of exclusion of amniotic fluid on intra-uterine healing of skin wounds in rabbit fetuses. J. Path. **107**, 127 (1972).

SOPHER, D.: The response of rat fetal membranes to injury. Ann. roy. Coll. Surg. Engl. **51**, 240 (1972).

SOPHER, D.: A study of wound healing in the foetal tissues of the cynomolgus monkey. In "Breeding Simians for Developmental Biology". Lab. Anim. Handbook **6**, 327 (1975).

STERZL, J., SILVERSTEIN, A. M.: Developmental aspects of immunity. Advanc. Immun. **6**, 337 (1967).

TOBIN, C. E.: The influence of adrenal destruction on the prenatal development of the albino rat. Amer. J. Anat. **65**, 151 (1939).

VALENTI, C.: Endoamnioscopy and fetal biopsy: A new technique. Amer. J. Obstet. Gynec. **114**, 561 (1972).

WOLFF, B.: Experimentelle Untersuchungen über die Entstehung extrauteriner Schwangerschaften und über die Möglichkeit operativer Eingriffe beim lebenden Säugetierfetus. Beitr. Path. Anat. **65**, 423 (1919).

New Aspects of Developmental Teratology

Increasing attention has been paid to abnormalites of development that are not associated with gross malformation. Dobbing has demonstrated the importance of a suitable environment in the late fetal period for achievement of the total potential of the central nervous system. In this section the well established teratological principle of selective sensitivity has been exploited to produce abnormalities of the brain with subsequent behavioural defects. Similar abnormalities may be induced by the activity of variable alleles which result in enzymatic polymorphism. The potential importance of this type of variation in man is described with particular reference to the development of the central nervous system. Such variability is inevitable in outbred populations, but its role in teratology has only recently been investigated. Finally, the effects of dysmorphogenesis on the wider unit, the family, are considered; these social implications of malformation provide the stimulus for all the basic investigations embodied in scientific teratology.

11. Morphological and Behavioural Abnormalities Caused by Insults to the CNS in the Perinatal Period

J. Langman, W. Webster, and P. Rodier

With 17 Figures

Introduction

During recent years teratologists have mainly concentrated on that period of development which is known as the time of organogenesis, and which in the mammalian embryo comprises the first third of gestation. Malformations can easily be produced during this phase of development and tend to be gross and easily recognizable. When the same teratogens are administered during the last third of intrauterine life, they do not cause major malformations and the fetus throughout this time period has generally been regarded as resistant to environmental and teratogenic influences. Hence, the last one-third of pregnancy has been virtually ignored as a period in which birth defects may arise.

Only recently has it been appreciated that this late period of development may be more dangerous than initially thought. Environmental teratogenic agents acting during this period, although not causing gross abnormalities, may interfere with cell proliferation, cell differentiation and/or cell migration and thus cause deficiencies of cell numbers, minute cellular abnormalities and cell dystopia, respectively. These anomalies might be difficult to detect morphologically, but might cause serious functional abnormalities in postnatal life.

In the central nervous system, in particular, certain regions continue to show high proliferative activity resulting in the formation of unique cell types until shortly before birth and in some areas even during postnatal life. Similarly, cell migration and neuronal differentiation in many regions continue throughout the last period of prenatal development. If environmental teratogenic agents were to interfere with these processes, it might be difficult to detect the abnormalities, even with the light microscope. Possibly they would reveal themselves only as behavioural abnormalities later in life. Of course, such abnormalities would not necessarily be restricted to the central nervous system, but might conceivably involve functional abnormalities in the endocrine system, immunological system or other systems.

During the last few years, an attempt has been made in our laboratory to explore the action of various drugs on the central nervous system of the mouse during the last trimester of pregnancy and shortly after birth and to evaluate their effects by morphological and behavioural studies.

CNS Development in Late Gestation and Early Postnatal Life

In the central nervous system of a 15-day mouse embryo cell proliferation is not seen in all areas, but is restricted to certain specific regions. By applying radioautographic techniques, it was found that large numbers of tritiated thymidine-labelled cells were present in the neuroepithelium of the lateral ventricles, in the corpus striatum and in the dorsal wall of the mesencephalon (Figs. 1 and 2). The neuroepithelium of other parts of the brain such as the myelencephalon, anterior mesencephalon and the diencephalon did not show proliferative activity at this stage and thus the cells were mainly unlabelled. This experiment emphasizes that not all

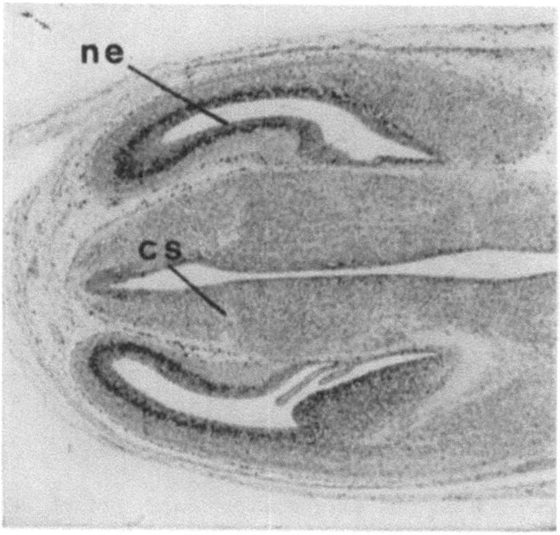

Fig. 1. Radioautograph of a coronal section through the head of a 15-day old embryo one hour after treatment with H^3-thymidine. Labelled cells of the neuroepithelium (ne) form a dark band around the lateral ventricles. In the corpus striatum (cs) labelled cells are seen scattered throughout

regions of the brain are developing at the same time. Some areas of the CNS have already their full complement of neurons on embryonic day 15 and will be unaffected by teratological agents interfering with proliferation, while others are at their peak of cell production and may be seriously affected.

In the neuroepithelial zone, which forms a pseudostratified layer of 5—7 cell rows, the nuclei of the proliferative cells replicate their DNA in the outer half of the layer and then move to the lumen to divide. At the same time the elongated neuroepithelial cells lose their external cytoplasmic processes and round up at the lumen. After cell division some of the daughter cells migrate out into the DNA synthetic zone to repeat the cell cycle, but many others leave the proliferative population and migrate beyond the neuroepithelial zone into the mantle layer, where they differentiate into adult neurons (Langman and Welch, 1967). The distance the cells migrate may be short, as in the mesencephalon, or very long as in the neocortex.

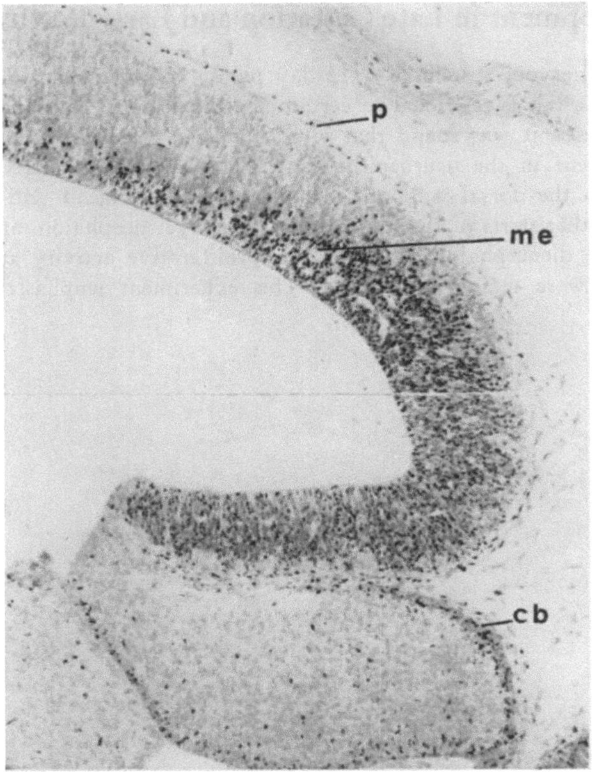

Fig. 2. Radioautograph of a sagittal section through the roof of the mesencephalon of a 15-day old embryo 16 hrs after treatment with H^3-thymidine. The neuroepithelium in the most caudal part of the mesencephalic roof is heavily labelled; more rostrally the neuroepithelium is almost inactive. p: pia; cb: cerebellum; me: mesencephalon

In the neocortex, the newly formed cells always take up a position superficial to all previously formed neurons of the cortical plate (ANGEVINE and SIDMAN, 1961; BERRY and ROGERS, 1965). Hence, the later a neuron is formed, the further it must migrate. Although in the mouse the distance the cells have to migrate is relatively short, in primates, particularly in man, it may be many millimeters (RAKIC, 1972, 1974). It has been suggested that during their migration from the proliferative layer to their ultimate destination the cells are guided by special radial glial fibers extending from the neuroepithelial layer to the superficial cortex (RAKIC, 1972).

The day a cell undergoes its final division is known as its "*birthday*". The cells whose birthdays fall on embryonic day 15 (E15), can be labelled with tritiated thymidine just prior to their final division and can be recognized in the adult brain as the most heavily labelled cells. Cells that underwent their final division before embryonic day 15 will be unlabelled and cells that undergo their final division on subsequent days will be more lightly labelled. Table 1 lists the location of the most heavily labelled cells seen in the adult mouse brain after labelling with tritiated

Table 1. Time of labelling

	Embryonic day 15	Embryonic day 19	Postnatal day 3
Cerebral Cortex	many cells in superficial layers caudally, slightly deeper layers rostrally	—	—
Hippocampus	many cells in pyramidal layer, especially CA 1	—	—
Dentate Gyrus	—	many granule cells	many granule cells
Corpus Striatum	many cells throughout	few cells, scattered throughout	—
Olfactory Tubercle	many small cells	—	—
Olfactory Bulb	many mitral cells	many internal granular layer cells, some glomerular layer cells	many glomerular layer cells, some internal granular layer cells
Hypothalamus	some clusters in ventral nuclei	—	—
Amygdala	some clusters, especially in medial cortical nucleus	—	—
Septum	some clusters in nuclei	—	—
Midbrain	some superficial clusters in inferior colliculus, a few in superior colliculus	—	—
Pons	some clusters in ventral nuclei	—	—
Cerebellar Cortex	—	internal granular layer and some cells around Purkinje cells, especially in vermis	internal granular layer and most cells around Purkinje cells, some basket cells
Retina	many labelled cells	many labelled cells	many labelled cells

thymidine on embryonic day 15, embryonic day 19, and postnatal day 3 (Rodier *et al.*, 1974).

If the labelling experiment is performed on E19, that is the day before birth, cell proliferation in the neuroepithelial layers has virtually ceased, but new areas of cell production are now visible. Labelled cells are seen in an extensive layer located between the quiescent neuroepithelial zone and the mantle layer around much of the lateral ventricles (Fig. 3). This layer is the subependymal layer and produces the granule cells of the dentate gyrus and olfactory bulb as well as most of the neuroglia of the forebrain (Smart, 1961; Altman, 1963). The second area of striking proliferation is the external granular layer of the cerebellum (Fig. 4). This layer lies over the cerebellar cortex immediately under the pia and will form the microneurons

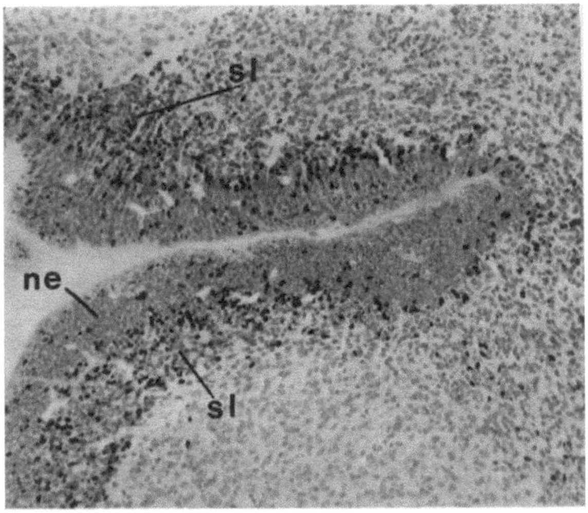

Fig. 3. Radioautograph of a section through olfactory region of a 19-day old embryo one hour after treatment with H^3-thymidine. Note the heavy labelling of the subependymal layer (sl); the neuroepithelium (ne) contains very few labelled cells

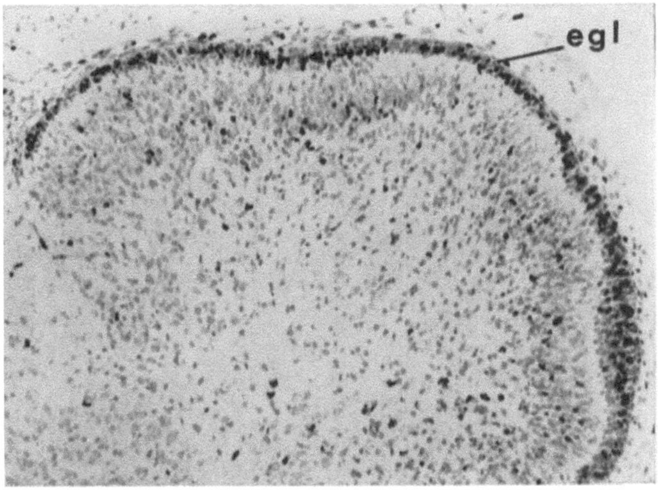

Fig. 4. Similar section through the cerebellum of a 19-day embryo. Note the heavy labelling of the cells in the external granular layer (egl)

(internal granule cells, basket and stellate cells) of the cerebellum (MIALE and SIDMAN, 1961; ALTMAN, 1969). The microneurons of the subependymal layer and the granule cells of the external granular layer migrate over considerable distances before they reach their final adult location. In the cerebellum the cells may be guided by glial fibers, while the subependymal cells are thought to follow fiber tracts, such

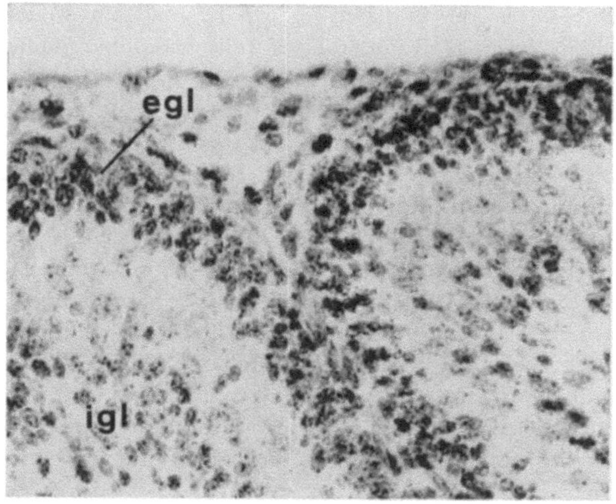

Fig. 5. Radioautograph of a section through a portion of the cerebellum of a mouse treated with H^3-thymidine on PN3 and killed 16 hrs later. Many labelled cells appear in the developing external granular layer (egl) and in the internal granular layer (igl)

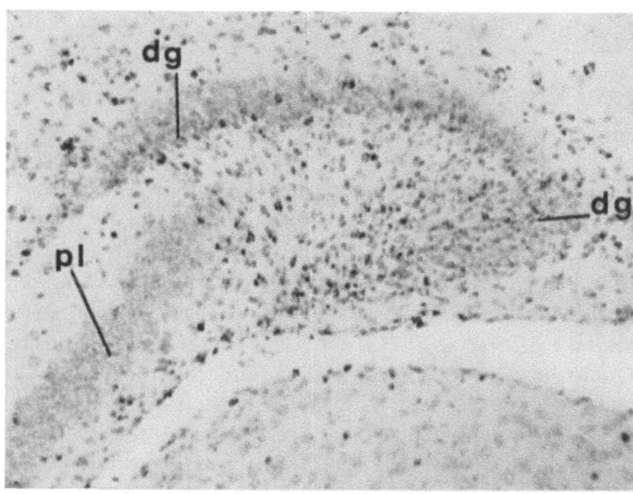

Fig. 6. Radioautograph of a section through the dentate nucleus treated with H^3-thymidine on E19 and killed 16 hrs later. Many labelled cells appear in the developing dentate gyrus (dg) and surrounding tissue. The earlier formed pyramidal cell layer (pl) of the hippocampus is free of label

as the corpus callosum (SMART, 1961; ALTMAN, 1963). The adult location of the cells formed on embryonic day 19 is listed in Table 1.

Tritiated thymidine injected on postnatal day 3 results in the presence of labelled neurons in essentially the same areas of the developing brain as seen on embryonic day 19 (Figs. 5 and 6). Obviously, the specific cells involved must be different, and some distinctions between the two periods can be made in adult animals. In the olfactory bulb, many internal granular layer cells and some glomerular layer cells are labelled on E19. Conversely, many glomerular layer cells and a few internal granular layer cells are labelled on PN3. The internal granular layer of the cerebellum is labelled on either day, but the earlier treatment results in the presence of labelled cells mainly in the vermis, while as a result of the later treatment labelled cells are found throughout the cerebellum. Treatment with tritiated thymidine on postnatal day 3 labels most of the glia around the Purkinje cells.

From the studies above, the following points should be emphasized. The cells of the CNS are formed over an extensive period of time during which they are potentially vulnerable to any agent or environmental condition which may interfere with proliferation, migration, or differentiation. However, the CNS must not be considered to be a uniform organ, but to consist of many parts, each with its own typical pattern of proliferation. At a given time, cell proliferation may be at its peak in some regions and thus be vulnerable to factors which interfere with division. Other parts, however, in which the activity has subsided, or is still to come, will be unaffected. It should therefore be clear that teratological agents, interfering with DNA-synthesis or mitosis on different days of development of the CNS will affect different proliferating populations and will result in cell deficits in different regions of the adult brain.

Morphological Effects of Prenatal and Postnatal Insults on the Developing CNS

It is presently known that a number of drugs and environmental agents can interfere with the proliferative activity in the developing CNS. Excess vitamin A has been shown to lengthen the cell cycle of the neuroepithelial cells resulting in a decrease in the number of cells formed during a given time (LANGMAN and WELCH, 1967). Other drugs such as 5-fluorodeoxyuridine (WEBSTER *et al.*, 1973), 5-azacytidine (LANGMAN and SHIMADA, 1971), methylazoxymethanol (SHIMADA and LANGMAN, 1970), hydroxyurea (SCOTT *et al.*, 1971), and colcemid (WEBSTER *et al.*, 1973) also have been shown to interfere with cell proliferation, mainly by killing many of the dividing cells. Similar results have been reported after X-irradiation (HICKS and D'AMATO, 1966; ALTMAN *et al.*, 1963) and viral infection (KILHAM and MARGOLIS, 1964; NARAYAN and JOHNSON, 1972). Zinc deficiency (HURLEY and SHRADER, 1972) and pre- or post-natal malnutrition (WINICK, 1968; WINICK and NOBLE, 1966) can also cause a reduction in brain cell numbers, although their actual mechanism of action is unknown. In addition to interference with cell proliferation, it is not unlikely that some of these factors also interfere directly with cell migration and differentiation. It is also possible, however, that changes in migration or differentiation occur as secondary effects in response to cell loss. Dystopia seen in the brains of severely retarded patients suggest that cell migration may be a vulnerable process (CROWE and STERN, 1972).

Thus far, many of the factors known to interfere with cell proliferation have not been systematically compared on several days and only a few attempts have been made to determine whether treatment on specific embryonic days results in specific cell deficits in the adult (Hicks *et al.*, 1959). To investigate this possibility pregnant mice were injected with 5-azacytidine on embryonic day 15 or 19 or on postnatal day 3 and the location of the cell deficits determined in adult brains (Rodier *et al.*, 1974).

If the damage in the embryo or the neonate is relatively small, it is often difficult to demonstrate cell deficits or structural disruption in the adult brains of the treated animals by microscopic methods. To help overcome this difficulty, we injected control mice with tritiated thymidine at the same stages of development when 5-azacytidine was administered to the experimental animals. Thus the cells labelled in controls should match the cells exposed to azacytidine in the experimental group, and indicate the regions where cell loss should occur after azacytidine treatment. Unlike the pyknotic nuclei produced by insult, which disappear within 48 hrs., the labelled cells are still available for study in adult animals.

Treating mice on E15 with 2 doses of azacytidine (4 mg/kg body weight), 6 hrs apart, results in extensive cell death in the areas identified by tritiated thymidine as the proliferative populations of the CNS (Figs. 7, 8, and 9). Surprisingly, the treated embryos do not die despite the extensive cell death, and are born after a normal length pregnancy. Examination of their brains, however, shows an extreme reduction in size, mainly due to a severe reduction of the cerebral cortex (Figs. 10 and 11). Other changes such as cell-free gaps and abnormal layering of the pyramidal cells in the hippocampus can be observed microscopically (Figs. 12 and 13). An overall reduction in the size of other regions, such as the corpus striatum (as expected from our labelling experiments) was also consistently observed. Other regions of the brain which had completed cell proliferation prior to treatment on embryonic day 15 were, as far as we could see, completely normal. Similarly, other cells of the brain, such as the granule cell population, which are formed after the period of treatment, appeared to be normal. Hence, the location of the damage in the CNS is determined by the areas where cells are proliferating at the time of treatment.

Mice treated with 5-azacytidine on E19 show damage to more restricted areas of the developing brain. Dead cells are mainly seen in the subependymal layer and the external granular layer of the cerebellum (Fig. 14). In the adult brain we did not see any evidence of cell loss, but this may be due to our inability to accurately estimate the vast numbers of small scattered neurons that are the descendants of the proliferative population seen on E19.

Treatment on PN3, although killing many of the proliferating microneurons and microglia (Fig. 15), did not result in obvious cell deficits in the adult brain. However, small changes in these cell populations might be undetected. For example, in a small sample of sections of control and experimental animals, considerably more light-nucleated cells were counted in the Purkinje cell layer of controls than in that of the azacytidine-treated animals (Figs. 16 and 17).

The lack of gross morphological damage after treatment on E19 or PN3 raises the question whether the microneuron populations can regenerate and make up for cell losses resulting from the treatment. Several studies have shown that the external granular layer does have considerable regenerative ability after postnatal insults. The layer must be almost completely destroyed to prevent its regeneration (Altman and Anderson, 1969). However, there is no evidence to suggest that such damage

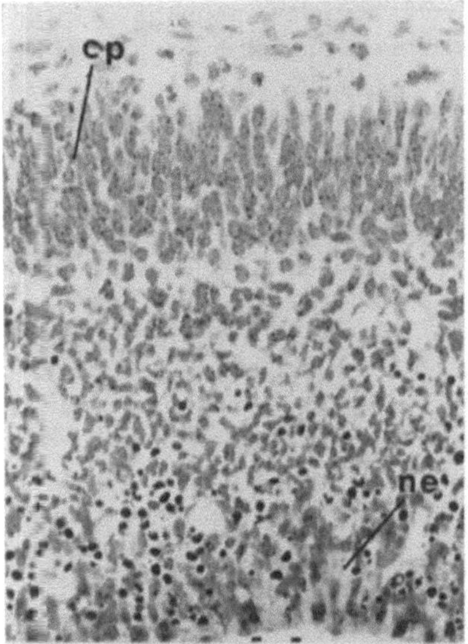

Fig. 7

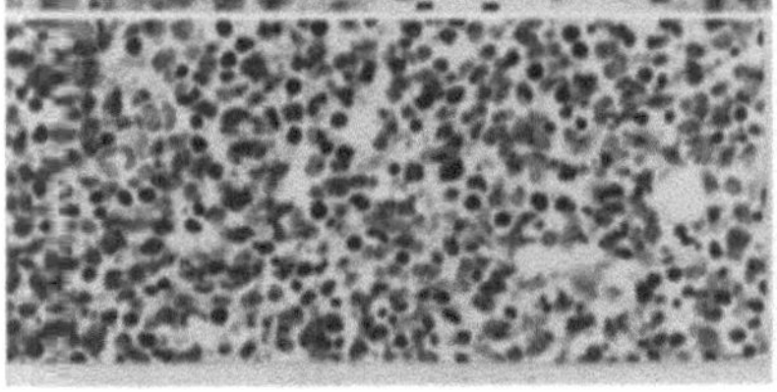

Fig. 8

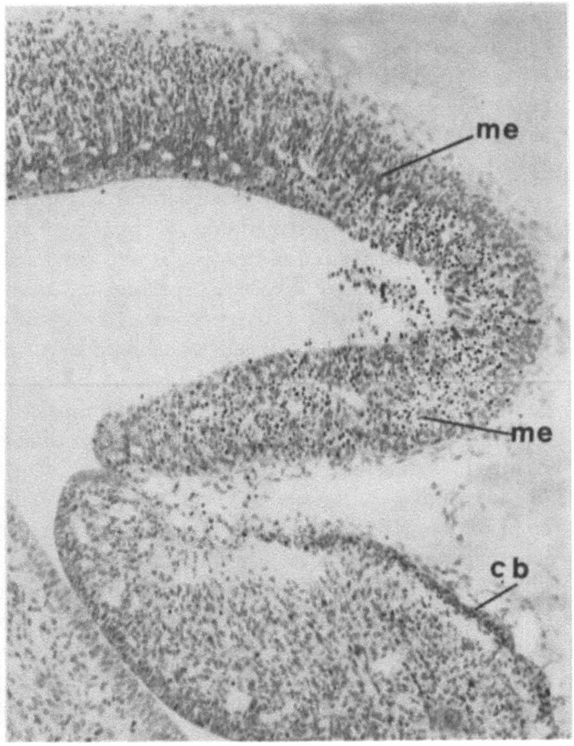

Fig. 9

Fig. 7. Section through the cerebral cortex of a 15-day old mouse embryo 16 hrs after treatment with azacytidine. Note the pyknotic nuclei in the neuroepithelial and subependymal layers. The lumen of the lateral ventricle is at the bottom of the picture. Cortical plate: cp; neuroepithelium: ne

Fig. 8. Similar section as in Fig. 7, but through the corpus striatum. Note the pyknotic nuclei throughout this structure (compare with Fig. 1) after treatment on E15

Fig. 9. Sagittal section through the mesencephalon of a 15-day old embryo 16 hrs after treatment with azacytidine. Note the many pyknotic nuclei in the caudal part of the roof of the mesencephalon. (Compare location of pyknotic nuclei with that of labelled nuclei in Fig. 2.) Mesencephalon: me; developing cerebellum: cb

is ever completely repaired. Although ANDREOLI *et al.* (1973) showed some repair and regeneration in the rhombic lip of the mouse embryo following treatment with 5-fluorodeoxyuridine, the process was incomplete and the treatment resulted in permanent cell loss. Similarly, any regeneration that occurred after 5-azacytidine treatment on embryonic day 15 was inadequate to prevent major cell deficits in the adult brain. Since functional abnormalities occurred after treatment on E15, E19, and PN3, it seems unlikely that repair was complete in any treated group.

Since throughout the body cells are being produced at the time of exposure to 5-azacytidine, it was to be expected that the overall body size would be reduced. At 5 days after birth the mean weight of the control newborn was 3.7 g, that of the

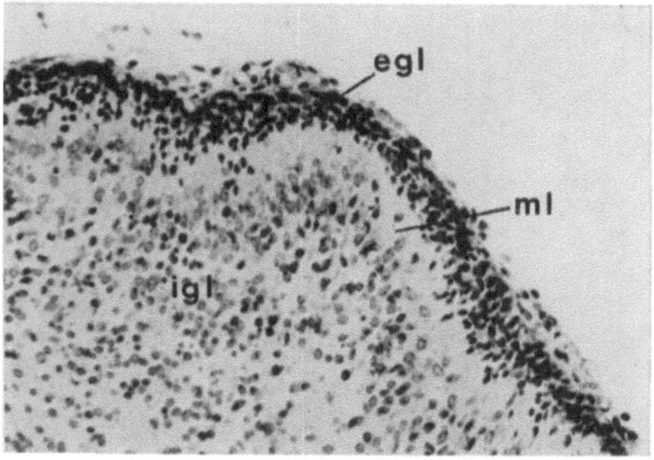

Fig. 10. Section through a portion of the cerebellum of a mouse treated with azacytidine on E19 and sacrificed 16 hrs later. Many pyknotic nuclei are present in the external granular layer (egl), a few in the molecular layer (ml) and internal granular layer (igl). Compare location of pyknotic cells to labelled cells in Fig. 4

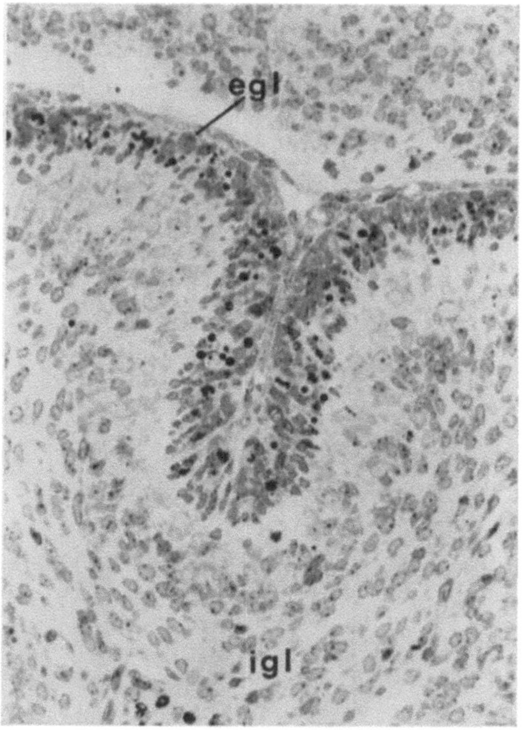

Fig. 11. Section through a portion of the cerebellum of a mouse treated with azacytidine on PN3 and sacrificed 16 hrs later. Pyknotic nuclei are present mainly in the external granular layer (egl), and a few are seen in the internal granular layer (igl). Compare location of pyknotic cells to labelled cells in Fig. 5

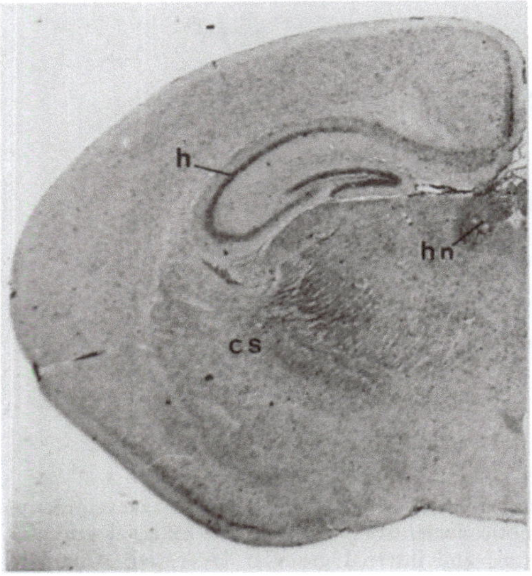

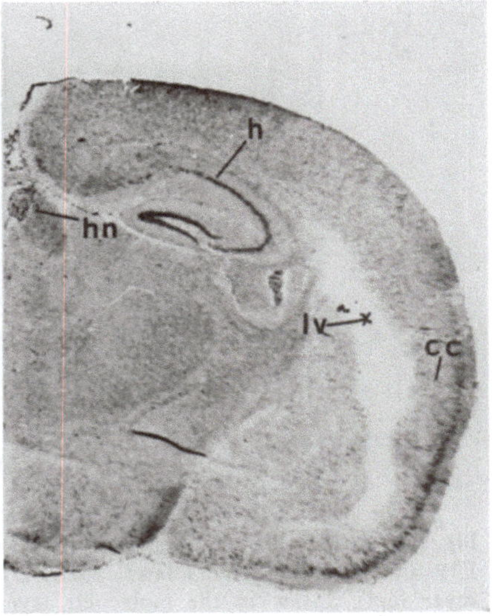

Fig. 12 Fig. 13

Fig. 12. Coronal section through the brain of an adult mouse treated with saline on embryonic day 15. Hippocampus: h; corpus striatum: cs; habenular nucleus: hn

Fig. 13. Coronal section through the brain of an adult mouse treated with azacytidine on day 15 of gestation. Note the small size of the brain, particularly of the cerebral cortex (cc) and hippocampus (h). The lateral ventricle (lv) is greatly enlarged. Habenular nucleus: hn

Figs. 12—17 have appeared in Morphological and behavioral consequences of chemically-induced lesions of the CNS. P. M. RODIER, W. WEBSTER, and J. LANGMAN. In Proceedings of the Seventh Annual Gatlinberg Conference on Research and Theory in Mental Retardation. N. ELLIS, Ed. published by Erlbaum Associates, Potomac, Maryland (1974).

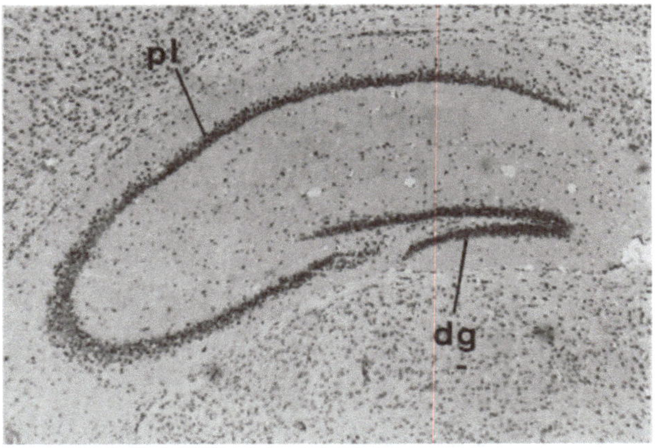

Fig. 14. Section through the hippocampus of an adult control mouse. Pyramidal cell layer: pl, dentate gyrus: dg

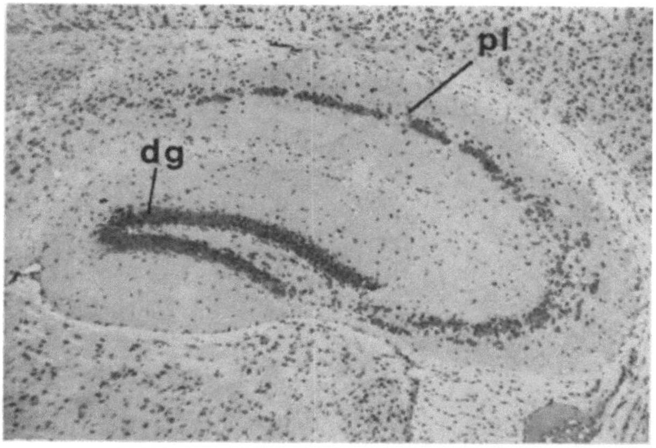

Fig. 15. Section through the hippocampus of an adult mouse treated with azacytidine on E15. Note the discontinuity of the pyramidal cell layer (pl) and the relatively normal appearance of the later-formed dentate gyrus (dg)

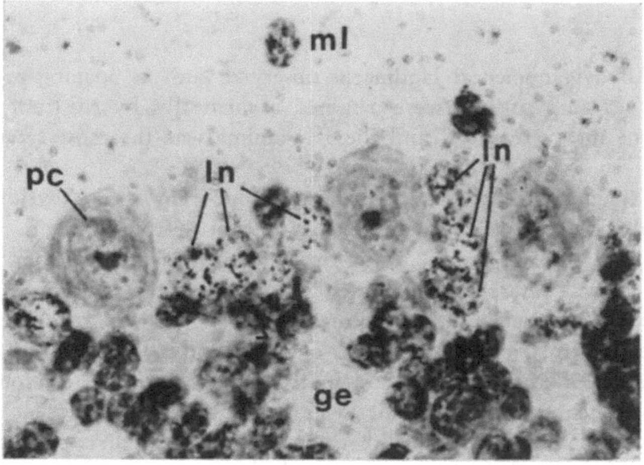

Fig. 16. Radioautograph through the cerebellum of an adult mouse injected with H^3-thymidine on PN3. Note the heavy labelling on light-nucleated cells (ln) in the Purkinje cell layer. Molecular layer: ml, Purkinje cells: pc, granule cells: gc

animals treated on PN3 was 3.5 g, that of the E19 animals was 2.9 g and of the E15 group 2.3 g. Each group differed significantly from the controls and the weight difference persisted into adulthood. For example, at 8 weeks the mean weights were 38.4, 35.8, 33.6 and 24.3 g, respectively. At this age, however, the weight of only the E15 animals was significantly different from that of the controls, but the pattern of slight weight reduction after later treatments was consistent. This stair-step ranking of the experimental groups characterized their physical development

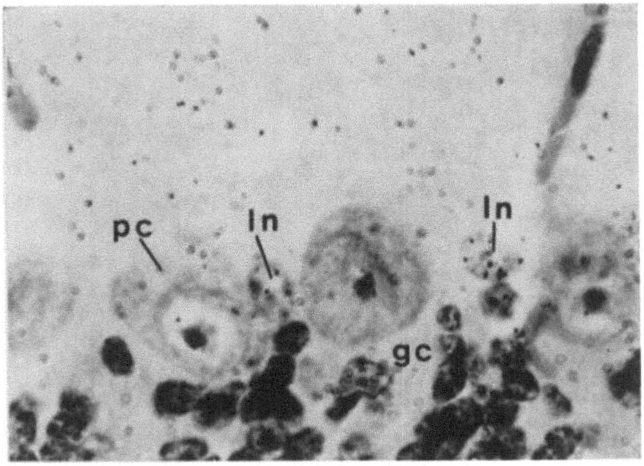

Fig. 17. Radioautograph through the cerebellum of an adult mouse injected with H^3-thymidine and azacytidine on PN3. Note the scarcity of light-nucleated cells (ln) and the light label on those present. Purkinje cell: pc, granule cells: gc

in general. All developmental landmarks observed, such as opening of the eyes and ears, and appearance of fur, were attained sequentially by the four groups, with controls as the most advanced and the E15 animals as the most retarded (RODIER et al., 1974).

Adult brain weights, like body weights, were reduced by the azacytidine treatment. Although only the E15 animals differed significantly from controls, mean weights were 0.555, 0.547, 0.534, and 0.413 g for control, PN3-, E19-, and E15-animals, respectively. It was interesting to note that when brain weight was considered as a percentage of body weight the ranking of the groups was reversed. That is, the brains of the controls make up 1.49% of their body weight, in the PN3 group 1.54%, in the E19 group 1.64%, and in the E15 group 1.77%. None of the differences is significant, but the trend is like that observed by other authors after treatments presumed to interfere with cell proliferation. For example, WINICK and NOBLE (1966) found only a 15% reduction in brain weight after caloric restriction of newborn rats as opposed to a 50% reduction in body weight. Apart from their size and slow development, no gross physical defects, external or internal, were seen in animals treated with azacytidine.

Behavioural Effects of Prenatal and Postnatal Insults on the CNS

Behaviourally, all three treatment groups differed from controls in several tests (Table 2). Perhaps even more importantly, they differed from one another. The differences were not only a matter of degree with earlier treatments leading to greater functional loss, but different categories of behaviour such as locomotor co-

Table 2. Time of treatment

Behaviours observed	Gestation day 15	Gestation day 19	Postnatal day 3
Gait	clumsy gait appears in second week, crossing of forelimbs, splaying and "high stepping" in hind limbs	normal gait	clumsy gait appears in first week, splaying and dragging of hindlimbs
Pivoting	excess pivoting persists into second week	normal pivoting	excessive pivoting ends after first week
Tremors	coarse axial tremors appear in second week, end by weaning	coarse axial tremors appear in neonates, end in third week	coarse axial tremors appear in neonates, end in third week
Righting	normal righting	slow righting at 6 days, normal by 9 days	slow righting at 6 days, normal by 9 days
Depth Perception	no evidence of depth perception until third week	slight delay?	slight delay?
Activity	hyperactive as adults	hypoactive as adults	normal as adults

ordination and general activity were altered by different treatments, suggesting that the behavioural abnormalities depend on the specific CNS structures damaged, rather than on the extent of cell loss (RODIER *et al.*, 1974).

When all groups were compared at six days of age, animals treated on E19 and PN3 differed from those treated on E15 and from the controls in their inability to right themselves from a supine position. Results from the labelling experiments indicated cerebellar damage in the groups treated on E19 and PN3, but not in the E15 group. Thus, the behavioural deficit in E19 and PN3 animals is exactly what would have been predicted from the lesion sites.

All treatment groups had suffered damage to CNS areas involved in motor function according to the labelling data. In the E15 animals damage was seen in the cerebral cortex and corpus striatum while in the other groups damage was done to the cerebellar cortex. The labelled cells in E19 animals were mainly in the vermis — a site that should influence axial motor control, but not necessarily coordination of the limbs. The cell types involved by treatment on PN3 were similar, but included more cells in the cerebellar hemispheres, where lesions tend to be associated with abnormal limb coordination (CHAMBERS and SPRAGUE, 1955). While we cannot explain the motor symptoms in detail, our observations do not contradict the projections made on the basis of the location of labelled cells.

Treatments involving the cerebellum led to pronounced intentional tremors during the first week of life. By postnatal day 10, the E15 animals also began to show coarse tremors. The difference in time of appearance of the tremors seems consistent with the idea that different lesions might underlie the malfunction in the different groups.

Locomotor development was uniquely affected by each of the three treatments. Azacytidine given on PN3 led to an abnormal gait characterized by splaying of the hind limbs and a tendency to pivot. Pivoting is an infantile form of locomotion in which the subject rests on a limp hind limb and paddles with its forelimbs with the result of spinning in place. This locomotor deficit was quite transient, while the abnormal gait was more persistent. Despite the apparent weakness of the hind limbs, the PN3 animals seemed to rear on their hind limbs effectively. Thus the malfunction may be better described as a coordination failure than as muscular weakness. In contrast, animals treated on E 19 were normal and even precocious in motor development. They pivoted rarely and displayed a well-coordinated gait. Animals treated on E15 at first appeared to have normal locomotor abilities, but then continued to pivot well beyond the time of the other groups. When walking they showed some tendency to cross the forelimbs — a pattern of behaviour rarely seen in any other group.

Since all treatments caused retinal damage, which has not been analyzed as yet, some visual deficits were expected. It was therefore of importance to determine whether the animals had sufficient visual capacity to allow later tests involving gross visual stimuli. Similarly, it was essential to rule out defective vision as the sole cause of locomotor deficits. In a visual cliff experiment, all treated groups eventually developed a preference for the "safe" side of the cliff. Thus, none of the treatments caused total blindness, and all animals had some depth perception by the time they reached maturity. Those treated on PN3 or E19 showed only a slight delay in the visual cliff test, possibly resulting from their delay in eye-opening. Animals treated on E15, however, did not begin to show visually-guided performance until the third week of postnatal life — a delay too long to be accounted for by late eye opening. This group had massive damage in the visual cortex and, according to the labelling experiments, some cell loss in the superior colliculus as well as in the retina. Hence, the malfunction could have been mediated by damage to any of these three areas.

The general activity of animals treated with azacytidine varied with the stage of development at which the drug was administered. Activity was measured in an open field using an Animex induction coil activity meter (LKB Farad). After weaning, E15 animals were hyperactive in repeated 2 min samples. Mice treated on E19 were hypoactive when compared to the controls. The PN3 group did not differ significantly from controls. Either damage to cerebral cortex or to the hippocampus or to both has often been associated with hyperactivity (JERRARD and BRUNNELL, 1968; DOUGLAS and ISAACSON, 1964) and thus it is not surprising that E15 animals were characterized by abnormally high activity. It is not clear why animals treated on E19 were hypoactive. Cerebellar damage is sometimes followed by a reduction in activity (WALLACE and ALTMAN, 1970), but this reduction is probably related to locomotor deficits, which were not observed in E19 treated animals. Some damage must have occurred in the dentate gyrus, subependyma, and olfactory bulbs of both E19 and PN3 animals. If one of these structures is related to the activity change, the critical damage in the two late treatment groups must be subtly different, since only the E19's differed from controls. Alternatively, it may be the combination of lesions that distinguishes one group from the other. In any case, the difference between the groups must be dependent on loss of specific cells, not on general damage to the several gross structures involved on both E19 and PN3.

In summary it may be stated that when mice are treated with azacytidine at different stages of fetal and postnatal life, the consequences are subtle alterations of neuroanatomy and not-so-subtle alterations of physical development and behaviour. Some of the behavioural effects are transient: normal righting reflexes appear in all animals in the second week of life, and all tremors disappear by weaning. Other deficits like the normal gait of PN3 animals are longlasting, but decrease greatly with time. Still other anomalies, such as activity differences, persist in adult animals. The importance of these deficits does not lie in their severity or persistance, but in the clear pattern by which different deficits are associated with different treatment days. The results suggest that a variety of "congenital brain damage" syndromes could be related to cell loss late in development.

Considering the many experiments involving agents known to produce cell loss, there is a wealth of evidence suggesting that our results are part of a general picture of interference with late neuronal development. Similar neuroanatomical alterations and similar behavioral changes have been produced before. Our work is original in a) demonstrating changes in anatomy and behaviour simultaneously, instead of separately; b) putting heavy emphasis on the temporal variable by using brief treatments and keeping the treatment constant; and c) using labelled controls to pinpoint sites of cell loss.

The period on or around E15 has been studied with several agents believed to interfere with cellular proliferation. Methylazoxymethanol treatment has been shown to cause deficiencies in motor tests with rats (CIOFALO *et al.*, 1971). X-irradiation of E15 rats produces hyperactive adults, as measured in tilt-cages (FURCHTGOTT and ECHOLS, 1958). In the same study, treatment on E15 led to low emotionality scores on several measures. (See p. 109 for discussion of emotionality). WERBOFF *et al.* (1962) also found significant hyperactivity and emotionality differences in rats irradiated on E15. Whlie our later treatment groups have not been rated on emotionality, significant differences between controls and those treated with azacytidine on E15 were observed. As with x-irradiation, the treated animals defecate and urinate less than controls. Several investigators have reported learning deficits in animals treated around E15 (HICKS, 1962; WERBOFF *et al.*, 1962; CIOFALO *et al.*, 1971; HADDAD *et al.*, 1969). All of these studies involved maze-learning tasks. On a passive avoidance task, the original group of azacytidine-treated animals showed no abnormalities at 4 months of age. However, a younger group was tested with surprising results. Only those treated on E15 differed significantly from controls and they were *superior* in performance. Since hippocampal lesions generally lead to inferior passive avoidance (MCCLEARY, 1961), this result is difficult to interpret, but both the maze-learning and passive avoidance differences suggest that some structures involved in learning are affected by treatment on E15. The reports including brain weights confirm that the reduction observed with azacytidine is also seen after methylazoxymethanol treatment and x-irradiation (HADDAD *et al.*, 1969; CIOFALO *et al.*, 1971; FOWLER *et al.*, 1962). Moreover, the specific structures affected are the same.

Less information is available for treatments that correspond to the E19 azacytidine treatment. In the irradiation experiments of FURCHTGOTT and ECHOLS (1958), the hyperactivity observed after treatment around day E15 gave way to hypoactivity on day E18 and after birth, just as in the present experiments.

The first week of life, including PN3, has been investigated extensively by ALTMAN and his colleagues. Although these studies involved more extensive damage because of repeated treatments with focal radiation damaging only the cerebellum, many of the behavioral results reported by these investigators are similar to those seen after azacytidine treatment. For example, irradiation of the cerebellum during the first week of postnatal life leads to tremor, righting difficulty and an abnormal gait characterized by poor coordination of the hind limbs (WALLACE and ALTMAN, 1970 a, 1970 b). These investigators also tested the possibility that hypotonia of the hind limbs could account for the locomotor deficits by comparing controls and treated animals in a weight-pulling experiment. As suggested by the azacytidine data, the deficits appear to be in coordination rather than in muscle strength. The irradiated rats were significantly hypoactive, unlike the groups treated with azacytidine on PN3. Whether this difference is due to timing, severity of damage or the inclusion of other brain structures resulting from the systemic azacytidine treatment is not clear. However, when BAYER *et al.* (1972) irradiated the dentate gyrus rather than the cerebellum of infant rats, hyperactivity resulted. It may be that the azacytidine treatment, which necessarily involves both areas, results in normal activity because the opposite effects of the lesions cancel each other out. In any case, focal damage to the cerebellum results in a behavioral syndrome very similar to that observed after azacytidine treatment on PN3.

Conclusions

Interference with cell proliferation may be well-tolerated by whole organisms or organ systems in which cell production contributes only to growth or replacement of cells. If proliferation is interrupted during periods when unique cell types are being produced, the loss may be permanent. The central nervous system produces special cell types throughout gestation and even after birth and since the cells for various CNS structures are produced at different times, a brief insult may damage some structures and spare others. Which structures sustain damage depends on the population of cells proliferating at the time of insult. Since the time of origin of cells can be ascertained by labelling techniques, it is possible to predict which regions will be damaged at any stage of development.

The varied lesions produced by interference at different stages are accompanied by different syndromes of behavioral abnormalities. Furthermore, the particular behavioral changes observed after azacytidine treatment can be produced by other agents at the same stages of development. The data suggest that late gestation and early postnatal life are not periods of resistance to teratological agents. Rather, insults at these times result in alterations of anatomy and function that are difficult to observe with standard teratological evaluation techniques.

All this might be of little relevance to the study of human birth defects, if no environmental factors had the property of interfering with cell proliferation in man. Unfortunately, DNA viruses, such as measles, do interfere selectively with proliferating cells. In fact, rat virus infection in suckling hamsters has been shown to damage the external granular layer, just as azacytidine and x-irradiation do (KILHAM and MARGOLIS, 1964). Like the other experimental treatments, the virus infection is followed by motor malfunctions. Thus, it is possible that a variety of abnormal behavioural syndromes might be caused by insults which interfere with cell proliferation during development.

Acknowledgements. This investigation was supported by NIH grant R01-NS06188. The authors wish to express their thanks to Mrs. MILDRED MARSHALL and Mrs. MARY DICKIE for their technical assitance, and to Miss PAMELA J. BAKER for assistance in the preparation of the manuscript.

References

ALTMAN, J.: Autoradiographic investigation of cell proliferation in the brains of rats and cats. Anat. Rec. **145**, 573—591 (1963).

ALTMAN, J.: Autoradiographic and histological studies of postnatal neurogenesis. III. Dating the time of production and onset of differentiation of cerebellar microneurons in rats. J. comp. Neurol. **136**, 269—294 (1969).

ALTMAN, J., ANDERSON, W. J., WRIGHT, K. A.: Gross morphological consequences of irradiation of the cerebellum in infant rats with repeated doses of low level x-ray. Exp. Neurol. **21**, 69—91 (1968).

ALTMAN, J., ANDERSON, W. J., WRIGHT, K. A.: Early effects of X-Irradiation of the cerebellum in infant rats: Decimation and reconstitution of the external granular. Exp. Neurol. **24**, 196—216 (1969).

ANDREOLI, J., RODIER, P. M., LANGMAN, J.: Influence of a prenatal trauma on formation of Purkinje cells. Amer. J. Anat. **137**, 87—101 (1973).

ANGEVINE, J. B., SIDMAN, R. L.: Autoradiographic study of cell migration during histogenesis of cerebral cortex in the mouse. Nature (Lond.) **192**, 766—768 (1961).

BAYER, S. A., BRUNNER, R. L., HINE, R., ALTMAN, J.: Behavioral effects of interference with the postnatal acquisition of hippocampal granule cells. Nature (Lond.) New Biol. **242**, 222—224 (1973).

BERRY, M., ROGERS, A. W.: The migration of neuroblasts in the developing cerebral cortex. J. Anat. (Lond.) **99**, 691—709 (1965).

CHAMBERS, W. W., SPRAGUE, J. M.: Functional localization in the cerebellum. I. Organization in longitudinal cortico-nuclear zones and their contribution to the control of posture, both extrapyramidal and pyramidal. J. comp. Neurol. **103**, 105—129 (1955).

CIOFALO, V. B., LATRANYI, M., TABER, R. I.: Effect of prenatal treatment of methylazoxymethanol acetate on motor performance, exploratory activity, and maze learning in rats. Comm. Behav. Biol. **6**, 223—226 (1971).

CROWE, L., STERN, J.: Pathology of Mental Retardation. p. 136, Baltimore: Williams & Wilkins 1972.

DOUGLAS, R. J., ISAACSON, R. L.: Hippocampal lesions and activity. Psychonom. Sci. **1**, 187 to 192 (1964).

FOWLER, H., HICKS, S. P., D'AMATO, C. J., BEACH, F. A.: Effects of fetal irradiation on behavior in the albino rat. J. comp. physiol. Psychol. **3**, 309—314 (1962).

FURCHTGOTT, E., ECHOLS, M.: Activity and emotionality in pre- and neonatally x-irradiated rats. J. comp. physiol. Psychol. **51**, 541—545 (1958).

HADDAD, R. K., RABE, A., LAQUEUR, G. L., SPATZ, M., VALSAMIS, M. P.: Intellectual deficit associated with transplacentally induced microencephaly in the rat. Science **163**, 88—90 (1969).

HICKS, S. P., D'AMATO, C. J.: Effects of ionizing radiations on mammalian development. Advances in Teratology, D. H. M. WOOLLAM Ed. p. 195—250. London: Logos Press 1966.

HICKS, S. P., D'AMATO, C. J., LOWE, M. J.: The development of the mammalian nervous system. I. Malformations of the brain, especially the cerebral cortex, induced in rats by radiation. J. comp. Neurol. **113**, 435—470 (1959).

HURLEY, L. S., SHRADER, R. E.: Congenital malformations of the nervous system in zinc deficient rats. Neurobiology of the trace metals zinc and copper. CARL C. PFEIFFER Ed. Int. Review of Neurobiology Suppl. 1 p. 7—51 (1972).

JERRARD, L. E., BRUNNEL, B. N.: Open-field behavior of hippocampal-lesioned rats and hamsters. J. comp. physiol. Psychol. **66**, 500—502 (1968).

KILHAM, L., MARGOLIS, G.: Cerebellar ataxia in hamsters inoculated with rat virus. Science **143**, 1047—1048 (1964).

LANGMAN, J., SHIMADA, M.: Cerebral cortex of the mouse after prenatal chemical insult. Amer. J. Anat. **132**, 355—374 (1971).

LANGMAN, J., WELCH, G. W.: Excess vitamin A and development of the cerebral cortex. J. comp. Neurol. **131**, 15—26 (1967).

MCCLEARY, R. A.: Response-modulating functions of the limbic system: Initiation and suppression. In: Progress in Physiological Psychology. I. E. STELLAR and J. M. SPRAGUE, Eds. New York: Academic Press 1966.

MIALE, I. L., SIDMAN, R. L.: An autoradiographic analysis of histogenesis in the mouse cerebellum. Exp. Neurol. **4**, 277—296 (1961).

NARAYAN, O., JOHNSON, R. T.: Effects of viral infections on nervous system development. I. Pathogenesis of bluetongue virus infection in mice. Amer. J. **68**, 1—14 (1972).

RAKIC, P.: Mode of cell migration to the superficial layer of fetal monkey neocortex. J. comp. Neurol. **145**, 61—83 (1962).

RAKIC, P.: Neurons in rhesus monkey visual cortex: Systematic relation between time of origin and eventual disposition. Science **183**, 425—427 (1974).

RODIER, P. M., WEBSTER, W. S., LANGMAN, J.: Effects of chemically-induced lesions on CNS morphology and function. In preparation. (1975).

SCOTT, W. J., RITTER, E. J., WILSON, J. G.: DNA synthesis inhibition and cell death associated with hydroxyurea teratogenesis in rat embryos. Develop. Biol. **26**, 306—316 (1971).

SHIMADA, M., LANGMAN, J.: Repair of the external granular layer of the hamster cerebellum after prenatal and postnatal administration of methylazoxymethanol. Teratology **3**, 119 to 125 (1970).

SMART, I.: The subependymal layer of the mouse brain and its cell production as shown by radioautography after thymidine-H^3 injection. J. comp. Neurol. **116**, 325—347 (1961).

WALLACE, R. B., ALTMAN, J.: Behavioral effects of neonatal irradiation of the cerebellum. I. Qualitative observations in infant and adolescent rats. Develop. Psychobiol. **2**, 257 to 265 (1970 a).

WALLACE, R. B., ALTMAN, J.: Behavioral effects of neonatal irradiation of the cerebellum. II. Quantitative studies of young-adult and adult rats. Develop. Psychobiol. **2**, 266 to 272 (1970 b).

WEBSTER, W., SHIMADA, M., LANGMAN, J.: Effect of fluorodeoxyuridine, colcemid and bromodeoxyuridine on developing neocortex of the mouse. Amer. J. Anat. **137**, 67—85 (1973).

WERBOFF, J., HAVLENA, J., SIKOV, M.: Effects of prenatal x-irradiation on activity, emotionality and maze learning ability in the rat. Radiat. Res. **16**, 444—452 (1962).

WINICK, M.: Cellular growth of the placenta as an indicator of abnormal fetal growth. Diagnosis and treatment of fetal disorders. p. 83 K. ADAMSONS, Ed. New York: Springer-Verlag 1968.

WINICK, M., NOBLE, A.: Cellular response in rats during malnutrition at various ages. J. Nutr. **89**, 300—306 (1966).

12. Polymorphisms: Their Lessons for Human Teratology

D. F. ROBERTS and J. BURN

With 5 Figures

This article aims to show how the techniques, facts and theory that have been accumulated in the study of human polymorphisms may be of relevance to understanding fetal maldevelopment. The genes that are transmitted on the parental chromosomes to the new organism at the moment of conception control the structures of all the proteins which the new organism makes, and are concerned in regulating their synthesis and their interaction with other substances, so that the biochemical make-up of each individual is essentially a reflection of his genetical constitution. Thus "one may anticipate that inherited differences ... whether they are expressed as differences in normal physical, physiological or mental characteristics, or as differences in the development of particular abnormalities, are likely to be a consequence of differences in enzyme or protein synthesis" (HARRIS, 1970). But development does not occur in a vacuum; it is a complex of gene-controlled synthetic processes proceeding in the environment provided by the cell cytoplasm. Error in this complex — in the gene, the gene control, or the environmental interaction as a result of insult — is to be seen as the primary lesion. Thus, as WADDINGTON (1963) pointed out, there is no difference in principle between situations in which the development of a phenotypic abnormality occurs in accordance with simple Mendelian laws of inheritance, and in which it is controlled by both environmental and hereditary factors.

A Model for Genetic Control

The Normal Haemoglobin Sequence

A model of how genetic control of fetal development (or maldevelopment) may be exercised, is provided by the haemoglobins. The globin of the normal adult haemoglobin molecule consists of two pairs of different polypeptide chains, two α chains and two β chains. A different gene specifies each chain, in which the sequence of constituents, respectively 141 and 146 amino acid residues, is controlled by the DNA base pair sequence. To each chain is attached a haem group so that the molecular weight of the total molecule is approximately 66,000. There is also a minor haemoglobin fraction (Hb A_2) consisting of two α chains and two δ chains, the latter again differing in structure from the α and β. These haemoglobins do not occur throughout life; there is instead a steady developmental sequence. In antenatal life, there first appears the principal embryonic haemoglobin Gower 1, and this consists of four identical polypeptide chains (ε_4). Early in embryonic development α and γ chains begin to be synthesised, and there occur next haemoglobin Gower 2 ($\alpha_2\, \varepsilon_2$) and haemoglobin Portland 1 ($\gamma_2\, \varepsilon_2$), and then the principal fetal haemoglobin, haemoglobin F ($\alpha_2\, \gamma_2$), which the adult form ($\alpha_2\, \beta_2$) gradually replaces during later fetal and early postnatal life. These chains are synthesised in different tissues. This means that since all cells contain identical genetic information, specific genes must be switched on and switched off at the appropriate point in development. That this is so is also suggested by the fact that fetal haemoglobin production, primarily taking place in the liver and spleen, can be artificially reactivated in adult bone marrow (HALL and MOTULSKY, 1968).

Variant Forms

Other variants occur at a given stage in the life cycle. In some human populations there are polymorphisms, in that there are variant forms, due to minor alterations in the base pair sequence, present in an appreciable number of individuals. These variant forms occur not only in adult haemoglobin (for example, haemoglobin S or haemoglobin C reach very high frequencies in some African populations), but also in fetal haemoglobin. Variants in sequence within the α, β and γ chains giving rise to structural variants of haemoglobin are well known. Most have relatively minor biological effect, but some are more severe; few homozygous Hb S infants survive. More severe, however, are conditions in which the switch mechanism is involved. Suppression, or deficiency of production, of a specific globin chain gives pure multimers (α_4, β_4 or γ_4), deleterious if present in more than trace amounts because of their malfunction (e. g. in oxygen transport, inability to combine with haptoglobin). In homozygous alphathalassemia, the defective haemopoiesis during development leads to the birth of infants with nonimmune hydrops fetalis showing hepatosplenomegaly and ascites as well as generalised hydrops (LIE-INJO *et al.*, 1962). One mutation in negroes causes failure of activation of the β and δ chains, so only fetal haemoglobin is synthesised even in the adult. Some chromosomal defects interfere with chain synthesis: in trisomy 13 disappearance of embryonic and fetal haemoglobin is delayed.

Glucose-6-phosphate dehydrogenase (G6PD) shows similar variant forms. This enzyme, involved in the shunt pathway of carbohydrate metabolism, requires a single structural gene for its synthesis, this time located on the X chromosome. The monomeric chain has a molecular weight about three times that of a haemoglobin chain, consists of about 350 amino acids, and over sixty variant forms are known. One group of variants causes chronic haemolytic disease, another group is associated with severe deficiency of enzyme activity, in which haemolytic reactions are precipitated by particular drugs. It is of course the interaction of the gene with the drug environment that is important, for the small minority of the population with the enzyme defect react adversely only if the drug is applied.

Implications

It therefore appears that intrinsic abnormalities in fetal development may arise by a) failure of the switching mechanism, or errors in its timing, b) errors in the substances synthesised. Search for variant substances, or deficiency of substances, as a cause of maldevelopment appears well worthwhile.

The precise biochemical defect is known in few abnormalities initiated antenatally, even among the number that are well established as being under simple genetic control. The law with regard to abortion has changed comparatively recently and it is only now that a sufficient amount of early fetal material has become available for study. For most fetuses from therapeutic abortions there is little reason to expect gross abnormality, but their investigation is worthwhile. Firstly, the information on the normal sequence of appearance of substances, and their activities at different stages of fetal growth, is incomplete, and it is necessary to establish the pattern of normal development against which findings from defective fetuses can be compared. Secondly, the material allows search for variant forms of substances against which minor variations in fetal development can be compared.

Some help can be gained in work of this kind from the much greater knowledge of biochemical defects in postnatal life and their effects, since fetal and postnatal phases of growth are temporally continuous in many respects and many processes initiated in fetal life continue postnatally. But there are a number of other difficulties. There are the problems of whether variant substances are true biological variants or whether they are due to artifacts of preparation of the material, storage of specimens, or indeed the result of the particular mode of pregnancy termination employed. One needs to be sure that the substances are indeed present at the time of differentiation and development of the relevant fetal tissues. Finally, it is necessary to know that the variant forms are genetically determined and here it is essential to draw to the attention of obstetricians the importance of the invesigation of successive fetuses that may become available from the same mother.

Enzyme Heterogeneity

The existence of multimolecular forms of enzymes, suggested over thirty years ago by Desreux and Heriott (1939) for the enzyme pepsin, was confirmed following technological advances. The emergence of electrophoretic methods, especially that using starch gel (Smithies, 1955), was particularly important and subsequent work has shown that many enzymes, if not the majority, possess multiple forms. These differ in varying degrees in their physiological and biochemical properties, and may thus be relevant in the field of teratology.

Markert and Moller (1959) coined the term isoenzyme to describe these different molecular species with closely related enzymatic and physical properties. The subsequent disagreement over definition and classification of the term was partly resolved by the International Commission (I.U.B., 1970) which recommended that

1. the term "multiple forms of the enzyme" should be used as a broad term covering all proteins possessing the same enzyme activity and occurring naturally in a single species;
2. the term "isoenzyme" or "isozyme" should apply only to those multiple forms of enzyme arising from genetically determined differences in primary structure and not to those derived by modification of the same primary sequence.

The Commission also produced a classification based on mode of production (Table 1), from which it appears that groups 1, 2 and 3 are 'true' isoenzymes, while those in groups 4—7 should be simply called 'multiple forms' since these represent essentially mechanisms of intracellular modification of the same polypeptide chain; their biological significance is not thereby diminished, of course, since they are just as much part of the intra-cellular milieu.

Table 1. Enzyme heterogeneity

Group	Reasons for multiplicity
1	Genetically independent proteins
2	Heteropolymers (hybrids) of 2 or more polypeptide chains, noncovalently bound
3	Genetic variants (allelic): common polymorphic rare mutants
4	Proteins derived from one polypeptide chain
5	Proteins conjugated with other groups
6	Polymers of a single subunit
7	Conformationally different forms
8	Artifacts of preparation

Of the genetic groups (1—3), *group 1* may be illustrated by the malate dehydrogenase enzymes of the mitochondrial and cytosol fractions of liver cells described by KAPLAN (1961). The two types of protein have the same enzymic activity, but are structurally quite different and each is under separate genetic control. *Group 2* may be illustrated by lactate dehydrogenase in which (like adult haemoglobin) two different types (A and B) of polypeptide chains occur, each under the control of a different gene. The whole normal enzyme molecule is composed of four of these polypeptide chains, the number of each type determining the electrophoretic mobility so that there are five different isoenzymes of lactic dehydrogenase separable on electrophoresis (one with four A chains, one with three A and one B, etc.). In *group 3* occur the common polymorphic variants such as erythrocyte acid phosphatase or phosphoglucomutase, in which each allele is responsible for the production of a particular band, or group of bands, on the zymogram produced after electrophoresis, most of which can be shown to have identifiable variation in physiological or biochemical properties. In this group there also occur the rare mutants, such as the variant forms of A or B chains of lactate dehydrogenase.

For teratology, though all structurally different proteins are of potential relevance, the variation in activity that so frequently occurs among isoenzymes of group 3 suggests that search for these may be particularly useful. But instead of a sharp dividing line between individual enzymes which show some functional overlap despite their control at separate loci, and multiple forms of the same enzyme with widely differing properties, it seems logical to postulate a continuous gradation of enzyme evolution. For instance, gene duplication may occur followed by progressive accumulation of base substitutions until the enzyme molecules (assuming molecular and biological viability) are sufficiently dissimilar for them to assume distinct functions, with negligible overlap. In variants of recent evolutionary history, the accumulation of base changes would be slight and functional overlap almost complete, giving perhaps little clinical effect.

Enzyme Heterogeneity and Clinical States

Evidence is increasing of the relationship of genetically determined abnormalities of antenatal onset to enzyme variation. Recent enzymic studies relating to the mucopolysaccharidoses provide an illustration (McKusick, 1974). The distinct clinical entities, Hurler's Syndrome (Mucopolysaccharidosis I) and Scheie's Syndrome (Mucopolysaccharidosis V) result from a defect in the same enzyme, alpha-L-iduronidase. One possible explanation is an allelic relationship between the genes responsible for these disorders, as exists between the Hb S and Hb C genes. Furthermore, a small number of cases have been identified in which the clinical features fall midway between the two conditions.

Further illustrations come from the lysosomal disorders (Spranger and Wiedemann, 1970). In generalised gangliosidosis and late onset GM-1 gangliosidosis there is a defect in β-galactosidase activity. In the former, all three isoenzymes (A, B and C) are missing while in the latter only B and C are defective, so permitting these diseases to be reclassified as GM-1 gangliosidosis types I and II respectively. Similarly, with the enzyme N-acetyl hexosaminidase, absence of the A isoenzyme results in GM-2 gangliosidosis type I (Tay Sach's Disease), loss of both A and B isoenzymes is seen in the clinically similar type II (Sandhoff's disease), while type III (late onset GM-2 gangliosidosis) results from a partial loss of the A isoenzyme only.

This interdependence of clinical and biochemical precision is seen more vividly in the case of arylsulphatase. This enzyme possesses 3 isoenzymes A, B and C. A defect in the first results in the disorder known as metachromatic leukodystrophy in which a massive demyelination occurs in the first few months of life. A deficiency of arylsulphatase B, on the other hand, results in the Maroteaux-Lamy syndrome, or mucopolysaccharidosis VII, in which there is a gross physical deformity with corneal clouding, joint stiffness and severe dysostosis. Finally, a total absence of arylsulphatase (A, B and C) produces juvenile sulphatidosis which shows features of both conditions. In these cases it is evident that the clinical features are closely related to the isoenzyme changes. That the majority can be diagnosed antenatally indicates that the biochemical lesion is already effective in fetal life, and is acting as an intrinsic teratogen.

Tissue Specificity of Isoenzymes

Many developmental disorders are highly localised, often showing tissue or cell type specificity. Defects in individual isoenzymes in such disorders likewise imply their tissue specificity. This is well established and can be illustrated by lactate dehydrogenase where different tissues exhibit a preponderance of either the isoenzymes with predominant A subunits or those with predominantly B subunits, and this, HARRIS (1970) suggests, is attributable to variations in activity of the two gene loci in different cell types. LDH 5 with four A subunits and LDH 1 with four B subunits differ in their kinetic properties, particularly in the inhibition of the latter by the accumulation of the substrate pyruvate. LDH 1 is predominant in tissues such as heart and brain, in which aerobic metabolism is continuous while LDH 5 is predominant in voluntary muscle, where anaerobic metabolism can occur. In fetal tissues, LDH 5 tends to predominate and it has been suggested that the relatively low tissue oxygen tension in the fetus may have a controlling influence, stimulating production of the A subunits and leading to the predominance of LDH 5. The ways in which such tissue specific patterns influence the clinical features of a disorder (and the methods for diagnosis) are well illustrated in some inborn errors of metabolism (Table 2). As an example, the enzyme phosphorylase is responsible for the separation of sugar groups from the storage molecule glycogen, in particular, in liver and skeletal muscle. Two clinically distinct conditions are attributed to an inherited defect of this enzyme. McArdle's disease (Cori Type 5) is characterised by the development of severe muscle cramps on exercise, and enzyme assay shows almost complete absence of muscle phosphorylase. In Her's disease (Cori Type 6) there is excessive deposition of glycogen in the liver associated with hypoglycaemia and acidosis, and in this disease liver posphorylase has been shown to be inactive. Here separate loci are responsible for phosphorylase production in muscle and liver and mutation at these sites is responsible for the specific symptoms of the two types of glycogenosis. The enzyme aldolase has three structurally distinct forms labelled A, B and C which are found particularly in muscle, liver and brain respectively. These isozymic proteins are tetramers and evidently differ in the structure of their characteristic polypeptide subunits, each of which is presumably determined by a separate gene locus. Each isoenzyme is responsible for the division of fructose sugars into two 3-carbon components in the pentose shunt pathway (RUTTER, 1968). In the inherited defect hereditary fructose intolerance, this division of fructose does not occur, leading to profound hypoglucosaemia when it is ingested. When the tissues are examined, this metabolic defect is seen to be present only in the liver where aldolase B is found, and the other isoenzymes act as normal.

The enzymes pyruvate kinase and hexokinase both show two isozymic forms produced by separate loci in red and white blood cells. A chronic haemolytic anaemia

Table 2. Spatial variation of isoenzymes as revealed by inborn errors of metabolism

Disorder	Enzyme	Enzyme normal in	Enzyme deficient in	References
Hexokinase deficiency	Hexokinase	W.B.C.	R.B.C.	VALENTINE *et al.*, 1967; KEITT, 1969; NECHELES *et al.*, 1970 a
Pyruvate kinase deficiency	Pyruvate kinase	W.B.C.	R.B.C.	BIGLEY, 1968; HARRIS, 1970
Phosphofructokinase deficiency	P.F.K.	R.B.C. (1 isoenzyme)	Muscle	WATERBURY and FRENKEL, 1969, 1972
Chronic granulomatous disease	Glutathione peroxidase	R.B.C.	W.B.C.	NECHELES, 1969
Fructose intolerance	Aldolase	Muscle	Liver	PENHOET, 1966, 1967; HERS and JOASSIN, 1961; FROESCH *et al.*, 1963
McArdle's disease	Phosphorylase	Liver	Muscle	SCHMID *et al.*, 1959; ROBBINS, 1960; DAWSON *et al.*, 1968
Hers disease	Phosphorylase	Muscle	Liver, W.B.C.	HERS, 1959; WILLIAMS and FIELD, 1961; HERS and VAN HOOF, 1968
Phosphorylase kinase deficiency	Phosphorylase kinase	Muscle	Liver, W.B.C.	HUG *et al.*, 1969, 1970; HUIJING and FERNANDES, 1969
Myeloperoxidase deficiency	Myeloperoxidase	Eosinophils	Neutrophils, Monocytes	LEHRER and CLINE, 1969; SALMON *et al.*, 1970
Oculocutaneous albinism	Tyrosinase	Adrenals	Melanocytes	FITZPATRICK and QUEVEDO, 1966
Hypophosphatasia	Alkaline phosphatase	Intestine	Bone, Liver, Kidney	RATHBURN, 1948; MCCANCE *et al.*, 1956; DANOVITCH *et al.*, 1968
Primary hyperoxaluria (type 1)	Alphaketoglutarate	Mitochondria	Cytoplasm	CRAWHALL, 1962; KOCH, 1967; MEDES, 1932; FELLMAN, 1968

has been attributed to a genetic defect in each of these enzymes and in both cases this has been found to be due to loss of the red cell isoenzyme specifically while the white cell isoenzyme is spared.

Interpretation of Spatial Variation

That different tissues possess distinct isoenzymes, one of which is specifically affected by a mutation, does not necessarily mean that these multiple forms must be coded for by separate gene loci. Tissue specific patterns may arise by any of the mechanisms outlined in Table 1, as well as the switch procedures (p. 202) activating different loci in different cell types. For example, the defects in many patients in the past identified as cases of Hers disease, on the basis of high liver glycogen and low liver phosphorylase levels, were subsequently shown to be due to a deficiency not in phosphorylase production, but in phosphorylase activation by the enzyme phosphorylase kinase. In these patients, now referred to as Cori type 8, homozygosity for the mutant kinase allele led to clinical signs closely resembling true Hers disease because this enzyme also shows tissue specificity.

Subcellular Variation

It is now well established that there exist considerable differences in the metabolism of the cytoplasm and the numerous organelles within it, and a number of the 'inborn errors' are now known to be specifically localised. Thus, among the glycolysis defects, the enzyme deficiency in Von Gierke's disease is microsomal, that in Gaucher's disease is lysosomal, that in propionic-acidaemia mitochondrial. If different isoenzymes were found in the various subcellular fractions, then different tissue fractionation would be necessary before any conclusions could be reached about the possible role of an enzyme in the pathogenesis of a disorder. In hyperoxaluria type 1, CRAWHALL (1962) and KOCH (1967) found that the deficient enzyme (α ketoglutarate: glyoxylate carboligase) showed normal activity in the mitchondrial fraction of liver, kidney and spleen, i. e. the inherited defect responsible for the raised oxalate production affected only the cytoplasmic isoenzyme. However, BROCK (1972) considers that this situation is not common. Most enzyme deficiencies have been investigated in whole tissue homogenates.

Temporal Variation during Development

In assessing the role of isoenzymes in teratogenicity it is necessary to know something of their availability or variation in activity at critical stages in development. Here information is again deficient. Our first example illustrates the interaction of a particular enzyme variant and an environmental insult. The insult was treatment by a drug which, like many others, freely crosses the placenta. If the variant had not been present at the critical moment, then the fetal defect would not have occurred. The enzyme glucose-6-phosphate dehydrogenase which is active antenatally (MESSINA, 1972) possesses many allelic variants, in some of which their suboptimal activity results in haemolysis when environmental stress, in the shape of certain drugs, is encountered. PERKINS (1971) reported on a stillbirth with hydrops fetalis. It was a negro male carrying the gene for the A^- variant of G6PD on the X chromosome, and was delivered at 36 weeks with severe erythroblastosis and anaemia, $2^1/_2$ weeks after the mother had taken a course of sulfisoxazole for a urinary tract infection. This drug, the only aetiological factor of note in the case, produces haemolysis in G6PD deficient adults so that the fetus appears to have suffered a drug-induced haemolytic crisis due to the presence of an allelic variant of G6PD. Among the numerous rare variants of G6PD, some are so severe as to cause spontaneous haemolysis, particularly Gd Chicago (KIRKMAN, 1964 b), Gd Oklahoma (KIRKMAN, 1964 a), Gd Duarte and Gd Albuquerque (BEUTLER, 1968) which are responsible for cases of congenital haemolytic disease. In these examples it is the fact of the availability of the isoenzymes that produces the disorder.

Many isoenzymes show quantitative and qualitative changes with development. This frequently involves an increase in the number of multiple forms due to increased intracellular complexity, and development of mature function. These changes apply particularly to those multiple forms which arise as a result of post-transcription modifications within the cell. A few systems, however, possess isoenzymes which disappear later in development. The isoenzymes of alkaline phosphatase which are specific to the placenta provide an obvious example, but a similar disappearance is also seen with fetal organs. For example, the activity of G6PD rises from a low level in early fetal life to a peak at 4—5 months, falling to the adult level by birth, and the enzyme molecule responsible for the early peak is distinct from the adult type, i. e. is an isoenzyme (MESSINA, 1972). In other systems the change is less dramatic. Thus, with lactic dehydrogenase in the brain, a relative excess of the M type subunit during fetal life and persisting three months after birth results in a changed electrophoretic pattern with the band LDH 3 being dominant (BONAVITA, 1962).

The lack of detailed observational data relating to developmental enzyme variations makes it difficult to offer explanations for their cause. Some, at least, must be causally related to the profound biochemical and structural changes which occur during differentiation. In such cases, combinations of inherited mutants occurring at the loci coding for these polypeptide chains could be manifest as a positive family history of lethal congenital defect without obvious postnatal biochemical abnormality. A proportion of unexplained fetal deaths may well be due to defects and variations in enzyme systems operating exclusively in early and very critical periods of life.

Non-Specific Esterases and the Developing Brain — An Example of Isoenzymatic Teratology

The esterase enzymes owe their name to their ability to hydrolyse various esters. They are closely related to the enzyme lipase, but differ in that the substrates of lipases have much longer acyl chains, i. e. their side chains contain more carbon atoms. Within the esterase group, several discrete enzymes with distinct physiological substrates have been recognised, particularly the cholinesterases. But also there are the "non-specific esterases", a category which refers to those polypeptide chains for which no natural substrate can be defined, and whose role remains obscure. For the purposes of investigation, the enzymes are made to act on artificial esters of naphthol formulated by NACHLAS and SELIGMAN (1949) liberating free naphthol which reacts with a diazonium salt to produce a water-insoluble pigment. In electrophoresis the deposition of this pigment marks the position of the esterase bands. Inhibitors such as E600, DFP, PCMB and eserine are used to subdivide the numerous electrophoretic zones present in most tissues. At present the two major groupings are the E600 resistant arylesterases, and the carboxylesterases which are sensitive to this inhibitor. In our study of the developing human brain, three artificial esters were employed: α naphthyl acetate (NA), α naphthyl propionate (NP) and α naphthyl butyrate (NB), whose acyl chains contain 2, 3 and 4 carbons respectively.

Figure 1 column A shows the typical electrophoretic pattern of non-specific esterases as seen in the adult human brain (grey matter). The 16 major bands marked agree with those described by BARRON and BERNSOHN and their associates (BERNSOHN 1959, 1964 a, b; BARRON 1961, 1962, 1963 a, 1966, 1968, 1972). These NA bands can be divided into two groups: the cathodal and lower anodal bands with band 8 are carboxylesterases, and bands 5, 6, 9 and 10 are arylesterases. The remaining bands are probably due to substrate overlap with cholinesterase and lipases and need not be discussed further. In addition to the bands shown, 3—4 additional bands lie between 8 and 9 which are visualised with the 3 carbon substrate NP. Like band 8, these resemble the carboxylesterase group.

When the early fetal pattern in Fig. 1 column B is compared with the adult brain pattern, the developmental changes are obvious. The major differences are firstly, the apparent absence of carboxylesterases from fetal brain and secondly the presence, in the fetal pattern, of a dense zone of activity which is referred to for the purposes of discussion as the 'F' band. When a series of some 60 brains extending throughout prenatal life was examined, it was found that the fetal pattern described was universally present in fetuses up to about 20 weeks. Thereafter, the carboxylesterases showed a progressive rise in activity, reaching adult levels by birth while the fetal band continued at about the same activity until 25 weeks in the cortex and fell gradually thereafter, reaching a low level by birth and disappearing by about 3 months postnatal age. Relating these temporal changes to present knowledge of the histological development of the brain, the rise in activity of the cathodal and lower anodal bands is associated with the period of neuronal maturation, axon and dendrite growth and glial cell proliferation. Since these enzyme bands show a widespread distribution in different tissues and species, however, and since this period of brain development is associated with widespread biochemical changes — Flexner's so-called 'critical period' — it seems likely that there is not direct causal relationship between these events, and that this case provides a good example of developmental isoenzyme changes associated with tissue and cellular maturation (p. 209).

This explanation cannot be applied to band 8, however, which together with the NP specific bands began to show increased activity in the last ten weeks of pregnancy, rising to a high level by 6 months postnatal age. These NP specific bands

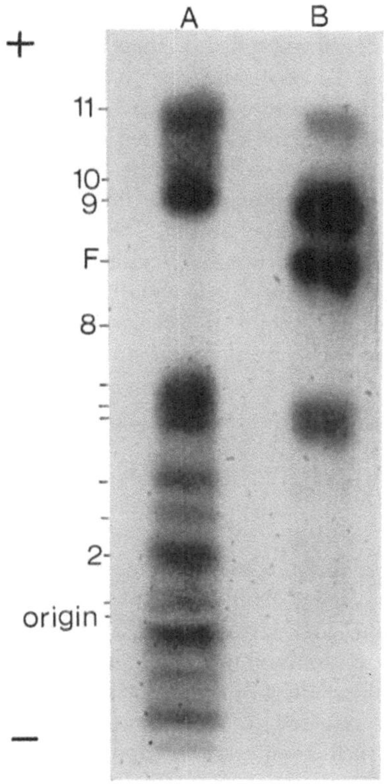

Fig. 1. Starch gel electrophoretic patterns of non-specific esterases in human brain: (A) normal adult; (B) early fetus

have been extensively studied by BARRON (1968, 1972), and have been found to react best with the 3 and 4 carbon substrates; only the most proximal band reacts with naphthyl acetate — band 8. The group as a whole are specific to the white matter of the central nervous system and are found in higher primates only. Biochemically they are characterised by their great sensitivity to organophosphorus inhibitors such as DFP, and their ability to hydrolyse 5 carbon esters. Thus they fall midway between the other esterases and the lipases.

There are clues to the possible significance of this isoenzyme group. These polypeptides seem to be closely associated with CNS myelin in their distribution. Their appearance in the cortex immediately precedes myelination according to the timing described by YAKOVLEV (1967), and Barron demonstrated that the activity of this group declined in the second postnatal year, after the majority of the cortex has completed its myelogenetic cycle. WENDER (1971) found, on histological examination of developing brain, a diffuse esterase activity in maturing neuroglia with accentuated activity in the myelination clusters of oligodendroglia. A similar raised activity was seen in the nerve fibres and this persisted into adult life while activity in the neuroglia subsided. It seems reasonable to suggest that this group of isoenzymes is closely involved in the production and maintenance of CNS myelin in man. Hence their pathological significance lies in their involvement with demyelination. In cases of multiple sclerosis BARRON and BERNSOHN (1963 b, 1965) showed that in plaque tissue the NP specific bands were absent, while RINNE (1968) showed that carboxylesterase activity is elevated in the cerebrospinal fluid of multiple sclerosis cases. Of more interest in the present context is the additional finding of BARRON and BERNSOHN of similar changes in a case of diffuse cerebral sclerosis, a condition which involves massive demyelination of the CNS in early childhood, often in the first year of life, sometimes with a familial tendency. While in the case quoted the esterase defect may well be secondary, it is equally possible that a genetic defect in, or environmental insult to, this group of isoenzymes could well result in defective myelin production and its early breakdown, and as such represent a teratogenic isoenzyme defect.

The F Band

The study of the F band provides a further example of the possible association between isoenzymes and teratology. Its biochemical properties show it to be similar to the arylesterases, being able to hydrolyse NA, NP and NB, i. e. up to 4 carbon esters, and being resistant to the inhibitor E600. In addition the band shows a relative resistance to the inhibitor PCMB, on the basis of which HOLMES and MASTERS (1968) and VOLPE (1970) referred to the fetospecific esterase as an acetylesterase, though the necessity for such a separate grouping appears questionable. Developmentally, this band persists at a constant level in the cortex until 25 weeks and thereafter fades. This timing can be correlated with the cessation of neuroblast division in the cortex (DOBBING, 1970). In adult brain, by using detergent to extract bound esterase, a band with the same mobility is faintly visible in the zymogram from grey matter, where the cortical neurones are located, but not in white matter. Furthermore, the electrophoretic data of KOKKO (1965) obtained using spinal ganglia which contain a high concentration of neuronal tissue also shows a band with the same mobility and inhibitor characteristics as the F band. It appears that this isoenzyme may be involved in the division of the immature neurones.

In some cases very close to the leading edge of the F band there appeared, after storage of the specimen, an additional band which could not hydrolyse NP, i. e. was specific to the 2 carbon substrate NA. This phenomenon may be explained if one accepts the subunit concept suggested by CHOUDHURY (1972) to account for the various properties of the non-specific esterases, and assumes that the F band comprises two subunits, labelled C2 and C4 on the basis of the maximum length of side chain they can accommodate. On storage these dissociate, and the free C2 subunits migrate further on electrophoresis so producing the extra band. This suggestion was supported by the findings on isoelectric focusing (PAPIHA and BURN, 1975). This technique separates protein molecules, using a stable pH gradient, on the basis of their isoelectric point, i. e. the pH at which the negative and positive charges on the protein are belanced. It was found that three bands corresponded to the fetal esterase (Fig. 3) which were labelled V, VII and VIII. It was shown that with a fresh sample

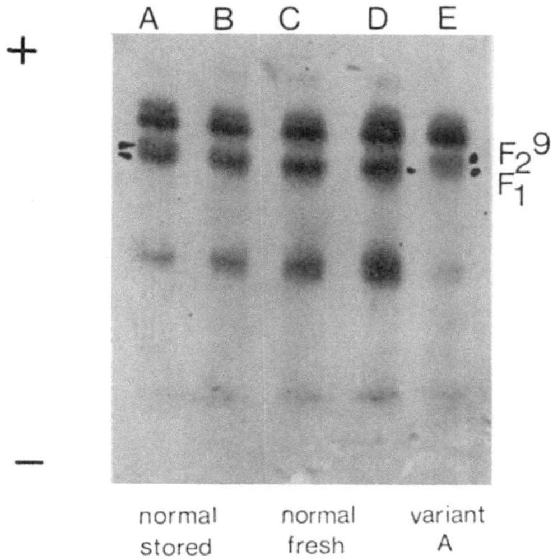

Fig. 2. Variations in fetal esterase pattern

band V was prominent, while an older sample showed reduced activity at position V and raised activity at VII and VIII. Since the latter reacted only with NA and band VII showed a prominent reaction with NP, it appeared that band V represented the complete enzyme and the other bands the two subunits.

F Band Variants

During this study three brains were analysed in which the electrophoretic properties of the F band were changed. The first variant observed, variant A, is shown in column F of Fig. 2; the normally dominant F1 band is virtually absent, while the F2 band is relatively prominent and, as in the other cases, was found to react only with the 2 carbon substrate, NA. The electrophoretic distinction was supported by isoelectric focusing, with bands V and VII absent and continued activity at position VIII (Column A, Fig. 3). These changes were attributed to some defect in the C4 component of the F band. Short-run electrophoresis (Fig. 4) demonstrated the presense of a defective unstable protein taken to represent an abnormal C4 subunit which, because of its altered properties, was unable to combine with the C2 subunits. All this evidence strongly suggests genetic determination of this variance, though there is no proof, in which case this 12 week fetus represents either a heterozygote or a homozygote for a mutant allele at the C4 locus. The two other specimens found which showed greater F2 and less F1 activity than normal and the presence of the mutant C4 band (variants B and C) were less extreme in their activity differences and may represent, on this genetic hypothesis, either heterozygotes for alleles of quantitatively different effect from that carried by variant A, or heterozygotes for the same allele as that for which variant A is homozygous. Fig. 5 summarises the electrophoretic findings relating to the fetal esterase band.

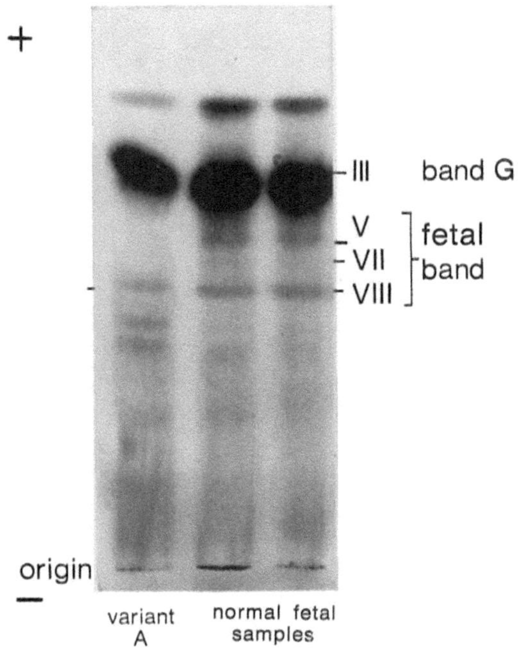

Fig. 3. Fetal brain esterases: patterns on thin layer isoelectric focusing

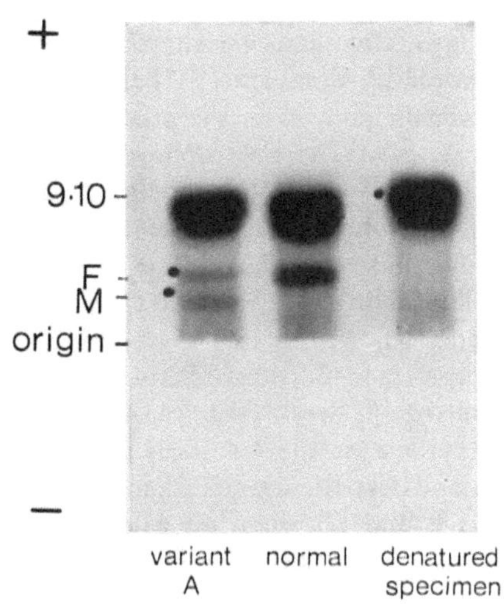

Fig. 4. Fetal brain esterase patterns: short duration electrophoresis. The fetal band F includes both F_1 and F_2. The new unstable protein in the variant (column A) is marked M

In view of the association between the F band and dividing neuroblasts, an F band defect could interfere with normal neurone division, and since the fetal brain in the first half of pregnancy is almost entirely made up of neuroblasts, any interference would probably affect total brain weight. The fetus providing variant A had a brain weight of 2.3 grams, which was more than 5 standard deviations below the age mean of 5½ grams (rather less than 50% of normal). Variants B and C were approximately 75% of mean brain weight falling on the lower 95% confidence limit. In all three cases the external size of the head remained within normal limits, the extra space being filled by CSF. These findings appeared to support the explanation of a genetically determined defect in a fetal isoenzyme specifically involved in neurone

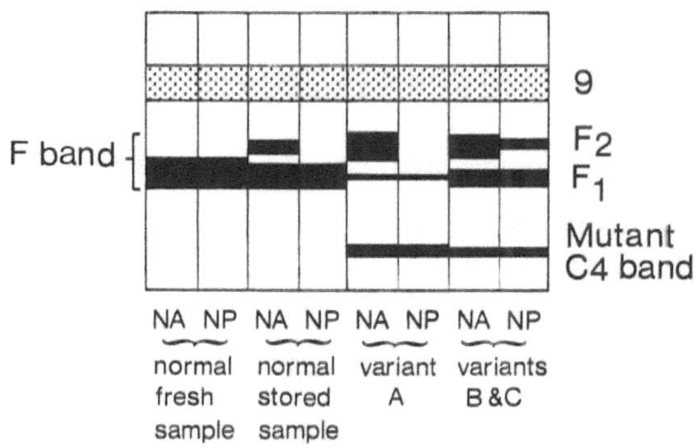

Fig. 5. Diagram of F band variation with NA and NP (2- and 3-carbon) substrates

division. Final support for the theory was provided by retrospective data relating to the social history of variant B. The mother of this fetus was found to have 14 sibs of whom 6 were mentally subnormal, 4 being housed permanently in institutions. An unspecified number of the remaining sibs were described as being 'borderline IQ' and the mother showed evidence of being in the lower range of normal IQ and being somewhat emotionally immature having had two abortions in two years to different consorts.

On clinical grounds, the affliction in this family would be described as 'simple mental retardation' owing to the absence of any obvious biochemical defect or associated structural deformity, this being the classification into which almost 50% of all retardates are placed (Walton, 1973). Dodge and Adams (1971) observed that such retardates are often born of dull or retarded parents, and that the term 'familial' was frequently justified. Furthermore, no evidence of physical abnormality, biochemical defect or gross brain growth defect is evident in these people. However, the present suggested association with neurone division means that the aetiological factor is specific to nerve cells. These represent less than 10% of the total weight at birth, and variation of the order here described is not detectable in the postnatal period. As Davison (1968) and Dobbing (1970) have shown, if neurone division is not completed in the given time, a permanent deficit results, and this would affect the higher centres most severely. Further, the lower cerebral structures such as the brain stem are not affected in these individuals.

While further work is necessary to corroborate these findings on non-specific esterase, they have been presented in some detail to provide illustrations of some of the many ways in which isoenzymes may be involved in both normal and abnormal development. Thus an enzyme or one multiple form may owe its appearance during development to tissue maturity and therefore not be involved in the process of differentiation. On the other hand, some multiple forms appear to be specifically involved in development, and either disappear completely or show much diminished activity once a particular stage is passed. It seems very likely that a closer examination for defects in such 'fetal' isoenzymes could well provide a biochemical and hence genetic answer to a number of hitherto unexplained inherited defects. It will also improve understanding of fetomaternal interaction in dealing with metabolites and drugs, as well as permitting the prediction of the onset of pathological effects (HAHN, 1971).

Other Applications of Isoenzyme Developmental Variation

The study of developmental changes in isoenzyme systems provides a sensitive index of the intracellular environment and may provide markers of disease whatever its cause. This approach has been usefully employed for general medicine, e. g. the diagnosis of myocardial infarction, using the serum isoenzyme patterns of lactic dehydrogenase (LDH) and creatine kinase (CPK) (LATNER and SKILLEN, 1968). Using the same isoenzymes in the study of Duchenne muscular dystrophy, EMERY (1964) and SCHAPIRA *et al.* (1968, 1970) showed that the normal developmental changes associated with maturity did not occur in dystrophic muscle. Normally with LDH, the M subunit becomes dominant by birth with an associated reduction in H subunit production, so that skeletal muscle at birth contains almost entirely LDH 5. In dystrophic muscle this change is retarded, with LDH 1 raised and LDH 5 reduced in both affected individuals and carriers. Similarly, creatine phosphokinase (CPK) comprises two subunits labelled M and B giving three isoenzymes BB, BM and MM. Normally, the B subunit is 'switched off' at about 5-months in skeletal muscle and only the M is produced thereafter. In all types of muscular dystrophy, however, this change is retarded and the other isoenzymes are seen in the muscle at birth. They presumably give rise to unusual serum isoenzyme patterns, e. g. the elevation of the CPK BM subunit in the serum of dystrophic patients (GOTO, 1974), to be related on this interpretation to developmental modification rather than the suggested subclinical heart damage (cardiac muscle being the chief normal source of the B subunit).

Schapira also found that the enzyme aldolase showed a 'fetal' pattern in dystrophic or atrophic muscle, with the persistence of C subunit production. This produced A, AC and C isoenzymes in the abnormal muscle instead of the usual A type only. Thus, the general effect in dystrophic muscle appeared to be a retardation of normal development and this was reflected in the isoenzyme system of muscle. Furthermore, these changes were present at birth so raising the possibility of early postnatal diagnosis in 'at risk' infants, before the clinical signs become apparent.

Another example of a diagnostic application is provided by the work of CAO and DE VIREILIIS (1971) who found that in cases of congenital hypothyroidism the serum isoenzyme pattern for CPK was abnormal. In congenital hypothyroidism the serum isoenzyme pattern shows an excess of the M type of subunit of this dimer, which is presumably related to the neuromyopathy and vacuolar change seen in the muscle of congenital hypothyroid cases. This example is seen to be directly analogous to the diagnostic approach in myocardial infarcts mentioned above.

In the condition of congenital biliary atresia, NATOLI *et al.* (1969) found a close association with changes in the serum isoenzyme pattern of the enzyme leucine aminopeptidase (LAP). This change involved the appearance of an additional band proximal to the usual single band in serum. The band was specific to all cases of atresia, being absent in 5 cases of neonatal hepatitis so providing a means of distinction between these conditions. There is no evidence to suggest this condition is directly caused by a defect in LAP, nor are there adequate data to show this extra band to be a fetal isoenzyme, though there is considerable developmental variation in different tissues (PATARYAS and CHRISTODOULOU, 1970).

Other Polymorphisms

The oldest known human polymorphisms, the human blood groups, give rise on occasion to the abnormalities associated with haemolytic disease of the newborn, perhaps the oldest known of intrauterine disorders arising as a direct result of genetic factors in the mother and fetus. IgG globulins which can cross the placenta are already present in the fetus before the twelfth week of gestation, and by this date passage of anti-Rh antibodies is documented (MOLLISON, 1972); by the age of 16—22 weeks, sufficient anti-Rh can cross the placenta to cause intrauterine death. Anti-A and Anti-B are also IgG red cell antibodies which are sometimes involved in the causation of a mild haemolytic syndrome and very occasionally severe haemolytic disease. Other blood group antibodies very rarely cause haemolytic disease, but blood group genes which have been implicated are c, E, K, k, Kp^a, S, s, M, Fy^a, Fy^b, Jk^a, Jk^b and many others. Some relatively common blood group antibodies, such as P1, do not cause haemolytic disease because they are primarily IgM.

Of other polymorphic systems usually used in population studies, transferrin bands are well established by the 17th week (PARKER and BEARN, 1962) and have been detected as early as eight weeks (GITLIN and BIASUCCI, 1969). Transferrin activity rises steadily through fetal life, and it appears that specific fetal components exist (PARKER *et al.*, 1963) which disappear shortly after birth.

Haptoglobin (Hp) types in early fetal life have been difficult to detect, though HIRSCHFELD and LUNELL (1962) found evidence for haptoglobin synthesis in fetuses from 17—30 weeks old. It required the development of immunological techniques to detect haptoglobin present in small amounts in the sera of 4 out of 50 fetuses between 8 and 16 weeks old (GITLIN and BIASUCCI, 1969). Activity is very low. The group specific components (Gc) in fetuses were first observed by HIRSCHFELD and LUNELL (1962) in 25-week fetuses, but again the development of radial immunodiffusion techniques was necessary before the small amounts present in early fetuses

could be detected (TOIVANEN *et al.*, 1969); the concentration increases during prenatal development.
Of the components of complement, C4 and C3 appear to have zero activity in early fetuses, but have been detected from the age of 15 weeks onwards, and thereafter the concentration of the two proteins increases steadily. They and the commoner C3 variants do not cross the placenta (PROPP and ALPER, 1968).
The studies of such polymorphisms in human fetuses have provided useful information on the quantitative development of some variant forms though few fetal variants of potential teratological relevance have been detected (perhaps because they have not been sought). These experiments have demonstrated the importance of immunoelectrophoretic procedures for the accurate estimations of the small amounts that may exist, and have shown how materno-fetal interaction can damage the fetus. They have provided useful information on the stages of gestation at which new proteins are released into fetal circulation, and on the origins and sites of synthesis of the proteins present in fetal blood (ADINOLFI, 1971). The polymorphic variants have provided useful information on which proteins cross the placenta, especially where that of the fetus differs from that of the mother. But fetal plasma proteins so far appear to be potentially less rewarding for teratology than the study of fetal isoenzymes.

Conclusion

This review, essentially speculative, has drawn upon the accumulated experience of human polymorphic systems to argue that search for variant forms of proteins in fetal tissue has much to contribute to the advancement of teratology and that enzymes are particularly worthy of study. A model for genetic control has been described, the meaning of enzyme heterogeneity investigated, and it is argued that for teratological relevance, tissue specificity of isoenzymes and availability at the appropriate stage in development are of fundamental importance. The argument is illustrated by a study of non-specific esterases in the developing human brain.
The data in support of this argument are scattered and limited; there is confusion of terminology, the lack of appreciation of which has meant that much information cannot be located by literature search. Many studies of inherited defects have undoubtedly omitted search for multiple forms of enzymes, and the present argument has been almost entirely restricted to such discrete forms. This is not to say that quantitative variation is not important, and indeed many studies of inherited defects have concentrated on this. The quantitative variation that occurs in fetal life is well illustrated in the plasma protein polymorphic systems.
Quantitative and qualitative variation are, of course, not mutually exclusive, and should ideally be studied together. In a forward-looking paper, MOTULSKY (1969) has postulated a quantitative model. Some 30% of all enzymes are known to be polymorphic, that is to have variant forms, some of which are present at appreciable frequencies in the population. Different variants of an enzyme may have different activities; for example the three genes that are commonly available for red cell acid phosphatase produce activities in the ratios 1, 1.5, 2; in adenylate kinase, the

two common genes produce an effect in the ratio 1 to 1.5. The distribution of enzyme activity in the population, therefore, depends upon the distribution of the genotypes, so that one homozygote is primarily responsible for all very low activities, of which some may be below the threshold for useful utilisation. In MOTULSKY's simple model, two such loci interact, and a specific birth defect occurs if the enzyme activity for both falls below the threshold, that is to say in those individuals who are double homozygotes. Here there is a clear pointer to the way in which a relatively simple genetic difference, affecting only one or two loci, may produce low frequency birth defects.

The type of investigation outlined here has much to offer for better knowledge of normal development, and of deviations from it. There are hundreds of enzymes with variant forms awaiting identification and activity quantification in different fetal tissues at different stages of development. The outlook for the advancement of teratology is bright.

References

ADINOLFI, M. A.: Genetic polymorphism and *in vitro* cultures in studies of the ontogenesis of human fetal proteins in BENSON, P. (ed.) "The biochemistry of development". London: Heinemann 1971.

BARRON, K. D.: Starch gel electrophoresis of brain esterases. J. Histochem. Cytochem. **11**, 139 (1961).

BARRON, K. D., BERNSOHN, J.: Separation and properties of human brain esterases. J. Histochem. Cytochem. **11**, 139 (1963 a).

BARRON, K. D., BERNSOHN, J.: Brain esterases and phosphatases in multiple sclerosis. Ann. N.Y. Acad. Sci. **122**, 369 (1965).

BARRON, K. D., BERNSOHN, J.: Esterases of developing human brain. J. Neurochem. **15** (4), 276—284 (1968).

BARRON, K. D., BERNSOHN, J., DOOLIN, P. F.: Subcellular localization of multiple forms of brain esterases. J. Histochem. Cytochem. **14**, 817 (1966).

BARRON, K. D., BERNSOHN, J., HESS, A. R.: Electrophoretic analysis of human brain esterases. Acta neurol. scand. Suppl. **1**, 61—62 (1962).

BARRON, K. D., BERNSOHN, J., HESS, A. R.: Abnormalities in brain esterases in multiple sclerosis. Proc. Soc. exp. Biol. (N.Y.) **113**, 521 (1963 b).

BARRON, K. D., BERNSOHN, J., MITZEN, E.: Nonspecific esterases of human peripheral nerve and centrum ovale. J. Neuropath. exp. Neurol. **31**, 562—568 (1972).

BERNSOHN, J., BARRON, K. D.: Multiple molecular forms of brain hydrolase. Int. Rev. Neurobiol. **7**, 297—342 (1964).

BERNSOHN, J., BARRON, K. D., NORGELLO, H.: 'Bound' and soluble esterases in human brain. Biochem. J. **91**, 24—26 c (1964).

BEUTLER, E.: In "Hereditary disorders of erythrocyte metabolism" E. BEUTLER (ed.), 114—124. New York: Grune & Stratton 1968.

BIGLEY, R. H., KOLER, R. D.: Liver pyruvate kinase (P.K.) isoenzymes in a P.K.-deficient patient. Ann. hum. Genet. **31**, 383 (1968).

BIGLEY, R. H., STENZEL, L. P.: Tissue distribution of human pyruvate kinase isoenzymes. Enzymol. Biol. Clin. **9**, 10 (1968).

BONAVITA, V., GUARNERI, R.: Lactic dehydrogenase isoenzymes in the nervous tissue: (1) The reaction of isozymes with DPN analogues and their inhibition by sodium meta-bisulfite. Biochem. Biophys. Acta **59**, 634—642 (1962).

BROCK, D. J. H., MAYO, O.: (ed.) The biochemical genetics of man. London & New York: Acad. Press 1962.

CAO, A., VIREILIIS, S. DE: Serum creatine phosphokinase isoenzymes in congenital hypothyroidism. J. Paediatrics 78, 134—135 (1971).
CHOUDHURY, S. R.: The nature of non-specific esterases. A subunit concept. J. Histochem. Cytochem. 20, 507 (1972).
CRAWHALL, J. C., WATTS, R. W. E.: The metabolism of (1-^{14}C)-glyoxylate by the liver mitochondria of patients with primary hyperoxaluria and non-hyperoxaluric subjects (1962). Clin. Sci. 23, 163 (1962).
DANOVITCH, S. H., BAER, P. N., LASTER, L.: Intestinal alkaline phosphatase activity in familial hypophosphatasia. New Engl. J. Med. 278, 1253—1260 (1968).
DAVISON, A. N., DOBBING, J.: Applied neurochemistry; Ch. 6, The developing brain (rat), 612. Oxford: Blackwell (Contemporary Neurology Series 4/5) (1968).
DAWSON, D. M., SPONG, F. L., HARRINGTON, J. F.: McArdle's disease. Lack of muscle phosphorylase. Ann. Intern. Med. 69, 229 (1968).
DESREUX, V., HERIOTT, R. M.: Existence of several active components in crude pepsin preparation. Nature (Lond.) 144, 287 (1939).
DOBBING, J., SANDS, J.: The timing of neuroblast multiplication in developing human brain. Nature (Lond.) 226, 639—640 (1970).
DODGE, P. R., ADAMS, R. D.: in Harrison's principles of internal medicine. 6th ed. ed. in chief, WINTROBE, M. M. (1971).
EMERY, A. E. H.: Electrophoretic pattern of LDH in carriers and patients with Duchenne muscular dystrophy. Nature (Lond.) 201, 1044—1045 (1964).
FITZPATRICK, T. B., QUEVEDO, W. C.: The metabolic basis of inherited disease. 1st ed. 324—340. ed.: J. B. STANBURY *et al.* New York: McGraw-Hill 1966.
FROESCH, E. R., WOLF, H. P., BAITSCH, H., PRADER, A., LABHART, A.: Hereditary fructose intolerance: an inborn defect of hepatic fructose-1-phosphate splitting aldolase. Amer. J. Med. 34, 151 (1963).
GITLIN, D., BIASUCCI, A.: Development of γG, γA, γM, β1C/β1A, C'1 esterase inhibitor, ceruloplasmin, transferrin, hemopexin, haptoglobin, fibrinogen, plasminogen, α_1-antritrypsin, orosomucoid, β-lipoprotein, α_2-macroglobulin and prealbumin in the human conceptus. J. clin. Invest. 48, 1433 (1969).
GOTO, I.: CPK isozymes in neuromuscular disorders. Arch. Neurol. 31, 116—119 (1974).
HAHN, P., SKALA, J.: Development of enzyme systems (human foetus). Clin. Abstract Gynae. 14, 655—668 (1971).
HALL, J. G., MOTULSKY, A. G.: Production of fetal haemoglobin in marrow cultures of human adults. Nature (Lond.) 217, 569 (1968).
HARRIS, H.: The principles of human biochemical genetics. North Holland, Amsterdam, London (1970).
HERS, H. G.: Etudes enzymatiques sur fragments hépatiques. Application à la classification des glycogénoses. Rev. int. Hépat. 9, 35—55 (1959).
HERS, H. G., HOOF, F. VAN: Carbohydrate metabolism and its disorders. ed. F. DICKENS, P. J. RANDLE and W. T. WHELAN, 2, 151—168. New York and London: Acad. Press 1968.
HERS, H. G., JOASSIN, G.: Anomalie de l'aldolase hépatique dans l'intolerance au fructose. Enzymol. biol. clin. 1, 4—14 (1961).
HIRSCHFELD, J., LUNELL, N. O.: Serum protein synthesis in foetus: haptoglobins and group-specific components. Nature (Lond.) 196, 1220 (1962).
HOLMES, R. S., MASTERS, C. J.: A comparative study of the multiplicity of mammalian esterases. Biochim. Biophys. Acta (Amst.) 151, 147—158 (1968).
HUG, G., SCHUBERT, W. K., CHUCK, G.: Deficient activity of phosphorylase kinase and accumulation of glycogen in the liver. J. clin. Invest. 48 (1969).
HUIJING, F., FERNANDES, J.: X-Chromosomal inheritance of liver glycogenosis with phosphorylase kinase deficiency. Amer. J. hum. Genet. 21, 275 (1969).
I.U.P.A.C. — I.U.B. Commission on biochemical nomenclature. The nomenclature of multiple forms of enzymes. Biochem. J. 126, 769—771 (1972).
KAPLAN, N. O.: in Mechanism of action of steroid hormones. ed. C. A. VILLEE and A. A. ENGEL. Oxford: Pergamon 1961.
KEITT, A. S.: Haemolytic anaemia with impaired hexokinase activity. J. clin. Invest. 48, 1997 (1969).

Kirkman, H. N.: "Chicago 1" variant of G6PD in congenital haemolytic disease. J. Lab. clin. Med. **63**, 715 (1964).
Kirkman, H. N., *et al.*: Functionally abnormal G6PD. Cold Spring Harbor. Sympt. Quart. Biol. **29**, 391 (1964).
Koch, J., Skokstad, E. L. R.: Deficiency of 2 oxoglutarate: glyoxylate carboligase activity in primary hyperoxaluria. Proc. nat. Acad. Sci. (Wash.) **57**, 1123 (1967).
Kokko, A.: Histochemical and cytophotometric observations on esterases in the spinal ganglion of the rat. Acta physiol. scand. **65**, Suppl. 261 (1965).
Latner, A., Skillen, A. W.: (eds.) Isoenzymes in biology and medicine. London and New York: Acad. Press 1968.
Lehrer, R. I., Cline, M. J.: Leukocyte myeloperoxidase deficiency and disseminated candidiasis: the role of myeloperoxidase in resistance to candida infection. J. clin. Invest. **48**, 1478—1488 (1969).
Lie-Injo Luan Eng, Lie, H. G., Ager, J. A. M., Lehmann, H.: Alphathalassaemia as a cause of hydrops foetalis. Brit. J. Haemat. **8**, 1 (1962).
Markert, C. L., Moller, F.: Multiple forms of enzymes: tissue, ontogenetic and species specific patterns. Proc. nat. Acad. Sci. (Wash.) **45**, 753 (1959).
McCance, R. A. *et al.*: Genetic, clinical biochemical, and pathological features of hypophosphatasia. J. clin. Med. **25**, 523—537 (1956).
McKusick, V. A.: Mendelian inheritance in man (4th edition). Baltimore: Johns Hopkins Press 1974.
Messina, A. M.: G6PD: Developing human liver. Proc. Soc. exp. Biol. (N.Y.) **139**, 778—782 (1972).
Mollison, P. I.: Clinical aspects of blood transfusion. Oxford: Blackwell 1972.
Motulsky, A. G.: Biochemical genetics of haemoglobins and enzymes as a model for birth defect research in Proc. 3rd Internat. Cong. Congenital Malformations, The Hague (1969).
Nachlas, N. M., Seligman, A. W.: The histochemical demonstration of esterase. J. nat. Cancer Inst. **9**, 415 (1949).
Natoli, G., Natoli, V. *et al.*: Leucine Aminopeptidase isoenzymes in neonatal hepatitis and biliary atresia. Lancet **1969 I**, 209, 25.
Necheles, T. F. *et al.*: Homozygous erythrocyte glutathione-peroxidase deficiency: clinical and biochemical studies. Blood **33**, 164 (1969).
Necheles, T. F., Rai, U. S., Cameron, D.: Congenital nonspherocytic haemolytic anaemia associated with an unusual hexokinase abnormality. J. Lab. clin. Med. **76**, 593 (1970).
Papiha, S. S., Burn, J.: Isoelectric focusing of non-specific esterases of developing human brain in thinlayer polyacrylamide gels. Biol. Neonate. In Press (1975).
Parker, W. C., Bearn, A. G.: Studies on the transferrins of adult serum, cord serum and cerebrospinal fluid: the effect of neuraminidase. J. exp. Med. **115**, 85 (1962).
Parker, W. C., Hagstrom, J. W., Bearn, A. G.: Additional studies on the transferrins of cord serum and cerebrospinal fluid: variation in carbohydrate and prosthetic groups. J. exp. Med. **118**, 975 (1963).
Pataryas, H. A., Christodoulou, C.: Leucine aminopeptidase variations in human foetal organs. Hum. Hered. 20 (**3**), 325—328 (1970).
Penhoet, E., Rajkumar, T.: Multiple forms of fructose diphosphate aldolase in mammalian tissue. Proc. nat. Acad. Sci. (Wash.) **56**, 1275 (1966).
Perkins, R. P.: Hydrops fetalis and stillbirth in a male G6PD deficient foetus possibly due to maternal ingestion of sulfisoxazole. Amer. J. Obstet. Gynec. **111**, 379—381 (1971).
Propp, R. P., Alper, C. A.: $C^{1}3$ synthesis in the human fetus and lack of transplacental passage. Science **162**, 672 (1968).
Rathburn, J. C.: Hypophosphatasia — a new developmental anomaly. Amer. J. Dis. Child **75**, 822—831 (1948).
Rinne, U. K., Riekkinen, P.: Esterase, peptidase and proteinase activities of human cerebrospinal fluid in multiple sclerosis. Acta neurol. scand. **44**, 156—167 (1968).
Robbins, P. W.: Immunological study of human muscle lacking phosphorylase. Fed. Proc. Fedn. Amer. Soc. exp. Biol. **19**, 193 (1960).
Rutter, W. J., Rajkumar, T. *et al.*: Aldolase variants: structure and physiological significance. Ann. N. Y. Acad. Sci. **151**, 102 (1968).

Salmon, S. E., Cline, M. J. *et al.*: Myeloperoxidase deficiency. New. Engl. J. Med. **282**, 250—253 (1970).

Schapira, F., Dreyfus, J. C., Allard, D.: Les isoenzymes de la créatine kinase er de l'aldolase du muscle foetal et pathologique. Clin. chim. Acta **20**, 439 (1968).

Schmid, R., Robbins, P. W., Taut, R. R.: Glycogen synthesis in muscle lacking phosphorylase. Proc. nat. Acad. Sci. (Wash.) **45**, 1236 (1959).

Smithies, O.: Zone electrophoresis in starch gels: group variation in the serum proteins of normal human adults. Biochem. J. **61**, 629 (1955).

Spranger, J., Widemann, H. R.: The genetic mucolipidoses, diagnosis and differential diagnosis. Humangenetik **9**, 113—119 (1970).

Toivanen, P., Rossi, T., Hirvonen, T.: The concentration of Gc globulin and transferrin in human fetal and infant sera. Scand. J. Haemat. **6**, 113 (1969).

Valentine, W. N. *et al.*: Hereditary haemolytic anaemia with hexokinase deficiency. Role of hexokinase in erythrocyte aging. New Engl. J. Med. **276**, 1 (1967).

Volpe, J. J. *et al.*: Regional distribution of isoenzymes of D. amino acid oxidase and acetylesterase in developing primate brain. Exp. Neurol. **28**, 76—87 (1970).

Waddington, C. H.: Principles of development and differentiation. New York: Macmillan & Co. 1966.

Walton, J. N.: Essentials of neurology, 3rd edn. London: Pitman 1971.

Waterbury, L., Frenkel, E. P.: Phosphofructokinase deficiency in congenital non-spherocytic anaemia. Clin. Res. **17**, 347 (1969).

Waterbury, L., Frenkel, E. P.: Hereditary nonspherocytic hemolysis with erythrocyte phosphofructokinase deficiency. Blood **39**, 415—425 (1972).

Wender, M. *et al.*: Histoenzymology of cerebral white matter in the developing rat brain. J. Hirnforsch. **13**, 223 (1971).

Yakovlev, P. I., Lecours, A. R.: The myelogenetic cycle of regional maturation of the brain. Regional development of the brain in early life. CIOMS Symposium (1967).

13. The Impact of Malformation on the Emotional Development of the Child and his Family

A. Bentovim

To understand the emotional responses of the family to the birth of a child with severe deformity and the subsequent difficulties in emotional development that occur with these children and their families, it is necessary to examine the normal processes that occur in parent and infant before and immediately after birth (Bentovim, 1972). Some aspects of this problem have been considered in association with particular abnormalities, e. g., spina bifida, hydrocephalus (Freeston, 1971), deformity of limbs (Pringle and Fiddes, 1970), Down's syndrome and mental handicap (Gath, 1972), cleft lip and palate (Dar *et al.*, 1974), syndactyly, cerebral palsy (Miller, 1958), congenital heart deformity (Bentovim, 1975), phenylketonuria (Bentovim *et al.*, 1970).

Emotional Developments during Pregnancy

During pregnancy, processes occur which prepare both men and women for the task of creating a family unit, enabling the mother to undertake her primary mothering tasks towards the future new-born infant, and the father to support her in them. She needs to be able to provide the right amount of contact for the baby, to provide movement or quiet, to be willing to act without demanding responses, and to allow the infant to dominate. She must respond to his needs as if they were her own.

This state has been called "primary maternal preoccupation" (Winnicott, 1958) an abnormal state of sensitivity and readiness to do what is necessary to meet an infant's demands at any time. Such a position is reached gradually during pregnancy, whilst the mother is focussing her attention on the infant growing inside her (Bibring, 1959). Accompanying these preoccupations are hopes for enrichment of "self" through the new child, perhaps fulfilling secret ambitions. At the same time, the mother has to cope with disturbing feelings that may arise when she is expecting her first child. She is beginning to adapt herself to the fact that she may be losing a job, skills, companionship and the security of her previous life. Now she may experience anger, and wish that she was not having a baby at all (Benedek, 1959). Following this sequence of feeling and thought, an understandable concern arises about whether the baby will be normal or damaged. If something does go wrong such ideas will themselves have acquired the status of an act and will be damaging. Quickening of the fetus is experienced as the beginning of an infant's independence and is accompanied by an awareness that the fetus is taking on its own existence culminating in birth and physical separation. The sensation of infant and mother being one continues, however, and these two feelings of identity and separateness are thought to be important in enabling the mother to give herself to the state of primary maternal preoccupation.

The Birth of an Infant with Malformation

The first question that the majority of mothers ask after birth is whether the baby is intact and if any deformity is present. Only then do they ask whether the baby is a boy or girl. Problems during pregnancy can affect the quality of the maternal state of mind at this time; follow-up studies of women throughout pregnancy and the puerperium indicate that excess excitement and anxiety, arising from conflicts during pregnancy, can result in more intense depressive symptoms during the puerperium. A study of children with psychosomatic gastro-intestinal disturbances related these to maternal crises during pregnancy (Brice-Pitt, 1968). Such crises include threatened miscarriages, previous stillbirths, marital or social difficulties, unresolved relationships with the mother's own parents, loss of a parent, move of the home, loss of security through father changing his job, or moving away from a familiar neighbourhood (Rose, 1961). All these factors may intrude into the relationship between mother and newborn and cause symptoms when the child is normal (Caplan, 1963). How much more so, then, even in a more happily supported situation, is the birth of a malformed infant a uniquely traumatic event.

The initial responses, as exemplified by interviews of mothers giving birth to children with spina bifida in South Wales (D'Arcy, 1968) are numbness, grief, disgust; waves of helplessness, rage or disbelief are felt. The expected perfect child is lost, and the feared, deformed child is born. This acts as a terrible blow to the parents' self-esteem; hopes for the future are shattered, loving feelings are lost, fears become real.

Immediately the question asked is: "What is wrong with me?" "What have I or my husband done wrong?" The disappointment can result in intense feelings of depression, loss and guilt (Lax, 1972). It has already been emphasised that the infant is felt to be part of and closely identified with the "self" of the mother throughout pregnancy, so that to find the infant damaged, deformed or malformed in some way is felt as an intense blow to the self: it is as if the mother is herself attacked, deformed or wronged. What is the response to this? The mother may deny the truth of what she sees: disbelieving it, she may time and again question the staff who have had to tell her the facts of the baby's condition. She may reject the baby, regarding it as something bad, something to be got rid of immediately. She might perhaps cover these feelings with an intense protective zeal, smothering rather than being neglectful, as a way of dealing with intense feelings towards the child who has caused her such pain. This is a substitution for self-hatred projected onto the child, and may also be manifest as excessive concern over cleanliness, and worries about the child being hurt by events which are clearly imaginary. Such anger can be directed towards the husband, his, or her family or the medical advisers and nursing staff. Her feelings can be amplified by her husband's response to the situation.

Professional intervention is necessary, since such feelings can interfere with the ability of a mother to perceive and respond to the cues from her baby and to care for him appropriately. The child is born with a whole repertoire of responses that teach the mother to meet his needs (RHEINGOLD, 1968). If she does not respond there may be serious consequences. Long-term disappointment, rejection, and depression can result in failures of holding, adaptation and attachment (BOWLBY, 1969). It is necessary for the paediatrician and his team to keep both parents informed and offer support and opportunities for discussion. It is not helpful to delay informing parents as this can lead to longstanding resentment (DAR *et al.*, 1974).

Gradually the process of mourning the loss of the normal child can be achieved, and the acceptance of the malformed child accomplished (SOLNIT and STARK, 1961). The continuing role of paediatrician, nursing staff, health visitor, social worker and general practitioner may be arduous and lengthy in the task of bringing mother and baby together under such circumstances, but is worthwhile for the future mental health of the child and family (KELLMER-PRINGLE, 1974).

Hospital Admissions and Malformation

One of the main problems in the early development of relationships between mother and infant arises in the hospital situation itself, perhaps in the obstetric or paediatric unit. Recent research (KLAUS *et al.*, 1972) in which differing amounts of contact were offered to mothers of newborn infants, has indicated that the mother needs to be able to explore, experience, hold and touch her baby during the first hours and days of life for a satisfactory attachment and bonding to take place between them. In the group of mothers with minimal contact less attachment took place. Observation and filmed records of feeding and caretaking showed that these mothers appear less responsive to the infants' cues, less preoccupied by him and less interested in his welfare. The time spent looking and smiling at the infant and in holding and caressing him is reduced, babies are held further away, eye-to-eye contact is not made as much during feeding, and the babies have more infections (KENNELL *et al.*, 1974). The infant does not have the feeling of security that is the basis for moving away from mother in order to explore the environment. Mothers who are deprived of early contact with their babies talk about feeling that they have lost them, and of not recognising the baby they have been given after the separation. These problems have been emphasised in studies of markedly premature infants that have spent long periods in incubators (BLAKE *et al.*, 1975), and will presumably apply to the malformed. The necessity for immediate operation on children with a major cardiac defect, with severe spina bifida, or a tracheo-oesophageal fistula may mean that the mother never has the opportunity of making that initial contact with her baby. It is significant that in a personal series of 100 children where abuse was suspected, approximately 30 had a major handicapping condition and 16 had needed a period in hospital for operative procedures or investigations at, or soon after, birth (BENTOVIM, 1974 a). A recent survey of 132 abused children showed that a significant number were handicapped (SMITH *et al.*, 1973). If initial bonding between mother and infant is not satisfactory then the inevitable frustration and anger which all mothers feel during the development of their children may be directed towards them, rather than away from them.

The implication of this recent research is that the previous supposition that babies could be separated without harm before the age of four months needs revision. The babies may not be affected so much at this time, but the mothers are. If mothers are to be the main source of rehabilitative therapy in the management of young handicapped children, then it is important that the relationship between mother and the infant needing hospitalisation should be fostered to the greatest extent. During this period it is important that the mother herself has skilled social-worker contact to help her deal with her own feelings of distress and distance, and to forge bonds with the infant.

Need for Emotional Working through of Initial Responses: its Relationship to Later Development

The importance of the proper working through of the intense feelings surrounding the birth of a malformed infant has been shown through studies which indicate that satisfactory emotional development of the malformed child depends more on the way in which the parents and the family relate to the child than to the extent of the handicap itself (DINNAGE, 1970, 1972, 1973; PRINGLE, 1964). It is now realised that long-term rejection or anxious over-protection, masking hostile feelings shown to a child over a number of years, markedly affect that child's degree of self-regard and self-confidence (RICHARDSON *et al.*, 1964).

Fortunately, in many cases the helplessness expected of an infant, and the hospital's fostering of an attachment, have helped to lessen the initial anxieties (D'ARCY, 1968). In those cases where, for example phenylketonuria can be successfully treated, cleft palate repaired, or a cardiac lesion corrected, hope is encouraged concerning the potential "rescue" of the child. It can become a problem when parental hopes are exaggerated and are greater than the expectations of medical advisers. Recent experience of the management of spina bifida has indicated that the bounds of reality must be repeatedly defined (LORBER, 1971).

When parents realise that development does not proceed as expected, fresh anxiety and concern is expressed. There may be disappointment when head control, sitting and standing are delayed, when speech does not develop, and when bladder and bowel control are not attained at the right time. Acutely painful feelings may recur at these times and a fresh attack on the adjustment and balance of the family is sustained. In work by HEWETT *et al.* (1970) where 100 children with cerebral palsy and their families were examined, it was found that at these times the parents had to accept the loss of the perfect child once more.

Such feelings are often experienced when children are taken to hospital for a routine visit, or when parents have to visit various specialists and retell the history. Other difficult times for parents include waiting for consultations, or when they are unable to ask questions, to get them answered, or to obtain the practical devices and social-work help that are necessary. In particular, problems arise when there is a feeling of insufficient coordination and communication between different departments of a hospital, or different hospitals and community clinics and agencies. They feel confused when different messages are given them by paediatricians, surgeons, general practitioners, or social workers. They are distressed when conflicting advice is given and covert disagreements are revealed, so that no one is trusted to take charge and all information is doubted and double-checked. Shopping around for opinions can occur in these circumstances. There may be insufficient information available, insufficient time from professional helpers to provide reassurance, insufficient case-work help from skilled social workers to deal with anger, negative feelings and practical wants. Numerous admissions to hospital may worsen an already precarious balance. In addition separations at toddler age become traumatic, so that insecurity and poor relationships are made worse by separation and a conviction arises on the child's part that he or she is really being rejected. The hospital dealing with the handicapped must care for the child and family and not consider the malformation as the only important focus of action. Without such help a precarious balance can be shattered. Rage, depression, fear of battering, strain, somatic aches and pains, financial difficulties, poor housing, marital strain or pressures from siblings may complicate the picture (TIZARD and GRAD, 1971). From these and other failures of development, a family's social life can be severely restricted, and the handicapped child has then to cope with the additional difficulties of withdrawn, preoccupied, depressed, angry and hopeless parents. The child with a malformation can thus be handicapped in many ways; by his deformity, by the response of his family, and by the responses of society itself.

Professional workers need to focus on a childs strengths as well as weaknesses, in order to preserve some sort of balance in the perceptions of the family. KOGAN *et al.* (1974) have shown the importance of this in a longitudinal study, where rejection of children was observed despite intensive professional intervention.

Early Emotional and Social Development, their Relationships to Malformation and Handicap

Having described aspects of mothering and some responses of the family, the emotional and social development of the infant and child need to be considered. There has always been much curiousity about what actually happens inside a baby's mind whilst he makes the steps of emotional development. How does the baby become aware that there is a world outside? He is clearly born with a capacity to respond to it. Video-recordings of mother-infant interactions soon after birth (BRAZELTON *et al.*, 1975) have shown the effectiveness of the adaptive behavior demonstrated. By his responses, the infant teaches what is necessary, for example feeding at one time and sleeping or playing at other times. In time infants learn to cope with their own tensions by thumb sucking, babbling, etc. (WINNICOTT, 1971). As increasing demands are made of the infant, he uses such movements and activities to cope with the frustrations of being aware that he has to sleep by himself, or has to share with other members of the family. Such activities enable him to cope, and integrate the different pictures that he has of those around him, so that his intense emotional feelings materialize as a sense of the real world.

In the first three to six months the infant seems to perceive the environment in a diffuse way, relating to balance, muscle tension, temperature, touch, warmth, smell, the feel of a mother's skin etc. Vision is not important until later, and it has been noticed that blindness may not be recognised during the first few months of life (FRAIBERG and FREEDMAN, 1964). Blind infants smile as normal infants (although not so persistently) and respond to touch, warmth and movement. They are often "good" babies, demanding little attention, and this, in turn, lessens the amount of attention they get from parents. Vision becomes important at about five to six months of age, and subsequent limitations mean that the blind child continues to rely on the earlier activities of body stimulation and movement for pleasure. He does not use objects and play materials. This prevents adaptive play and restricts knowledge of the world around him: the familiar is reassuring, the outside unknown and dangerous (WILLS, 1970).

Similar responses are found in other children who are deprived of information and stimulation as a result of malformation, whether they be blind, deaf or exhibit a reduction in movement through muscle paralysis, or skeletal malformation (FREEDMAN, 1972). Such infants and young children prefer the familarity and predictability of body-stimulation and care, rather than new stimuli which may be stubbornly rejected. They may cling to familiar situations in a rigid and ritualistic manner, resembling autism. The mother may adapt and be relieved not to have to amuse a baby whom she has rejected. If the infant does not push to become independent, but clings to a world of his own, he may be left in this "happy" state.

The malformed child who is blind perceives no smile to relieve an angry word, hence the idea of a consistent outside person is developed later than usual (WILLS, 1970). As a result, normal assertiveness or aggressiveness is inhibited for fear of provoking some punishment. A degree of deafness, or difficulty in comprehending or understanding language, means that the child, feeling his world to be incomprehensible, rejects it angrily. His parents become frustrated at their attempts to communicate, which leads to mutual rejection and tantrums. The child reacts to the birth of a sibling, a separation that he cannot understand and growing up generally, by furious outbursts. He may bully other siblings (WILLIAMS, 1970).

Problems of the Older Child and Adolescent

During development, a child is expected to modify his imperious demands and to adapt socially. It is hoped that a child will grow up to control himself through inner-directed constraints and not have to rely on other people to stop him (BENTOVIM, 1971). He needs to be able to do this without tension or shame. Children need to develop adequate trusting relationships, whether with the teacher who takes their class, the physiotherapist who works with them, or the surgeon or paediatrician who sees them regularly. It is expected that the child will be able to distinguish between the omnipotence of early thought, fantasy and pleasure-seeking, and be able to make reality-based observations and adjust to the world around him.

The boy or girl also needs to have a clear sense of maleness or femaleness and an adequate sense of individuality within the family group (RUTTER, 1971). Many of these functions are very much affected by the malformation and the induced responses both in the young child and the family. It has been found that longstanding contact with mothers involving close bodycare over a prolonged period may mean that a boy may tend to adopt a passive feminine role for himself rather than an assertive masculine one. Frequent surgical or medical procedures, the use of applicances, callipers, or urinary bags may also provoke a feeling of being damaged or mutilated, emphasing feelings of being different (BERGMAN, 1960). Expectations of parenthood in both sexes may be reduced (BERGMAN and FREUD, 1965).

In making contact with other children the handicapped child may use his appliance or special diet to gain prestige, but he may meet rejection, fear and disgust, particularly in adolescence (DORNER, 1973). In middle childhood when physical excellence and skills signify high status the handicapped child feels a failure, and has a low position in the hierarchy of relationships with other children (RICHARDSON *et al.*, 1964). At this time he begins to feel that instead of being love-worthy in his family, he should be respect-worthy in the community of children and adults. Such children may talk a great deal about aggression but do not enter the rough and tumble of school life, they may focus on their bodies and their evident shortcomings, feel ugly and useless, and in need of care from mother instead of being able to face competition. Alternatively, in adolescence, there may be a complete denial of difficulty with foolhardy rebellious behaviour.

Another area affected is the family's ability to provide a system which matches the needs of its members. Meeting a handicapped child's needs can impose great strain. As well as ensuring the personal development of all children, a family has to provide for the adult needs of sexual satisfaction and a mutually supportive relationship with another adult (LIDZ, 1964). The parents of normal children find meeting each others demands a considerable strain, whilst still trying to satisfy the children (RICHMAN *et al.*, 1974). When a family also has to give special attention and devotion to the child with a malformation, the balance of relationships within the family can be distorted. In a study of 20 cerebral palsied individuals the whole family was sometimes found to have focussed around the handicapped child ignoring their own needs. Marital stresses were often denied and a myth of togetherness fostered, which if exposed might result in family breakdown (SCHAFFER, 1964). Other siblings have to bear this burden: the family exists for them, but often they are made to feel of secondary importance by a parent who seems to have a special relationship with the handicapped child. This attitude may result in overestimation of the potential of the handicapped child (TEW *et al.*, 1974). As a result the normal sibling may become depressed and angry, or rebellious, complaining of aches and pains of their own, to try to gain attention. Sometimes the sibling is used as a way of diverting feelings and is made a scapegoat. Consequently the normal sibling feels that the problems of the handicapped child are his fault. He may expect punishment and therefore provoke it, or become anxious or depressed. In addition older girl sibs frequently help to bear the family's physical burden (GATH, 1974).

Marital strains may result from family size limitation after the birth of a handicapped child (STEVENSON and STEVENSON, 1970). Genetic counselling for such problems may require several consultations to "work through" the mutual blaming and bitterness, particularly if there is a high genetic loading. It is always painful to face such facts and someone has to be blamed, whether it is onself, a marital partner, the medical profession, or some specific event, fantasy or fact. The alternative is to live in a world which is uncontrollable and randomly hostile.

A study of the families of 319 children with congenital heart disease has shown that the special position of the handicapped child means that he is always without fault and the most important member of the family (BENTOVIM, 1974 b). The child may then fail to develop an empathic appreciation for the feelings of others in the family and may act in a manner more appropriate to a younger child. He has to make sense of his own state of existence, his pain, his discomfort, his clumsiness, or his failure to comprehend and be understood. He also has to accept the fact that his appearance may be different from other children (LANSDOWNE, 1974). He may attribute such problems to actions of his parents, or other children in the family, or to his own badness. A variety of problems arise out this difficulty; fearfulness, over-aggressiveness, or obsessional behaviour. It is often necessary to talk to the child about his problems so that he can begin to accept himself as he is, rather than add to what he sees with ideas from his inner world.

Prevention of Unnecessary Handicap

To prevent future emotional disturbance adding to physical handicap, early intervention is essential. In general, young children with malformations should remain with their parents rather than be separated for special educational help. For a child without parents the substitution of a foster-home or family group home is preferable to an institutional placement. Separations or medical intervention should be reduced to a minimum and parents should accompany their children whenever possible. Facilities must be made available, not only for the child with a specific handicap, but also to help the family to participate in the process of treatment, although disappointment can be realised when no magical improvement occurs (KOGAN *et al.*, 1974).
To achieve this broad-based treatment a multidisciplinary professional team is often necessary (HOLT and REYNELL, 1965, 1967). Initially a paediatric clinic and later a district assessment centre should accept this task. The community of general practitioner, area health authority and welfare clinic, social services and voluntary societies have to provide an extended family network, enriching the family's own resources. These different professional groups need to be aware of tensions arising in families. Nurses, doctors, social workers, and health visitors should note the quality of relationships as they develop between child, mother, father and siblings (BENTOVIM, 1974 a).
Crises have to be faced and help given to deal with long-standing difficulties by workers skilled in this field. There is merit in making sure that both parents are seen in a crisis, and the families are put in touch with a source of support. Frequently professional workers involved with families find additional skills by co-operating and meeting together. The regular clinic where a number of parents attending with specific problems meet provides an opportunity for the formation of self-help parent groups. The growth of voluntary societies, whether for autism, cystic fibrosis, the mentally handicapped, or other groups, can help channel the powerful feelings aroused in families to constructive, reparative ends. There is a risk that excessive hope can be generated by these activities and that normal grief and mourning might not be expressed, thus denying the feelings of helplessness, anger and rage that are present.

Ultimately the parents must accept the child if the best in him is to be developed. The ultimate aim is to prevent the malformed child becoming unnecessarily handicapped.

Conclusion

The impact of a handicap on the normal processes of development through pregnancy, infancy, childhood and adolescence have been traced. It is impossible to think of the child in isolation; he and the family are one inseparable unit. The professions involved in care must orientate themselves towards the family unit so that the development of children can be fostered within it. Only in this way is effective treatment of the conditions likely to be achieved with minimal damage to the child's ability to proceed from the family to the outside world. Providing the individual with an independent place in society should be the aim when helping the child and family with a malformation (Younghusband *et al.*, 1970).

References

Benedek, T.: Parenthood as a developmental phase. J. Amer. psychoanal. Ass. **7**, 389 (1959).

Bentovim, A.: Psychological and Social Aspects of Cardiac Disease in Children. In: Congenital Heart Disease in Children. Ed. Graham, G. R. In Press.

Bentovim, A.: Emotional Disturbances of Handicapped Pre-School Children and their families. Brit. Med. J. **3**, 579 and 634 (1972).

Bentovim, A.: Treatment: A Medical Perspective in The Maltreated Child. ed. Carter, J. London: Priory 1974.

Bentovim, A.: Early Emotional Development and its relationship to children with handicaps and the family. Proc. of Conf. of Special Education, 1974.

Bentovim, A., Clayton, B., Francis, D. E. M., Shepherd, J., Wolff, O. H.: The use of an amino-acid mixture in treatment of Phenylketonuria. Arch. Dis. Childh. **45**, 640 (1970).

Bergmann, T.: Application of analytic knowledge to children with organic illness in Recent Developments in Psychoanalytic Child Therapy. Ed. Weinreb. New York: Int. Univ. Press 1960.

Bergmann, T., Freud, A.: Children in Hospital. New York: Int. Univ. Press 1965.

Bibring, G. L.: Some considerations of the psychological processes in pregnancy. Psychoanal. Stud. Child **14** (1959).

Blake, A., Stewart, A., Turcan, D.: Parents of babies of very low birth-weight, a Long-term follow-up. The Parent-Infant relationship — Ciba symposium, Elsevier, 1975.

Bowlby, J.: Attachment and Loss, Vol. 1 and 2. London: Hogarth 1969 and 1973.

Brazelton, T. B., Tronick, E. C., Adamson, L., Rivinus, H., Wise, S.: Early mother-infant reciprocity. The Parent-Infant Relationship — Ciba symposium, Elsevier, 1975.

Brice-Pitt, J.: Atypical Depression following childbirth. Brit. J. Psychiat. **114**, 1325 (1968).

Caplan, G.: Prevention of Mental Disorders in Children. London: Tavistock 1963.

Dar, H., Winter, T. S., Tal, Y.: Families of Children with Cleft Lips and Palates: Concerns and Counselling. Devel. Med. Child Neurol. **16**, 513 (1974).

D'Arcy, E.: Congenital defects, mother's reactions to first information. Brit. Med. J. **3**, 796 (1968).

Dinnage, R.: The Handicapped Child. Research Review, Vol. I, II and III, London, Longman and the National Bureau of Co-operation in Child Care, 1970, 1972, 1973.

Dorner, S.: Psychological and Social Problems of Families with an adolescent spina bifida patient. Devel. Med. Child Neurol. Suppl. **29**, 24—27 (1973).

Fraiberg, S., Freedman, D. A.: Studies in the ego development of the congenitally blind. Psychoanal. Stud. Child **19** (1964).

Freedman, D. A.: On the limits of the effectiveness of psychoanalysis: early ego and somatic disturbances. Int. J. Psycho-Anal. **53,** 363 (1972).

Freeston, B. M.: An enquiry into the effect of a spina bifida child upon family life. Devel. Med. Child Neurol. **13,** 456 (1971).

Gath, A.: The Effects of Mental Subnormality on the family. Brit. J. Hosp. Med. **147** (1972).

Gath, A.: Sibling reactions to mental handicap: A comparison of the brothers and sisters of mongol children. J. Child Psychol. **15,** 187 (1974).

Hewett, S., Newsom, J. and E.: The family of the handicapped child. Univ. Nottingham Press, 1967.

Holt, K. S., Reynell, J. K.: Assessment of Cerebral Palsy, Vol. I and II. London: Lloyd-Luke 1965 and 1967.

Kellmer-Pringle, M.: The needs of children. Hutchinson, 1974.

Kennell, J. H., Jerauld, R., Wolfe, H., Chesler, D., Kreger, N. C., McAlpine, W., Steffa, M., Klaus, M. H.: 'Maternal behaviour after one year of extended post partum contact.' Develop. Med. Child Neurol. **16,** 172 (1974).

Klaus, M. H., Jerauld, R., Kreger, N. C., McAlpine, W., Steffa, M., Kennell, J. H.: Importance of the 1st 5 post-partum days. New Engl. J. Med. **268,** 460 (1972).

Kogan, K. L., Tyler, N., Turner, M.: 'The Process of interpersonal adaptions between mothers and their cerebral palsied children.' Develop. Med. Child Neurol. **16,** 518 (1974).

Lansdowne, R., Pollak, L.: The forgotten people: a study of the psychological effect of facial deformity. Child Care, Health and Develop. I, 85 (1975).

Lax, R. L.: Some aspects of the interactions between mother and impaired child. Mother's narcissistic trauma. Int. J. Psycho-Anal. **53,** 339 (1972).

Lorber, J.: Results of treatment of myelomeningocele. An Analysis of 524 cases, with special reference to possible selection for treatment. Develop. Med. Child Neurol. **13,** 279 (1971).

Miller, E.: Cerebral palsied children and their parents. Exceptional children **24,** 298 (1958).

Pringle, M. L. K.: The emotional and social adjustment of physically handicapped children. Occ. Publ. No. 10, N.F.E.R. Slough, Bucks., 1964.

Pringle, M. L. K., Fiddes, D. O.: The Challenge of Thalidomide Studies in Child Development. Nat. Bureau for Coop. in Child Care. Longman, 1970.

Rheingold, H.: The Social and Socialising infant in D. A. Gaslin (ed.) Handbook of Socialisation theory and research. Rand McNally, 1968.

Richardson, S. A., Hastorf, A. H., Dornbush, S. M.: Effects of physical disability on a child's description of himself. Child Develop. **35,** 893 (1964).

Richman, N., Stevenson, J. E., Graham, P. J.: Prevalance of Behaviour Problems in 3 year old children: an epidemiological study in a London Borough. J. Child Psychol. (In press) 1975.

Rose, J. A.: Prevention of mothering breakdown associated with physical abnormalities of the infant. In: Prevention of Mental Disorders in Children. ed. Caplan, G. (Tavistock), 1961.

Rutter, M.: Normal Psycho-sexual Development. J. Psychol. Psychiat. **11,** 285 (1971).

Schaffer, H. R.: Families of Handicapped Children. Int. J. soc. Psychiat. **10,** 266 (1964).

Smith, S. M., Hanson, R., Noble, S.: Parents of Battered Children: A Controlled Study. Brit. Med. J. **4,** 338 (1973).

Solnit, S. J., Stark, M. H.: Mourning and the birth of a defective child. Psychoanal. Stud. Child **15** (1961).

Stevenson, A. C., Stevenson, B. C. C.: Genetic Counselling. London: Heinemann 1970.

Tew, B., Laurence, K. M., Samuel, P.: Parental Estimates of the Intelligence of their physically handicapped child. Devel. Med. Child Neurol. **16,** 494 (1974).

Tizard, J., Grad, J. C.: The mentally handicapped and their families. Oxford: Univ. Press, 1961.

WILLIAMS, C. E.: Some psychiatric observations on a group of maladjusted deaf children. J. Child Psychol. 11, **1** (1970).
WILLS, D. M.: Psychological development of blind children. Psychoanal. Stud. Child **25** (1970).
WINNICOTT, D. W.: Through Pediatrics to Psycho-analysis. London: Tavistock 1958.
WINNICOTT, D. W.: Transitional Objects and Transitional Phenomena in Playing and Reality, Tavistock 1971.
YOUNGHUSBAND, E., BIRCHALL, D., DAVIE, R., PRINGLE, M. L. K.: Living with handicap. National Bureau for Cooperation in Child Care, 1970.

Subject Index

(Page numbers in *italics* refer to tables in the text)

MIX
Papier aus verantwortungsvollen Quellen
Paper from responsible sources
FSC® C105338

If you have any concerns about our products,
you can contact us on
ProductSafety@springernature.com

In case Publisher is established outside the EU,
the EU authorized representative is:
Springer Nature Customer Service Center GmbH
Europaplatz 3, 69115 Heidelberg, Germany

Printed by Libri Plureos GmbH
in Hamburg, Germany